Life events and psychiatric disorders:
controversial issues

Life events and psychiatric disorders:

controversial issues

EDITED BY HEINZ KATSCHNIG

The right of the University of Cambridge to print and sell all manner of books was granted by Henry VIII in 1534. The University has printed and published continuously since 1584.

CAMBRIDGE UNIVERSITY PRESS

Cambridge

London New York New Rochelle

Melbourne Sydney

Published by the Press Syndicate of the University of Cambridge
The Pitt Building, Trumpington Street, Cambridge CB2 1RP
32 East 57th Street, New York, NY 10022, USA
10 Stamford Road, Oakleigh, Melbourne 3166, Australia

First published 1986

Printed in Great Britain by the University Press, Cambridge

British Library cataloguing in publication data

Life events and psychiatric disorders: controversial issues.

1. Psychology, Pathological. 2. Stress (Psychology)
I. Katschnig, Heinz
616.89'071 RC455.4.S87

Library of Congress cataloguing in publication data

Main entry under title;
Life events and psychiatric disorders.

1. Life change events. 2. Stress (Psychology)
3. Mental illness – Etiology. I. Katschnig, Heinz.
[DNLM: 1. Life Change Events. 2. Mental Disorders – etiology.
3. Stress, Psychological – complications. WM 172 L722]
RC455.4.L53L54 1986 616.89'07'1 85-19000

ISBN 0521 255961

UP

CONTENTS

CONTRIBUTORS

Dr P. Bebbington
MRC Social Psychiatry Unit
Institute of Psychiatry
De Crespigny Park
Denmark Hill
London SE5 8AF, England

Professor A. M. Becker
Spitalgasse 19
A-1090 Vienna, Austria

Professor G. W. Brown
Medical Research Council
Department of Social Policy and Social Science
Bedford College and Royal Holloway College
(University of London)
11 Bedford Square
London WC1B 3RA, England

Professor B. Cooper
Zentralinstitut für Seelische Gesundheit
Postfach 5970
D-68 Mannheim 1, J 5, Germany

Dr Eva Egger-Zeidner
Psychologische Beratungsstelle für Studierende
Merangasse 23
1A-8010 Graz, Austria

Dr Tirril Harris
Medical Research Council
Department of Social Policy and Social Science
Bedford College and Royal Holloway College
(University of London)
11 Bedford Square, London WC1B 3RA, England

Professor H. Katschnig (Editor)
Psychiatrische Universitätsklinik
Währinger Gürtel 18–20
A-1090 Vienna, Austria

Professor M. Lader
Institute of Psychiatry
De Crespigny Park
Denmark Hill
London SE5 8AF, England

Dr G. Pakesch
Psychiatrische Universitätsklinik
Währinger Gürtel 18–20
A-1090 Vienna, Austria

Dr G. Turpin
Plymouth Polytechnic
Drake Circus
Plymouth
Devon PL4 8AA, England

PREFACE

Everyone's personal experience seems to support the notion that stressful life events not only make people unhappy, but also sick. This popular belief is expressed and obviously reinforced by common popular sayings such as that of a 'broken heart'. In addition, world literature is full of examples which show that stressful events may disturb people's health. When, in the tales of the 1001 nights, King Shahzaman is betrayed by his wife, the story teller relates that 'his face became pale and his body sickened'. However, while disturbances of our psychological and physical health can be rather regularly predicted after extremely disruptive events of a catastrophic nature, the situation is much less clear in the case of those life changes which are a normal ingredient of life. Health disorders following, for instance, retirement, birth of a child, or loss of a job may be more frequent than expected among people who do not experience these events, but we are still far from being able to predict the occurrence of such health consequences. And predictability is at the heart of scientific knowledge.

This book deals with the possibilities and limitations of life event research to increase our scientifically supported knowledge of the causes of functional mental disorders. However, uncertainties and professional controversies about how to define the dependent variables – functional mental disorders – and also the many difficulties in measuring the independent variable – non-catastrophic life event stress – still prevent one from finding a simple and definite answer to the question of a possible causal relationship between life stress and functional mental disorders. Consequently, the articles contained in this volume not only deal with the possible nature of the relationship between life stress and functional mental disorders (Chapters 2, 3, 5, 6) but also with specific diagnostic issues (Chapters 1 and 7) and with the problems of measuring life stress (Chapters 4 and 5). In the concluding chapter (8) some recommendations for future research on the relationship between life stress and mental disturbances are formulated. The contributions are not merely of academic interest, since they are all concerned with psychiatric disorders of a clinical order and with practical research problems and limitations inherent in studying psychiatric populations. Basic psychological research on how normal people cope with life stress is outside the scope of this book, although we are certainly in need of a better understanding as to how perception, attitude and attributional style bear on the pathogenic effect of life stress.

The book starts with a historical review by Brian Cooper dealing with the development of the concept of reactivity in relation to the diagnosis of functional mental disorders. This topic is taken up again at the end of the book when Katschnig, Pakesch & Egger-Zeidner discuss current views on the concept of reactivity in relation to defining and studying subtypes of depressive disorders. These diagnostic issues are of utmost importance, since all arguments and conclusions about the aetiological relevance of life event stress are heavily influenced by the definition of the dependent variable, or, in other words, by the selection of a study population. In Kahlbaum's (1866) words: 'Before embarking upon aetiological research we must know the various manifestations and specifications of a subject matter'. It is astonishing how careless some research workers are when they deal with diagnostic issues and how frequently, for example, simple commonsense judgments are used for dividing a depressive population into a 'reactive' and an 'endogenous' group. It will be shown how large the confusion is already on the terminological level and what cures are possible for this deplorable state of psychiatric diagnosis in relation to life event research.

The problems surrounding the measurement of life event stress are not less serious. Here, from the very beginning of the new era of life event research – i.e. starting with Holmes & Rahe's (1967) publication of the 'Schedule of Recent Experience' (SRE) – a global and simplistic approach has dominated, which clearly contrasts with the complex and motley theories of psychoanalysis. Obviously the fascination of quickly providing – by the use of a self-rating list, e.g. the SRE – a quantitative measure of life stress has swept away more sophisticated thinking and has left many students of life stress and illness with a skeleton of figures without the meat of life. Selye's (1946) classical concept of 'stress', with its emphasis on the non-specificity of the stressor, has certainly contributed to this oversimplified approach of the early life event researchers. It is somehow understandable that the checklist approach is still very popular in life event research, since it is infinitely easier to use self-rating lists such as the SRE with its predetermined 'Life Change Units' than to collect, in a lengthy interview, a wealth of information, and evaluate *a posteriori* the specific 'threat' entailed upon a specific person in a given social context (which corresponds to the approach of the London 'Life Event and Difficulty Schedule' by Brown & Harris, 1978). In the contributions by Katschnig on the measurement of life stress and by Brown & Harris on the Bedford College studies of depression, a clear position is taken against the self-rating technique and the 'checklist' approach. It is argued in these articles that for measuring stressful events of a non-catastrophic nature, no easier way exists than cumbersome interview methods with trained interviewers which guarantee both a detailed description of an event and its context and a high reliability of measurement. Quantification may be one important issue of life event research, but 'qualification', i.e. the detailed description of what really happened, must not be neglected. Arnold Toynbee's formulation of the dilemma of all human science, 'the price of quantification is the ignoring of uniqueness', is also inherent in life event research.

Four chapters deal with the possible causal links between life stress and functional mental disorders. In contrast to classical social epidemiology, with its search for correlations between mental disorders and categorical social variables, life event research is directly concerned with the dynamics of the 'before' and 'after' of life stress and illness and should thus provide a better possibility of increasing our knowledge of pathogenetic processes than the static epidemiological approach. It is on the problems of the nature of the causal links between life event stress and specific functional mental disorders that the sharpest controversies might be expected; however, a rather conciliatory tone prevails in the chapters concerned with these causal links. Alois Becker deals with the possible psychological mechanisms of the pathogenic effect of life events, whereas Graham Turpin and Malcolm Lader outline the presently conceivable biological mechanisms through which life events may exert a pathogenic effect on the development of functional mental disorders; both contributions consider biological as well as psychosocial variables. In addition Paul Bebbington of the Institute of Psychiatry and George Brown and Tirril Harris of Bedford College in London, known to be long-standing opponents, in some sense hold similar positions, since both groups have adopted a vulnerability model of one or the other kind. This model implies that life events are pathogenic only in conjunction with psychosocial and/or biological vulnerability factors, although the emphasis may be put on one or the other side of the scale. In all these chapters it is shown that merely looking for simple correlations between life stress and illness onset is not enough. In Brown & Harris' and

Turpin & Lader's contributions, in particular, it becomes clear how complex the theoretical models of the relationship between life stress and illness onset must be if they are both to accommodate existing research results and serve as a stimulating framework for future research. There is no doubt that such future research will need all the methodological sophistication available today and will consequently be rather cumbersome. Also in life event research there is no easy way around the complexities of life.

Acknowledgements

This book could not have been produced without the help of many of my teachers, colleagues and friends. Professor Hans Strotzka of the Institute of Psychotherapy of the University of Vienna has encouraged me to leave the narrow path of ideology and to try to reconcile phenomenological, biological, psychological and social aspects of mental illness. Professor Peter Berner of the Psychiatric Clinic of the University of Vienna, has always furthered my scientific interests and activities, especially in the field of psychiatric diagnosis. To Professor Frederic Redlich and the Foundations' Fund for Research in Psychiatry I am particularly indebted for the possibility of spending two fruitful years in Great Britain, where I made acquaintance with the problems of life event research. Professor George Brown and Tirril Harris of Bedford College in London introduced me to the subtleties of life event research and Professor Michael Shepherd and Professor John Wing of the Institute of Psychiatry, London, were helpful in many ways. Dr Norman Kreitman of the MRC Unit for Epidemiological Studies in Psychiatry in Edinburgh paved the way for carrying out my first life event study at the Regional Poisoning Treatment Centre of the Royal Infirmary in Edinburgh, where all staff members showed the utmost kindness when I interfered in their daily routine in carrying out my research. Marie Moyer, Geraldine Fuchs-Robetin, Andrea Brandl-Nebehay, Eva Egger-Zeidner and Monika Vyslouzil did the life event interviewing in the various studies carried out in the UK and in Austria. Rainer Strobl, Gerd Eichberger, Hans Schanda and Detlev Nutzinger, as well as Peter Sint and Peter Seelig, took part in my own studies in one way or another. The 'Deutsche Forschungsgemeinschaft (Bonn)' and the 'Fonds zur Förderung der Wissenschaftlichen Forschung (Wien)' provided grants for these studies. I am also indebted to the publishers Urban & Schwarzenberg, Munich and Baltimore, for allowing me to use parts of a book edited by myself in German (*Sozialer Stress und psychische Erkrankung: Lebensveränd-ernde Ereignisse als Ursache seelischer Störungen?* Munich and Baltimore, 1980). William Kieffer, Meera Sarin, Brian Cooper and Keith Chester helped with the translation. I am especially indebted to Johanna Bewry who typed and endlessly retyped my manuscripts. To Hildegard, Michael, Isabelle and Tamara I am most grateful for their understanding and tolerance.

Vienna, May 1985 Heinz Katschnig

References

Brown, G. W. & Harris, T. O. (1978). *Social origins of depression: a study of psychiatric disorder in women.* London: Tavistock Publications. New York: Free Press.

Holmes, Th. H. & Rahe, R. H. (1967). The Social Readjustment Rating Scale. *Journal of Psychosomatic Research,* **11**, 213–18.

Kahlbaum, F. J. (1866). Die Sinnensdelirien. Ein Beitrag zur klinischen Erweiterung der psychiatrischen Symptomatologie und zur physiologischen Psychologie. *Allgemeine Zeitschrift für Psychiatrie,* **23**, 1–86.

Selye, H. (1946). The General Adaptation Syndrome and the diseases of adaptation. *Journal of Clinical Endocrinology,* **6**, 117–230.

1

Mental disorder as reaction: the history of a psychiatric concept

BRIAN COOPER

And it was not disease or crime
Which got him landed there,
But because they laid on My Mother's Son
More than a man could bear.

What with noise, and fear of death,
Waking, and wounds and cold,
They filled the Cup for My Mother's Son
Fuller than it could hold.

Kipling's lines about a mentally sick soldier express what seems to most people a self-evident truth – that a man may be driven mad by his experiences. Yet, paradoxically, the significance of life events for the phenomena of mental illness remains one of the central, unresolved issues of psychiatry. Above all, the notion of psychiatric disorder as a *reaction*, as a direct response to environmental change, continues to be a subject of vigorous debate.

The forefathers of modern psychiatry saw no reason to withhold judgment on this question. Among the causes listed by Pinel, in his tabulation of cases treated at the Bicêtre in Paris, were acute fever, sunstroke, childbearing, alcoholic excess and loss of property (Pinel, 1962). His successor, Esquirol, published a table of 'moral and physical causes', based on extensive clinical material collected at three clinics (Table 1.1). Here, the emphasis is placed firmly on environmental factors: genetic inheritance is cited in only 10% of the pooled cases, compared, for example, with domestic difficulties in 15%.

In Table 1.1, the distribution of cases is set out as though the individual causes were mutually exclusive. Esquirol's comments in the text show, however, that he did not hold this simplistic view of the matter. The proximal or exciting causes could, he affirmed, give rise to illness only if the necessary predisposition was present. Given the existence of such an underlying tendency, a random stressful event could then serve as the igniting spark.

This simple general model, according to which individual cases of mental disorder result from the combination in varying strengths of predisposing and precipitating factors, has been accepted as adequate for their purposes by many leading figures of psychiatry, from Esquirol's time to the present day. It was given firm definition by Wilhelm Griesinger (1867), in the first edition of his famous textbook.

Table 1.1 *Table of moral and psychological causes of insanity*

Causes	Salpetrière 1811–12	Privat Institution 1811–12	Bicêtre 1808–13
Domestic trouble	105	156	99
Unhappy love	46	25	37
Jealousy	18	8	—
Shock	38	8	—
Anger	16	—	—
Injured self-esteem	1	16	—
Disappointed ambition	—	12	78
Poverty and mishaps	77	14	116
Excess of studying	—	13	49
Political events	14	31	82
Misanthropy	—	2	—
Fanaticism	8	1	55
Inherited tendency	105	150	—
Fever	13	12	—
Apoplexy	60	10	157
Head injuries	14	4	—
Sunstroke	12	4	—
Epilepsy	11	2	118
Syphilis	8	1	—
Abuse of mercury	14	18	—
Abuse of strong drinks	26	3	106
Worm infestation	24	4	—
Masturbation	10	14	21
Harlotry	33	6	—
Menstrual disorders	55	19	—
Uterine cramps during pregnancy	11	4	—
Consequences of childbearing	52	21	—
Menopause, climacteric	27	11	—
Advanced age	60	4	36
All cases	858	573	954

Source: Esquirol (1827).

Griesinger's aetiological model

Griesinger has come to be regarded as the leading nineteenth-century exponent of organic psychiatry, and his name to be associated with a doctrine – that of the unitary psychosis – which does not now command wide support. This is unfortunate, since it has led to neglect of his views on other topics. The chapter on aetiology in his textbook is remarkably modern in tone; indeed, when one reflects that Griesinger was only 28 at the time and had had little experience in clinical psychiatry, it represents a striking intellectual achievement.

He begins by declaring that the causes of insanity comprehend the internal states which predispose to its development; the external circumstances with which its appearance tends to be associated and the various forms of trauma of which it may be a consequence. The way in which these factors operate to produce mental disease may be far from clear, but the task of aetiology in the strict sense is to identify the causes of illness, not to explain their mode of action. He then goes on:

> A closer investigation of the aetiology of insanity soon shows that, in the great majority of cases, it was not a single specific cause under the influence of which the disease was finally established, but a combination of several, sometimes numerous, causes, both predisposing and exciting...
>
> The difficulty lies in the proper appreciation of the influence which each one of these circumstances has on the production of the disease. We must endeavour by every means to keep the mind unbiased by this or that theory, and from one-sided preference for one or for certain series of causes; for example, the somatic or the mental...
>
> An influence of causation can naturally be attributed with most certainty to those circumstances whose mode of action can be clearly traced, and whose effects may therefore be considered as physiological necessities: or, where this is not the case, to those whose influence is established by reliable statistics... We should always bear in mind that anything, to be a cause, must really precede the presumed effect... (Griesinger, 1867; 127–30).

There follow many acute observations on the aetiology and pathogenesis (including psychogenesis) of mental disorders, which cannot be quoted here. Three aspects of Griesinger's formulation deserve to be underlined because of their relevance for modern causal research. First of all, he attempts no division of mental disorders into some due to external events and others which arise internally. It is implicit in his schema that events may play a part in the genesis of any mental illness, and that the relative importance of external and internal factors should be assessed in each individual case. Secondly, though he considers psychological causes to be the most frequent, Griesinger makes no distinction in principle between events of emotional or symbolic significance (e.g. bereavement, loss of social status) and those with a direct physical or physiological impact (e.g. head injury, acute infection). Whilst accepting that psychological experiences are important, both as predisposing and as precipitating causes, he does not concern himself with the illnesses provoked by them as a special category. Finally, he is modest but firm in the requirements he makes for judging the causal significance of an event. Indeed, only two criteria are stipulated: the event must precede the onset of illness and must be linked with the illness, either by a clearly demonstrable pathogenesis (e.g. brain damage, intoxication) or by a positive statistical association, or both.

Empirical versus rational

Griesinger's aetiological concepts, as here expounded, are not those of an extreme organicist; on the contrary, they are so broadly eclectic as to be acceptable, in principle, to adherents of many different schools. Their main weakness is that they offer no guidance to classification, and hence to precise diagnosis. For this reason, models of the type proposed by Griesinger have always tended to appeal most strongly to those physicians whose interests lie primarily with the manifestations and course of disease in the individual patient, and who are less concerned with problems of classification. Griesinger himself subscribed to the notion of the 'Einheitspsychose', first propounded by Zeller and subsequently developed by Neumann (1859): a doctrine which has continued to attract some supporters up to the present day, but which in the latter half of the nineteenth century was virtually forgotten in the renewed search for psychiatric disease entities.

Kendell (1975) has suggested that attitudes towards diagnosis and classification in psychiatry tend to correspond to the two great philosophical traditions, Aristotelian and Platonic, whose struggle for dominance is represented in medical history by the dialectic between two opposing concepts of disease: in the words of Baisette (1931), '. . . un rhythme que nous retrouvons dans les alternances: Cos et Cnide, hippocratisme et galenisme, vitalisme et organicisme, médicine synthétique et médicine analytique . . .'. Thus, because they were writing in a period when the Aristotelian, or Hippocratic, tradition was uppermost, Pinel, Esquirol and the young Griesinger adopted an empiricist standpoint. Soon afterwards, however, as the pendulum began to swing back and medicine entered a new Platonic era, physicians became increasingly concerned with questions of nosology.

The view of history as a cyclical process is itself Platonist in spirit and relies upon oversimplification. Not only do the two broad tendencies always co-exist, but the various components which enter into each (functionalist versus structuralist, empiricist versus rationalist, dynamic versus static, biographical versus ontological, etc.) do not fit together as neatly as is often supposed. To take an example from psychiatry, Kraepelin, the great classifier, was in some respects much closer to empiricism than any of the leaders of the 'dynamic' psychoanalytical school.

More cogent explanations can be offered for the preoccupation with nosology and classification which characterized psychiatry during that era. The prevailing conservatism of Europe's political and social climate, following on the events of 1848, tended everywhere to favour deterministic concepts of human behaviour at the expense of dynamic theories, and not least in psychiatry (Güse & Schmacke, 1979). At the same time the rapid progress of scientific medicine and, in particular, the great strides being made in organic pathology, stimulated attempts to identify corresponding disease entities underlying mental disorder, each with its own characteristic aetiology, pathology, symptom constellation and clinical course. The results, embodied in the work of Falret, Baillarger, Kahlbaum, Hecker, Kraepelin and others, form a major part of the heritage of modern psychiatry (Zilboorg & Henry, 1941) and require no discussion here. One important side-effect, however, should be noted: although the quest for specific causes was largely unsuccessful, the tendency to equate descriptive with aetiological classification – to assume that a characteristic clinical picture denotes a certain type of causation – was perpetuated in psychiatric teaching.

New diagnostic constructs

By the end of the nineteenth century, trends in classification and system building had already outstripped advances in psychiatric knowledge. The need to demarcate and to categorize, in those large areas where causation and pathology remained mysterious, led to the coining or adaptation of a number of terms which were linked, explicitly or implicitly, with diagnostic constructs. Of those which were to gain wide usage, three have special relevance in the present context; namely, *psychogenic*, *exogenous* and *reactive*.

Psychogenic

Lewis (1972) commented with justice on the word 'psychogenic' that:

> The role of this concept in the theoretical discussion of almost all forms of mental disorder is so widespread, so loosely interpreted, and so intimately entangled with assumptions about causation and psychopathology that concise review is impossible.

It was from the outset an imprecise term. Sommer (1894), who introduced it, intended to denote a group of disorders contained within the broad category of hysteria. These morbid conditions were, he maintained, both evoked and influenced by ideas. He did not try to explain where or how the ideas in question arose, but since he placed great emphasis on the role of predisposing factors (including organic disease) and of abnormal suggestibility, one may infer that he thought of external events as having only a triggering, or catalytic, effect.

This is, indeed, the sense in which the term psychogenic became assimilated into the psychiatric literature. Kraepelin, who revised his classification with each successive edition of his textbook, used the neutral appellation 'general neuroses' in earlier editions, but switched to 'psychogenic neuroses' in the seventh.* The group included, besides hysterical states, shock reactions and anticipatory anxiety. Kraepelin was careful to stress that the root cause of such disorders must always be sought in the mental predisposition.

The concept of psychogenesis was extended to other neuroses by Bonhoeffer (1911) and to the psychoses by Hoch (1907). Discussion gradually came to centre less and less on questions of aetiology and classification; more and more on the endopsychic processes which were thought to underly these various forms of mental disturbance. Psychogenic seemed at times to be equated with comprehensible. Thus Maier (1912), Kretschmer (1918) and others traced the origins of delusional illness in the patient's life history and personal experiences, while Birnbaum (1923) showed how the features of a psychosis could be conditioned by pathoplastic factors, some of which were socioculturally determined. These illuminating studies served incidentally to expose the weakness of the term psychogenic as a diagnostic label, since it became increasingly clear that psychogenesis in the broad sense entered into the development of every mental illness.

* Menninger (1963) has suggested that this change was a result of Kraepelin's move from Heidelberg to Munich, where he came into contact with a different type of patient.

Reflecting on these ambiguities and shifts of meaning, Lewis (1972) concluded that the word should be given '... decent burial, along with some of the controversies whose fire it has stoked.' His advice is unlikely to be followed so long as clinicians find it convenient to distinguish between 'psychogenic' and 'organic' symptoms. As a diagnostic adjective, however, there is little doubt that psychogenic would be better dropped.

Exogenous

More promising at first sight is the term exogenous which, being by definition concerned with factors outside the organism, refers unequivocally to aetiology, as opposed to pathogenesis. It was introduced into psychiatry, together with endogenous, as the basis of a dichotomous classification (Möbius, 1893), and to that extent appears suitable for taxonomic purposes. Closer scrutiny, however, reveals some serious defects.

If the two categories, exogenous and endogenous, are treated as jointly exhaustive, they may serve merely as a cloak for ignorance, in much the same way that the terms organic and functional may do. If they are treated as mutually exclusive, they do less than justice to clinical experience, which teaches that the causes of mental illness can be both internal and external, and that neither need be obviously primary. If the classification is treated as descriptive rather than aetiological, this ignores the fact that a given syndrome may be endogenous in some instances and exogenous in others; thus a typical 'endogenous' psychosis may be due to developing neurosyphilis or to medication with steroids. How the classification is applied will depend on the operational definitions employed: exogenous, for example, can be taken to mean 'outside the body' or 'outside the brain'. It will also depend on how far back the causal chain is traced; for example, genetic mutations may be due to exposure to radioactivity.

In view of these drawbacks, it is somewhat surprising that the words exogenous and endogenous should have been so quickly accepted and so widely used in psychiatric terminology. The explanation seems to be that hardly any attempt was made to grapple with the taxonomic problems. Instead, endogenous became a label for chronic mental illness of unknown origin, and as such equated, or closely linked, with other terms such as constitutional, hereditary and even degenerative (Lewis, 1971). Exogenous, on the other hand, became associated with acute illness episodes, and hence with the terms reaction and reactive.

Reaction and reactive

A fascinating historical account of the introduction of these terms during the nineteenth century, first into medicine and then into psychiatry, has been given by Starobinski (1977). By the end of the century, the word reaction was common currency, both in biology and in experimental psychology (where stimulus–response psychology, for example, became in German Reiz–Reaktions-Psychologie). It was taken up and used by psychiatrists, at first as a psychological concept (changes in mental function or behaviour, in response to psychological stimuli), and then as a biological concept (changes in brain function resulting from environmental or metabolic change). Of these two usages, the former was to prove the more influential.

At first, reaction was used to refer to psychological correlates or antecedents of neurosis, rather than to the clinical phenomena themselves. Sommer (1894) wrote of the reaction of the patient's personality on compulsive drives. Breuer & Freud (1955: p. 8) described the part played by reactions in the genesis of hysteria:

> The most important of these is *whether there has been an energetic reaction to the event that provokes an affect*. By 'reaction' we here understand the whole class of voluntary and involuntary reflexes – from tears to acts of revenge – in which, as experience shows us, the affects are discharged. If this reaction takes place to a sufficient amount a large part of the affect disappears as a result...If the reaction is suppressed, the affect remains attached to the memory.

An abnormal reaction is here conceived as a faulty response to emotional stimuli, which does not in itself constitute a neurosis, but which helps to lay the foundations for a neurosis. It may occur long before the appearance of clinical symptoms, and thus forms part of that predisposition thought to be necessary for the development of any mental illness. This concept of reaction was to become widely accepted in the psychoanalytic movement, and to be incorporated into such formulations as Freud's 'reaction formation' and Jung's 'reaction systems'.

In general, psychoanalytic writers did not pay much attention to problems of taxonomy and clinical classification, their attitude remaining basically that expressed by Freud in his celebrated essay on 'Little Hans': '...that our conception of 'disease' is a purely practical one and a question of summation, that predisposition and the eventualities of life must combine before the threshold of this summation is overstepped,...' (Freud, 1909). The notion that the clinical phenomena of mental disorder might themselves represent a form of reaction crystallized only slowly. As soon as it did so, it was seen to present a contrast to the degeneration and disease process hypotheses, and thus to offer a possible axis of classification. Some authors – for example, Ziehen (1894) – had already referred to reactive psychosis, reactive mania, etc., but with no causal implication: they conjectured that the manic phase of a circular psychosis might in some sense be a reaction to the depressive phase, and vice versa. Now Hellpach (1904) proposed that the milder forms of mental illness ('...the neurasthenic, nervous, hypochondriacal and phobic disorders') should be divided into two main groups, the reactive and the productive. The former would comprise disorders with a well-defined onset, occurring in previously normal persons as a response to events, and having a favourable prognosis. The latter would include milder analogues of manic-depressive and other psychoses, some of which might indeed be triggered off by events such as child-birth, bereavement or loss of money, but whose clinical course and severity were quite independent of the event: 'The abnormality carries within itself the seeds of its own future development; it is productive.'

Hellpach made a spirited, if not altogether convincing, attempt to show that this proposal represented an improvement on the exogenous–endogenous dichotomy of Möbius. After discussing the weaknesses of the latter, summarized above, he went on to say that '...this dualistic concept is not compatible with an important aspect of causation; it is restricted to the question of onset'. His own suggestion, on the other hand, would conform well with the descriptive criteria set out by Kahlbaum, Hecker and Kraepelin, and thus ensure that '...the question "how?" should be at the focus of interest; not, however, solely in relation to the onset, but rather to the whole manifestation of being ill'. The point is valid if the descriptive clinical groupings do indeed correspond to Hellpach's proposed dichotomy, but not otherwise.

The first clear definition of a group of reactive disorders was made by Eduard Reiss of Tübingen, in his monograph on affective illness (Reiss, 1910). From the study of an extensive clinical material, he reached the conclusion that life events had not infrequently played a critical role in aetiology, and hence that it was justifiable to speak of purely reactive depression. Reiss was, however, well aware of the inherent fallacy of *post hoc ergo propter hoc*. Certain conditions, he declared, must be fulfilled before an illness can be classed as reactive. The preceding events must be serious in nature and of a kind to distress the affected person deeply (here, however, the individual personality should be borne in mind). The onset of illness must follow directly on the traumatic events and must be abrupt rather than insidious in character; subsequent remission may occur either rapidly or slowly, and will be influenced by external circumstances. The content of the morbid ideas must be connected with the causal events, or at any rate must be understandable in terms of the person's character and background. Ideas of guilt, for example, need not speak against a diagnosis of reactive depression, if they are in keeping with the person's self-image. The duration of illness should not be greatly prolonged, but no precise limit can be fixed: the curve of remission varies too much from case to case. Not seldom, added Reiss, does one see patients whose symptoms have persisted for weeks or months after the external cause has been removed.

Perhaps the most impressive feature of Reiss' monograph is his ability to identify a group of purely reactive depressive states, yet at the same time to insist on the essential continuity of the range of depressive illness:

> Everywhere we find connections and transitions; it is possible without the least difficulty to arrange the very widely-differing individual cases in a long, unbroken chain, ranging from the simple, reactive mood-changes of the constitutional depressive to hysterical psychoses on the one hand, and on the other hand to periodic endogenous depression, and thence to typical cyclothymic disorders.

This observation was highly significant, since it at once suggested that labels such as reactive, exogenous, etc., on the one side, and productive, endogenous, etc., on the other, were referring to differences of degree, rather than of kind, in the causation of mental disorders. Reiss' conclusions in this regard were influential on the thinking of some British and American psychiatrists, but much less so on the European continent. Here, the word reaction came more and more to denote a qualitative difference and to be applied only to certain carefully defined groups of conditions. Two main categories of reaction were distinguished: the one psychological (psychogenic reactive) and the other biological (exogenous reactive).

The psychogenic reaction

Karl Jaspers (1965), following the lines laid down by Hellpach, Reiss and others, defined reaction as a psychological concept. He went a good deal further, however, in stipulating criteria for what was acceptable as a reactive state. In essence, there were three requirements:

> In conclusion let us once more summarise the factors common to all *genuine reactions*. There is a *precipitating factor*, which stands in a close time-relationship with the reactive state and has to be one which we can accept as adequate. There is a meaningful connection between the *contents* of the experience and those of

> the abnormal reaction. As we are concerned with a reaction to an experience, any abnormality will lapse with the course of time In particular, the abnormal reaction comes to an end when the primary cause for the reaction is removed (regaining one's freedom, the return of the homesick girl to her people). Reactive abnormalities are therefore a complete contrast to all morbid processes which appear spontaneously.

It is noticeable that although Jaspers, in contrast to Reiss, did not adduce any clinical material in evidence, his general tone is more dogmatic – almost, indeed, as though he were pronouncing ontological truths, rather than simply trying to construct a useful working model. The weakness of this position becomes at once apparent when one considers the disorders which, in Jaspers' submission, show such a strong polarity with the main body of psychiatric illness. They include prison psychoses, compensation neuroses following industrial injury, psychoses following earthquakes and other natural disasters, homesickness reactions, war psychoses and psychoses due to isolation (as, for example, among deaf persons or those living in foreign-speaking populations). Not only is this a heterogeneous collection, but the clinical picture within each group may vary widely. Moreover, Jaspers is forced by his own criteria to exclude those disorders, such as post-partum psychosis, whose morbid content and subsequent course may be unrelated to the precipitating event.

Despite these grave flaws, Jaspers' formulation has had widespread and lasting influence. Kurt Schneider, a great admirer of Jaspers, adopted his criteria and used them in defining the 'abnormal reaction to experiences' (Schneider, 1927). He sharpened the distinction between such reactions and the main body of mental disorders, by insisting that the former were meaningfully motivated and should not be considered as forms of illness, but rather as 'abnormal characteristics of sane mental life'. In 1950, Schneider wrote a brief account of his views for the benefit of American psychiatrists, in which he gave the schema set out in Table 2. Here, abnormal reactions to experiences are grouped together with intellectual and personality deviations, and do not come under the rubric of illness. Schneider explained that he preferred to restrict the words illness, psychosis and pathological to conditions where there was evidence of organic pathology or developmental defect. The same point had been made repeatedly in his German publications: 'The term "illness" is quite inapplicable in this context. We have repeatedly confined "illness" to psychic disturbances with a somatic etiology, and we can find no such basis here. Since there is no question of illness, treatment involves psychotherapy only and no medication, apart perhaps from the smallest possible conservative support.' (Schneider, 1950*b*). Schneider's classification was thus perfectly consistent with his own theoretical premises. It gives rise, none-the-less, to a number of awkward questions. To begin with, what exactly is being classified? It cannot be only mental illness, since the first category would then be excluded. If, as seems probable, Schneider was simply trying to classify the scope and content of psychiatric practice in his day, then we need to know which 'abnormal varieties of sane mental life' qualify for psychiatric attention: though not, apparently, for medical treatment. What is psychotherapy, if not a form of treatment? And since affective disorders (cyclothymia) and schizophrenia have no known organic pathology, should they not logically be placed in the first, rather than the second, category?

The arguments propounded by Schneider have been carried to their logical conclusion by some latter-day psychiatrists – notably Szasz (1961) – who hold that only disorders with a known organic pathology can legitimately be classed as mental illnesses and hence qualify for medical treatment. Most clinicians who use the term 'abnormal reaction'

Table 1.2. *Schneider's classification*

1. Abnormal varieties of sane mental life	
Abnormal intellectual capacity (predisposition)	
Abnormal (psychopathic) personalities	
Abnormal reactions to emotional impressions	
2. Results of illness and developmental defects	
Somatological (aetiological) grouping:	Psychological (symptomatological) grouping:
Intoxications	
Paresis	Acute: clouding of consciousness
Other infections	
Other somatic illnesses	Chronic: personality deterioration
Abnormal brain development	(congenital: arrested personality
Brain injuries	development) and dementia
Cerebral arteriosclerosis	Cyclothymia
Senile brain diseases	
Other brain diseases	
Genuine epilepsy	Schizophrenia
?	
?	

Source: Schneider (1950*a*).

continue to behave in practice as though this were a medical diagnosis, and to offer the patients concerned not only psychotherapy, but also medication and whatever other forms of treatment they believe to be indicated.

Reactive (psychogenic) psychoses

In Schneider's classification, all psychoses are assumed to have a somatic pathology, and by definition are not reactive. A very different approach has been adopted in the Scandinavian countries, where a distinct group of psychogenic, or reactive, psychoses is recognized. Although the monograph by August Wimmer (1916), who first described this category, has not been translated, the clinical features of the reactive psychoses have been lucidly summarized by Strömgren, both in English and in German (Strömgren, 1972, 1974).

Wimmer's definition ran as follows:

> As psychogenic psychoses we designate . . . the various, clinically independent psychoses, the main feature of which is that they – usually on a definite predisposed foundation – are caused by mental agents ('mental traumata'), and in such a way that these pathemata determined the moment for the start of the psychosis, the fluctuations (remissions, intermissions, exacerbations) of the disease; very often also its cessation. Likewise the form and the content of the psychosis are more or less directly and completely ('comprehensibly') determined by the precipitating mental factors. To these criteria can, finally, be added the predominant tendency of these disorders to recovery and, more specifically, that they never end in deterioration (Strömgren, 1974).

The criteria indicated here are obviously similar to Jaspers', although Wimmer is applying them specifically to psychotic states. Strömgren (1968) considered it unlikely that Wimmer had been influenced by Jaspers, pointing out that Wimmer's ideas were first set out in a paper published in 1913, the same year in which the first edition of *Allgemeine Psychopathologie* appeared.

The consequence of Wimmer's teaching was the demarcation of a group of disorders which would otherwise have had to be distributed among the existing categories of psychosis. The emphasis on psychogenesis and on the good prognosis suggests overlap with the 'schizophreniform states' of Langfeldt (1939) and the 'Emotionspsychosen' of Staehelin (1947) and Labhardt (1963), though the category is clinically more heterogeneous than either. According to Strömgren, it comprises three main syndromes: (1) emotional reactions (mainly depressive); (2) confusional states, with clouding of consciousness; (3) paranoid reactions. Definition of the category is thus based, not on the clinical features, but on a distinctive mode of onset and course.

Strömgren and his colleagues have tried, by means of careful clinical investigation, to establish the validity of this diagnostic concept. Faergeman (1963), at Strömgren's suggestion, carried out a 15–20-year follow-up study on patients who had been diagnosed by Wimmer and his staff, during the years 1924–26, as having psychogenic psychoses. Of 170 patients, all but 10 were successfully followed up (53 who had died in the intervening years being assessed on the basis of the medical history). The original diagnosis was confirmed in 79 cases, or just under 50%; 56 (35.0%) were now considered to have been misdiagnosed, while in the remaining 25 (15.6%) the diagnosis remained uncertain. Most of the misdiagnosed cases turned out to be schizophrenic psychoses.

In a subsequent study, McCabe & Strömgren (1975) examined the family history of 40 patients with a diagnosis of reactive psychosis, consecutively admitted to two Danish hospitals. They calculated the morbid risk for reactive psychosis, manic-depressive psychosis and schizophrenia among the parents and siblings of the probands, and compared the estimated risk of each condition among the siblings with corresponding estimates based on Stroñgren's own earlier studies of affective psychosis and schizophrenia (Strömgren, 1938). Among the parents, the morbid risk for reactive psychosis, manic-depressive psychosis and schizophrenia was estimated at 4·0, 7·4 and 0·0%, respectively. The findings for the siblings are summarized in Table 1.3.

Table 1.3. *Reactive psychosis: morbid risk among probands' siblings, compared with siblings of manic-depressive and schizophrenic patients*

Type of psychosis	Probands' siblings		Siblings of manic-depressives[b]		Siblings of schizophrenics[b]	
	Cases	Bz[a]	Cases	Bz[a]	Cases	Bz[a]
Reactive	7	104	1	177	6	328
Manic-depressive	2	82	13	163	2	299
Schizophrenic	1	125	3	188	27	371

[a] Bz (Bezugsziffer) = adjusted population, estimated by Strömgren's method.
[b] Cross-section material from Strömgren (1938).
Source: McCabe & Strömgren (1975).

The morbid risk for reactive psychosis was significantly higher among the siblings of the probands than among the other groups; moreover, their morbid risk for schizophrenia was low. It would appear that, despite some overlap with manic-depressive psychosis, the reactive psychoses display their own pattern of familial risk. The morbid risk for psychosis generally was as high among the probands' siblings (3.2%) as among those of manic-depressive and schizophrenic patients (3·2% and 3·5%, respectively). According to Strömgren (1968), the morbid risk for reactive psychosis in the general population is about 1%, which is similar to that for schizophrenia. While it is not possible from these data to estimate the 'heritability' of reactive psychosis, it would appear that familial predisposition is of roughly equal importance in this group and in schizophrenia. This raises a question as to what contribution environmental factors make to the aetiology of reactive psychosis, over and above any part they may play in the causation of 'endogenous' psychoses such as schizophrenia.

It may be that the genotype is associated with a form of increased sensitivity which manifests itself in exaggerated or abnormal responses to environmental stimuli, which for most people are innocuous. Minor life events and experiences would then have, for the affected individuals, the same pathogenic significance as pollen and house dust for those who are allergic to them. The difficulty with this kind of model is that, if environmental pathogens are ubiquitous, and the vulnerable persons thus constantly exposed to them, one would expect the resulting illness to run a chronic or recurrent course: a pattern to which schizophrenia conforms more closely than reactive psychosis.

A further criticism concerns the implied equation, reactive = psychogenic. Slater (1964), in a detailed review of Faergeman's (1963) monograph, pointed out that organic illness had probably played an important part in 16 cases (10.0%), while no psychogenic factors were reported for a further 9. It is, of course, possible for psychological and physical noxae to interact and reinforce one another; but in that event one cannot assume that the former are always of primary significance and the latter secondary. In this context, it may be relevant that about 15% of reactive psychoses take the form of delirious reactions or states of clouded consciousness (Strömgren, 1974). These are conditions more usually associated with cerebral or systemic disease than with purely psychic causes, so that the question of differential diagnosis, as between psychogenic and organic reactions, is evidently an important one.

The organic reaction type

In the foregoing discussion, a reaction is conceived of as a response of the person to his environment. In the biophysiological sense of this term, it is not the individual but his brain that reacts. Mental disorder as a consequence of brain disease, systemic illness or intoxication has been recognized throughout the history of psychiatry, but its definition and description were limited, until the present century, by the lack of any unifying principles. Large numbers of conditions were reported, corresponding to the underlying causes: thyrotoxicosis, myxoedema, infectious fevers, head injury, sunstroke, pellagra, surgical operations, etc. It was the achievement of Karl Bonhoeffer to bring order to this confused scene, by delineating the principal organic psychosyndromes and by demonstrating that each could be due to a variety of causal agents.

In his earlier papers, Bonhoeffer (1908; 1909) referred to this group of conditions as symptomatic and exogenous psychoses. He did not differentiate firmly between those which resulted from acute infection or trauma, and hence could be labelled exogenous in the narrow sense, and those which resulted from metabolic or endocrine disease. Indeed, he considered the distinction artificial from a clinical standpoint, as the following passage makes clear:

> From a general overview of the symptomatic mental disorders, one point seems to me to stand out with particular clarity. The wide variety of the underlying disease processes is in sharp contrast to the great similarity of the clinical pictures. One has the impression that we are dealing with typical psychic reaction-types, which are relatively independent of the specific forms of noxious agent. Infective diseases, debilitating systemic illnesses, auto-intoxication arising from the most various kinds of organic disorder; all result in essentially similar forms of mental impairment. One is justified in speaking of exogenous psychological reaction-types, since chronic intoxication, severe brain damage or cerebral oedema can all manifest similar acute clinical pictures (Bonhoeffer, 1910).

The principal forms of reaction designated by Bonhoeffer were delirious states, twilight states, epileptiform excitement, disorientation, Korsakow-type dysmnesia and paranoid hallucinatory states. In order to explain the generic relationship between various kinds of trauma or intoxication and the ensuing mental disorder, he postulated intermediate metabolic products, which were directly responsible for the altered functioning of the brain.

What Bonhoeffer attempted was, therefore, nothing less than an integrative synthesis of organic mental states, comparable to that of Kraepelin for the 'endogenous' psychoses. To a large extent, he was successful. The organic psychosyndromes recognized in modern psychiatry – clouding of consciousness, delirium, confusional states, dysmnesic syndrome, organic neurasthenia – correspond fairly well to those named by Bonhoeffer (Kennedy, 1949; Conrad, 1972). Insofar as they have demonstrable neuropathological correlates, these syndromes can be accepted as valid in a sense that psychopathological or purely descriptive groupings cannot. Yet a final synthesis has proved elusive, and some doubts persist.

Part of the trouble stems from Bonhoeffer's choice of terms. 'Exogenous' is a dubious label for a group of conditions which may arise (*a*) from physical or chemical trauma to the brain; (*b*) from primary cerebral disease; (*c*) from cerebral dysfunction secondary to systemic disease; (*d*) from effects of malnutrition, drug abuse, etc. 'Reaction' is also a questionable term if the organic syndrome proves to be the manifestations of a developing, possibly irreversible, disease process. Prognostic criteria, corresponding to those stated by Jaspers for psychological reactions, would if applied in the field of organic psychiatry automatically rule out many of the symptomatic disorders.

A further source of difficulty is that typically 'endogenous' psychoses may occur in association with cerebral or other forms of physical disease (Bleuler, 1951). At times, the mode of onset leaves the clinician in little doubt that the mental disorder is secondary to somatic disease. Should such conditions be classed as 'exogenous reactions', even though the clinical features do not correspond? Cases in point are the manic or paraphrenic psychoses which may herald Dementia paralytica, the schizophreniform picture of amphetamine psychosis (Connell, 1958) and the schizophrenia-like psychoses of epilepsy (Slater, Beard & Glithero, 1963).

There can be little doubt that predisposition is important for the genesis of many symptomatic psychoses. Kleist (1920) found evidence of recurrent episodes among patients with post-infection psychoses, which he ascribed to an underlying 'symptomatic lability'. As with the reactive psychoses discussed above, the familial tendency appears to be non-specific. Beck (1930) reported a definite family history of psychosis in one fifth of his probands, but only a fraction of the affected relatives had had symptomatic psychoses. Formanek (1939), investigating the records of 117 patients with this diagnosis, found a history of psychosis in 25 siblings; of these, 16 had been diagnosed as schizophrenic. The distinction between symptomatic and endogenous psychoses is anything but clearcut, in terms either of the clinical picture, of the medical history or of the family history. Further difficulties arise in assessing the evidence, since most of the milder forms of delirium, confusional state and secondary affective disorder are never seen by psychiatrists, but are dealt with by general physicians and surgeons. The series reported in the psychiatric literature are, therefore, highly unrepresentative.

Despite its limitations, Bonhoeffer's concept has proved of great clinical and paradigmatic value. He demonstrated that certain morbid conditions, well defined as to pathology, symptomatology and – up to a point – course and response to treatment, were not specific disease entities, but could be caused by a variety of agents, external or internal, acting singly or in combination. This at once gave rise to the question: if an organic reaction type, then why not a schizophrenic or a manic-depressive reaction type? Should perhaps all the major psychoses be regarded not as nosological entities, but rather as pathological states, analogous to congestive heart failure or uraemia, each resulting from the action of various aetiological agents along a final common pathway?

The psychobiological model

These implications were clearly in Bleuler's mind when he transmuted the Kraepelinian concept of Dementia praecox into 'the group of schizophrenias' (Bleuler, 1911); on balance, however, he rejected them. Psychological stress, he opined, could cause a flare-up of symptoms when the disease was already present, much as physical exertion could cause a haemoptysis in someone whose lungs were already affected by tuberculosis. But, he added, the analogy was not exact, since the symptoms of schizophrenia, unlike those of tuberculosis, did not betoken tissue damage, but rather '. . . a reaction under altered circumstances, not differing in principle from a normal reaction' (p. 281).

An altogether firmer disavowal of Kraepelinian notions came from the United States, where in the years 1903–11 the Swiss-born psychiatrist Adolf Meyer published a series of influential papers setting out his theory of psychiatric reaction types. Meyer believed that, in the state of knowledge at that time, attempts to explain hysterical fits, delusional systems, etc., in terms of cellular pathology were futile. If, on the other hand, these phenomena were viewed as faulty responses or attempts at adjustment, the way was opened to a search for modifiable determining factors, and thence possibly to preventive action. Meyer was unwilling to relegate the precipitating causes of illness to a subordinate role:

> We do well to point to the constitutional peculiarity – a lack of immunity. Since there are cases in which we cannot find any precipitating factors, we are apt to spread ourselves on a statement of heredity and possibly degeneracy of make-up, of possible lesions, etc., and to over-emphasize these issues. What we actually know is that this patient is apt to react with a peculiar depressive reaction where others get along with a fair balance. The aetiology thus involves: (1) constitutional make-up, and (2) a precipitating factor . . . It is my contention that we must use *both* facts and that, of the two, for prevention and for the special characterization of the make-up, the precipitating factor is of the greater importance because *it* alone gives us an idea of the actual defect and a suggestion as to how to strengthen the person so that he may become resistive. It is a problem of index of resistance with regard to certain difficulties of mental adjustment. (Meyer, 1908).

Meyer was here writing about a case of depression, but he regarded the point as valid for all forms of mental illness. In the simple system of classification he developed, all the categories were described at first as reaction types (schizophrenic, affective, organic, etc.) and then subsequently as 'ergasias' (parergasia, thymergasia, anergasia, etc.). In this schema, the notion of specific disease entities was virtually abandoned.

Over the years, Meyer's concepts evolved into a 'psychobiological' theory of illness, according to which the phenomena of mental disorder can be understood only in relation to the genetic endowment, life history and social adaptation of the individual patient. Meyerian 'commonsense' psychology is essentially normative in its implications, insisting that both the occurrence of a psychosis and its content can be understood if one knows enough about the patient. Great importance is to be placed, therefore, on detailed anamnesis, and on the biographical correlates of mental illness. This approach was entirely in keeping with the philosophy of a man who, throughout his life, was concerned as much with humanitarian reform as with medical science; who pioneered the development of out-patient psychiatry and of psychiatric social work, and who foresaw the community mental health centre half a century before its appearance.

Meyer's typology was, in some respects, a distinct advance on the narrower formulations of Jaspers, Bonhoeffer and Bleuler. Contrasts between exogenous and endogenous, psychogenic and organic, reactive and productive, fell into place as motifs in a larger pattern. The way seemed open at last for the construction of a general theoretical model, which would incorporate the aetiology of both physical and mental illness. In one sense, indeed, this was true, since Meyer's psychobiological theory provided a template for use in anthropological and psychosomatic medicine (Weizsäcker, 1951; Selye, 1956). Yet within the main corpus of psychiatry, and especially in European psychiatry, Meyer's concepts were to have relatively little influence. Why should this have been the case?

One explanation is simply that his terminology was not acceptable. Attempts at neologistic classification are not uncommon in psychiatry, and tend for the most part to be greeted with some reserve. Terms such as 'dysergasia' and 'parergasia' conveyed nothing to most clinicians. More serious was the criticism that Meyer's formulation was over-inclusive. A theory which is broad enough to explain everything in general can explain nothing in particular. Slater & Roth (1969) no doubt had this weakness in mind when they wrote of 'the unproductive generalities of Meyerian psychobiology' and opined that his approach had proved heuristically sterile. It is certainly true that, in the half century following Meyer's early papers, little attempt was made to render the concept of the reaction types operational in a scientific sense, so that it might be subjected to empirical testing.

Modern concepts and classifications

The years 1880–1914 were remarkably productive in psychiatric theory. We still rely to a great extent, in clinical description and diagnosis, on the conceptual tools forged during that period. Most of the psychiatric classifications in use today would be readily intelligible to the leading authorities of the 1914 era.

The concept of reaction is a case in point. By that year, most of the important theories had been stated, the protagonists of the different schools – organicist, phenomenological, psychoanalytic, psychobiological – had taken up their respective positions and established their ground. Nothing that impinged on psychiatry in the next two generations – neither experience of military and civilian casualties in two world wars (Meyer, 1961*b*), nor the slow accumulation of evidence from epidemiological and ecological research (Cooper & Shepherd, 1970), nor the growth of psychological and sociological theories of behaviour – exercised any profound influence on the thinking of psychiatrists about this issue. Purely casuistical studies appeared to have achieved all that was possible in that direction; so that when, for example, Lewis (1934) wrote his classic papers on melancholia, those who agreed with him that depressive illness was a single broad entity were now doubly convinced, whilst those who did not remained sceptical as before.

The advent of computer technology seemed for a time to offer promise of a more refined, scientific approach to the problems of diagnostic classification. By and large, this promise has not been fulfilled (Kendell, 1975). In any case, the results of multifactorial analysis must depend on the selection of 'input' data, and it is self-evident that an input restricted to clinical descriptive items can yield no information bearing directly on aetiology. Factor analysis, principal components analysis or cluster analysis may be of help in deciding whether or not psychotic and neurotic depression are distinct entities; what they cannot do, with the kind of input so far provided, is to distinguish between reactive and endogenous types.

Uncertainty and confusion on this issue continue to be reflected both in psychiatric textbooks and in systems of classification. The diagnostic schemata in use in many different countries up to about 1960 were ably reviewed by Stengel (1959) for the World Health Organization, by Meyer (1961*a*) and by Menninger (1963). Their reports supply much information on modern psychiatric concepts of reaction and reactive states.

The influence of Adolf Meyer was still strongly apparent in the Diagnostic and statistical manual of the American Psychiatric Association – DSM-II (American Psychiatric Association, 1965), which listed schizophrenia, manic-depressive psychosis, psychoneuroses, etc., as reactions, and added that 'to each category of "Chronic Brain Disorders" one of the following qualifying phrases can be added: (i) with psychotic reaction; (ii) with neurotic reaction; (iii) with behavioral reaction'. In this schema, 'Acute Brain Syndrome' (which corresponds roughly to Bonhoeffer's exogenous reaction type) is one of the few categories *not* classed as reactive. The Canadian system cited by Stengel differed from the American, in that neurotic disorders were classed as reactions (anxiety, hysterical, obsessive-compulsive, etc.), but psychoses were not.

As might be expected, the term 'reaction' has featured less prominently in European systems of classification. It does not occur in the French standard system. The pre-war German system (the so-called Würzburg scheme) included a category of 'abnormal reactions', which was later expanded to 'abnormal reactions and developments', and lumped various neuroses together with paranoid reactions, induced psychoses, prison psychoses, etc. Here the influence of Jaspers and Schneider can be detected. Attempts to improve on this schema were made by Kleist (1953), Conrad (1956) and Leonhard (1957). In all three classifications, the emphasis is on somatogenic, or endogenous, causation. Kleist has a group of 'abnormal predispositions with psychogenic reactions', consisting mainly of psychopathic states; Conrad has a group labelled 'reactions to inner conflict', which comprises neuroses and psychosomatic disorders.

The Scandinavian classifications pay much more attention to reactivity. The Danish Psychiatric Society developed a scheme which included both (*a*) psychogenic mental disorder (affective, confusional and paranoid psychoses) and (*b*) 'isolated abnormal reactions' (affective, hysterical, paranoid, etc.). An elaborate Norwegian classification lists several forms of reactive psychosis, and also differentiates between neuroses and neurotic reactions.

The concept of reactive psychosis has gained recognition in a number of other countries. In the Soviet Union, a group of psychogenic mental disorders is described, which includes 'reactive psychoses' as well as various neuroses; schizophrenia and manic-depressive psychosis are listed separately and are not thought of as reactions. In Japan also, the term 'reactive' is employed in a restricted sense, the main psychoses being classed explicitly as 'endogenous'. Here, psychogenic psychoses comprise a distinct group, apparently corresponding to the Scandinavian concept.

The need for an internationally agreed classification has become increasingly apparent over the past two to three decades, and the system developed by the World Health Organization has been adopted by professional bodies in many countries. In the successive revisions of this scheme, the word 'reaction' has been used less and less in a broad, Meyerian sense, more and more with firm aetiological connotations. This trend has doubtless helped to make the classification as a whole more acceptable to European psychiatrists, but has also served to underline the difficulties of aetiological classification.

In the current glossary, based on the ninth revision of the *International Classification of Diseases* (ICD) (World Health Organisation, 1978), a category of 'other non-organic psychoses' is listed, restricted to 'the small group of psychotic conditions that are largely or entirely attributable to a recent life experience. They should not be used for the wider range of psychoses in which environmental factors play some (but not the *major*) part in aetiology.' The subgroups of this category, 'depressive type' and 'excitative type' are noted to be similar in their symptoms to the depressed and manic forms of affective psychosis, but unlike these to be provoked by emotional stress. No attempt is made to define emotional stress, other than in very general terms – bereavement, severe disappointment or frustration. The diagnostic decision rests, therefore, with the individual psychiatrist, on the basis of his history taking and his notion of what constitutes an adequate causal stress.

Anomalies of this kind can be avoided only by means of bi- or multiaxial systems of classification in which the clinical features and the supposed causal agents are grouped on separate axes. This conclusion was reached by Essen-Möller & Wohlfahrt (1947), who sketched the outline of a biaxial system nearly 40 years ago. Any given syndrome (for example, a manic psychosis) could be linked with one or more of a range of possible causal factors (for example, cerebral syphilis, systemic infection, puerperium, mental trauma, heredity). Though the principle was sound enough, many of the suggested categories were idiosyncratic and the system as a whole never gained wide clinical acceptance. Nevertheless, Essen-Möller persisted in advocating a biaxial form of classification (Essen-Möller, 1961, 1971) and in recent years his call has been echoed in a number of countries (Wing, 1970; Helmchen, 1971; Ottosson & Perris, 1973).

A move in the direction of biaxial classification is apparent in ICD-9, in which psychoses secondary to organic disease are listed in Section V (Mental disorders), whilst the primary organic disease can be coded separately under one or another of the remaining sections. Childhood psychiatric disorders can be similarly linked with organic disease or with mental retardation. An experimental trial of a multiaxial system for classifying child psychiatric disorders illustrates some of the difficulties to be overcome. Whereas the experimental schema proved superior to the conventional system (as represented by ICD-8) for defining clinical syndromes, the agreement between psychiatrists in coding aetiological – and especially psychosocial – factors of illness was poor (Rutter, Shaffer & Shepherd, 1973).

A more ambitious and radical revision of a standard schema was undertaken by the American Psychiatric Association's Task Force on Nomenclature and Statistics, in producing the DSM-III (American Psychiatric Association, 1980; Spitzer, Williams & Skodol, 1980). There is no need to dwell here on the merits of this system, whose use of operational diagnostic criteria represents, in the eyes of one observer: '. . . a breakthrough that is as obvious, necessary, fundamental and important as the corresponding breakthrough in obstetrics and surgery when Semmelweiss, Oliver Wendell Holmes and, later on, Lord Lister, demanded that obstetricians and surgeons wash their hands before operating on the human body'

(Feinstein, 1977). One may, however, venture to remark that breakthroughs achieved with the aid of numerous committees are apt to be attended by a spirit of compromise, and in this respect DSM-III is no exception. Thus, while in theory, Axis I (Clinical syndromes) is essentially descriptive, aetiological factors being coded on Axis III (Physical disorders and conditions) or Axis IV (Severity of psychosocial stressors), in practice this distinction is not entirely upheld. Axis I includes 'Brief reactive psychosis', which by definition always follows a psychosocial stressor and has a duration of less than 2 weeks. (If it persists beyond 2 weeks, a diagnosis of schizophreniform disorder must be considered). In addition, there is the category of Adjustment Disorder, which '. . . is characterized by a maladaptive reaction to an identifiable psychosocial stressor occurring within three months of the onset of the stress. . . It is assumed that the disturbance will eventually remit after the stressor ceases, or when a new level of adaptation is reached.' While, therefore, DSM-III is undoubtedly an important step towards the separation of the phenomenological and causal aspects of psychiatric classification, there is still some way to go before that goal is achieved.

Conclusion

After nearly 90 years, the psychiatric concept of mental disorder as reaction remains nebulous, and its value in classification uncertain. The foregoing historical sketch has adumbrated some of the misconceptions and sources of confusion which exist in this field, and which require closer examination. Leaving aside the question of obscure terminology ('exogenous' meaning exopathic, 'endogenous' for cryptogenic, 'stress' instead of strain, etc.), ambiguity can be detected in four areas: (1) the concept of illness; (2) the concept of aetiology; (3) the basis of classification; (4) the strategy and methods of investigation.

The concept of illness

The notion of mental disorder as a reaction was introduced at a time when medicine was dominated by the disease entity theory of illness. This viewpoint required a sharp division between reactions and 'real' illness. In the intervening period, and especially in the past 30 years, medical models of illness and health have undergone radical revision (Kendell, 1975), though this fact appears to have escaped the notice of some psychiatric theorists and of many behavioural and social scientists. A wide range of morbidity, physical as well as psychiatric, is now seen as representing pathological and statistical deviation from established norms; hence, there is no good reason not to regard mental disorders as being, in Kurt Schneider's phrase, 'abnormal varieties of sane mental life'. The essential criteria of illness lie, not in its relationship to underlying organic disease, but rather in the distress and handicap suffered by the affected individual; in the impairment of normal physiological or psychological functioning; and in the consequent biological and social disadvantage. Any 'reaction' which fulfils these criteria qualifies to be considered as an illness, whatever its causation.

The concept of aetiology

The nineteenth-century preoccupation with specific disease entities strongly influenced psychiatric thinking about aetiology. It was argued that, before a mental illness could be classified as exogenous, a necessary and sufficient external cause must be demonstrable in every case; if the external factors exercised a merely quantitative, or contributory, effect, then the primary cause must be internal and the disease an endogenous one. This line of argument inevitably weighted the scales in favour of an endogenous hypothesis, since the prediposing internal factors did not have to be demonstrated, whereas any supposed external factors did: in all cases of doubt, the onus of proof rested with the environmental hypothesis.

Here again, medical thinking and attitudes have changed radically during the present century. Not only are the postulates of Henle and Koch inapplicable to multifactorial causal models but, even for such specific diseases as pulmonary tuberculosis, it is now widely accepted that the single, necessary and sufficient causal agent is an oversimplification. The occurrence and spread of any form of disease within a population can be fully comprehended only in terms of an ecological system which incorporates host and environment as well as agent (Susser, 1973).

The concept of multifactorial aetiology has great importance for psychiatric theory. It removes the need for any basic division between reaction and illness, or between those illnesses which are thought to be reactive and those which are not. The role of environmental factors may extend far beyond those categories at present labelled exogenous or reactive. We do not yet know, in point of fact, if the types of environmental stress that precipitate an acute anxiety neurosis differ, qualitatively or quantitatively, from those which may be implicated in acute schizophrenic psychosis – or for that matter in myocardial infarction or duodenal ulceration. The only safe assumption at present is that environmental factors of some kind play a part in the causation of any mental disorder, unless it has been shown to have a concordance rate of 100% in monozygotic twins.

A related point concerns the nature of the causal link. Environmental agents need not be thought of only as stimuli, which trigger off abnormal responses (reactions) in certain predisposed individuals. Relatively few of the life events and experiences said to be pathogenic actually conform to the stimulus model. Some have a traumatic or noxious effect, directly or indirectly, on the brain: the resulting mental and behavioural changes can hardly be called reactive. Others, whose operation is psychologically mediated (bereavement, personal crises, loss of property or status, etc.) commonly pose problems of readaptation. If one considers the kind of experience often cited as the paradigm of a psychological trauma – involvement in an earthquake or other communal disaster – little imagination is required to grasp what misery and hardship may await the survivors. Pure 'shock' situations, uncomplicated by any continuing threat or problems of readjustment, are seen only rarely in psychiatric practice. Indeed, the psychiatrist does not as a rule see patients immediately after they have suffered a psychological trauma, but only later, when the altered life situation has begun to have its effect. Not until this stage is reached are individual responses likely to be recognized as morbid or maladaptive.

The basis of classification

We have seen how expressions such as reactive and endogenous, originally introduced to imply types of causation, come gradually to be employed as descriptive labels for conditions of unknown aetiology. If it were true, as Kahlbaum, Kraepelin and others postulated, that the major syndromes of psychiatry represented discrete nosological entities, each with its own characteristic aetiology and pathology, such a shift of meaning would not be so important. All the evidence, however, is against this belief. The clinical features of many so-called reactive conditions are not clearly distinct from those classed as endogenous; the one group is not known to be more closely linked with environmental change and stress situations than the other; neither is there any firm basis in population genetics for such a dichotomy.

The diagnostic classifications in use throughout medicine are to some extent illogical, in that they bring together on a single axis conditions defined in aetiological, pathological, descriptive and prognostic terms. This situation is at its worst in psychiatry, because here aetiology and pathology are still so weak. Although attempts at radical revision are unlikely to prove wholly successful as long as these weaknesses persist, the development of biaxial or multiaxial systems of classification offers some hope of progress. For the present, the best strategy in clinical practice must be to keep to descriptive diagnosis unless or until the aetiology of the condition has been firmly established, and to avoid labels such as 'reactive' whenever more suitable descriptive terms are available.

Strategy and methods of investigation

Two broad research strategies lend themselves to investigation of the causes of disease: the clinical and the epidemiological. Contrasts between the two should not be drawn too sharply, since they are complementary and each to some extent overlaps the other. Nevertheless, in the present context the differences are of some importance.

The clinical approach concentrates on individual patients who come under medical care. It attempts by means of detailed investigation to discover the nature of the underlying morbid process; to establish how the patient's symptoms and disabilities have been caused. The method is essentially rational, seeking to establish connections which the clinician can accept as meaningful and can use as guides to treatment and prognosis.

The epidemiological approach concentrates on representative groups of the general population. It attempts by means of extensive enquiry to establish important characteristics of healthy and of sick people within this population. It is not primarily concerned with the nature of the morbid process, but rather with associations between the occurrence of illness and the strength of biological or environmental factors. The method is essentially empirical, seeking to establish connections which the scientist can accept as valid and can use, both to construct hypotheses and to make recommendations for possible preventive action.

An important practical consequence of the choice of research strategy concerns the interpretation of disease distributions. The clinical approach will tend to support the view that a given morbid condition is sharply differentiated from the normal, or that two diagnostic categories are clearly distinct from one another. The epidemiological approach, by including all 'borderline' and intermediate states in proportion, will tend to support that view that a given morbid condition merges imperceptibly into the normal range, or that two diagnostic groups merge one into another. The characteristic distribution pattern derived from clinical studies will thus be bimodal; that derived from epidemiological research will be a skewed unimodal curve. Figure 1.1 illustrates three hypothetical distributions derived from clinical and epidemiological research; it emphasizes that the difference between the former and the latter may be pronounced to a greater or a lesser extent.

Until about 20 years ago, almost all investigations of the precipitating causes of mental illness relied exclusively on the clinical approach. All the theoretical formulations and classifications discussed in this review were derived, whether at first or at second hand, from the examination of

Figure 1.1. (*a*) Clinical and (*b*) epidemiological interpretations of distributions of quantitative biological characteristics (Cochrane, 1971). The shaded areas represent pathological values of the characteristic measured.

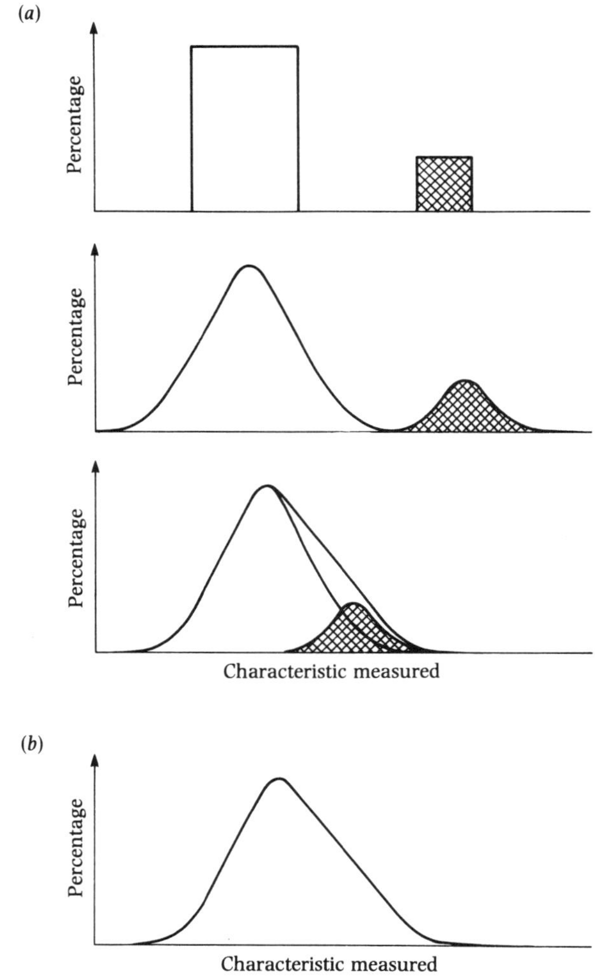

patients who came under psychiatric care. The results bear witness to the great strength and suppleness of the clinical research strategy, but they also reveal its limitations when not used in conjunction with the epidemiological. Fortunately, as some of the other contributions to this volume testify, determined efforts are now being made to restore the balance and to ensure that, in the future, our knowledge of the relationship between life events and mental illness will rest on firm scientific foundations.

References

American Psychiatric Association (1965). *Diagnostic and statistical manual for mental disorders – II (DSM-II)*. Washington: APA.

American Psychiatric Association (1980). *Diagnostic and statistical manual for mental disorders – III (DSM-III)*. Washington: APA.

Baisette, G. (1931). *Hippocrate*, vol. 1. Paris: Grasset.

Beck, E. (1930). Zur Frage des Erbfaktors bei den symptomatischen Psychosen. *Msch. Psychiat. Neurol.*, **77**, 38.

Birnbaum, K. (1923). *Der Aufbau der Psychose*. Berlin: Springer.

Bleuler, E. (1911). *Dementia praecox, oder die Gruppe der Schizophrenien*. Leipzig & Wien: Deuticke.

Bleuler, M. (1951). Psychiatry of cerebral diseases. *Br. Med. J.*, **2**, 1233.

Bonhoeffer, K. (1908). Zur Frage der Klassifikation der symptomatischen Psychosen. *Berlin klin. Wschr.*, **45**, 2257.

Bonhoeffer, K. (1909). Zur Frage der exogenen Psychosen. *Zentr. ges. Neurol. Psychiat.*, **20**, 499.

Bonhoeffer, K. (1910). *Die symptomatischen Psychosen im Gefolge von akuten Infektionen und inneren Krankheiten*. Leipzig & Wien: Deuticke (pp. 124–25).

Bonhoeffer, K. (1911). Wie weit kommen psychogene Krankheitszustände und Krankheitsprozesse vor, die nicht der Hysterie zuzurechnen sind? *Allg. Z. Psychiat.*, **68**, 371.

Breuer, J. & Freud, S. (1955). *Studies on Hysteria*. Standard edition of the complete psychological works of Sigmund Freud, vol. 2. London: Hogarth.

Cochrane, A. L. (1971). *Effectiveness and efficiency: random reflections on health services*. London: Nuffield Provincial Hospitals Trust.

Connell, P. H. (1958). *Amphetamine psychosis*. Maudsley Monograph No. 5. London: Chapman & Hall.

Conrad, K. (1956). Beitrag zur Diagnosenstatistik. *Fortschr. Neurol.*, **24**, 231.

Conrad, K. (1972). Die symptomatischen Psychosen. In *Psychiatrie der Gegenwart*, vol. 2, *Klinische psychiatrie*, ed. K. P. Kisker, J. E. Meyer, M. Müller & E. Strömgren, pp. 1–70. Berlin: Springer.

Cooper, B. & Shepherd, M. (1970). Life change, stress and mental disorder. In *Modern trends in psychological medicine*, vol. 2, ed. J. H. Price, pp. 102–30. London: Butterworth.

Esquirol, E. (1827). *Pathologie und Therapie der Seelenstörungen*. Leipzig: Hartmann.

Essen-Möller, E. (1961). On classification of mental disorders. *Act. Psychiat. Scand.*, **37**, 119.

Essen-Möller, E. (1971). Suggestions for further improvement of the international classification of mental disorders. *Psychol. Med.*, **1**, 308.

Essen-Möller, E. & Wohlfahrt, S. (1947). Suggestions for amendment of the official Swedish classification of mental disorders. *Act. Psychiat. Scand. Suppl.* **47**, 551.
Faergeman, P. (1963). *Psychogenic psychoses.* London: Butterworth.
Feinstein, A. R. (1977). A critical overview of diagnosis in psychiatry. In *Psychiatric diagnosis*, ed. V. M. Rakoff, H. C. Stancer & H. B. Kedward, pp. 189–206. New York: Brunner/Mazel.
Formanek, R. (1939). Zur Frage der symptomatischen Entstehung von Psychosen. *Z. ges. Neurol. Psychiat.*, **165**, 78.
Freud, S. (1909). *Analysis of a phobia in a five-year-old boy. Standard edition of the complete psychological works of Sigmund Freud*, vol. 10. London: Hogarth (1955).
Griesinger, W. (1867). *Mental pathology and therapeutics* (transl. C. L. Robertson & J. Rutherford). London: New Sydenham Society.
Güse, H. G. & Schmacke, N. (1979). Aufstieg und Zerstörung der wissenschaftlichen Psychiatrie in Deutschland. In *Jahrbuch für kritische Medizin*, vol. 4, pp. 161–91. Argument – Sonderband AS 37. Berlin: Argument-Verlag.
Hellpach, W. (1904). *Grundlinien einer Psychologie der Hysterie.* Leipzig: Engelmann.
Helmchen, H. (1971). Problems in the use and acceptance of an international glossary to ICD 8. Fifth World Congress of Psychiatry, Mexico City, 1971. Unpublished manuscript.
Hoch, A. (1907). The psychogenic factors in the development of psychoses. *Psychol. Bull.*, **4**, 161.
Jaspers, K. (1965). *Allgemeine Psychopathologie* (8th edition). Berlin: Springer. (English translation, 1963, *General psychopathology*, transl. J. Hoenig & M. W. Hamilton. Manchester: Manchester Univ. Press.)
Kendell, R. E. (1975). *The role of diagnosis in psychiatry.* London: Blackwell.
Kennedy, A. (1949). The organic reaction types. In *Modern practice in psychological medicine*, ed. J. R. Rees, pp. 316–56. London: Butterworth.
Kleist, K. (1920). *Die Influenzpsychosen und die Anlage zu Infektionspsychosen.* Berlin: Springer.
Kleist, K. (1953). Die Gliederung der neuropsychischen Erkrankungen. *Psychiat. Neurol.*, **125**, 526.
Kretschmer, E. (1918). *Der sensitive Beziehungswahn.* Berlin: Springer.
Labhardt, F. (1963). *Die schizophrenie-ähnlichen Emotionspsychosen.* Berlin: Springer.
Langfeldt, G. (1939). *The schizophreniform states.* Copenhagen: Munksgaard.
Leonhard, K. (1957). *Aufteilung der endogenen Psychosen.* Berlin: Akademie-Verlag.
Lewis, A. J. (1934). Melancholia: a clinical survey of depressive states. *J. Ment. Sci.*, **80**, 277.
Lewis, A. J. (1971). 'endogenous' and 'exogenous': a useful dichotomy? *Psychol. Med.*, **1**, 191.
Lewis, A. J. (1972). 'Psychogenic': a word and its mutations. *Psychol. Med.*, **2**, 209.
McCabe, M. & Strömgren, E. (1975). Reactive psychoses. A family study. *Arch. Gen. Psychiat.*, **32**, 447.
Maier, H. W. (1912). Uber katathyme Wahnbildung und Paranoia. *Z. ges. Neurol. Psychiat.*, **13**, 555.
Menninger, K. (1963). *The vital balance.* New York: Viking Press.
Meyer, A. (1908). The role of the mental factors in psychiatry. *Am. J. Insan.*, **65**, 39.
Meyer, J. E. (1961*a*). Diagnostische Einteilung und Diagnosenschemata in der Psychiatrie. In *Psychiatrie der Gegenwart*, vol. 3, 1st edition, ed. H. W. Gruhle *et al.*, pp. 130–80. Berlin: Springer.

Meyer, J. E. (1961*b*). Die abnormen Erlebnisreaktionen im Kriege bei Truppe und Zivilbevölkerung. In *Psychiatrie der Gegenwart*, vol. 3, 1st edition, ed. H. W. Gruhle *et al.*, pp. 574–619. Berlin: Springer.
Möbius, P. J. (1893). *Abriss der Lehre der Nervenkrankheiten*. Leipzig: Abel.
Neumann, H. (1859). *Lehrbuch der Psychiatrie*. Erlangen: Enke.
Ottosson, J. O. & Perris, C. (1973). Multidimensional classification of mental disorders. *Psychol. Med.*, **3**, 238.
Pinel, P. (1962). *A treatise on insanity*. History of Medicine Series No. 14, Transl. D. Davis. New York: Hafner.
Reiss, E. (1910). Konstitutionelle Verstimmung und manisch-depressives Irresein. *Z. ges. Neurol. Psychiat., Orig.* II, 347.
Rutter, M., Shaffer, D. & Shepherd, M. (1973). An evaluation of a proposal for a multi-axial classification of child psychiatric disorders. *Psychol. Med.*, **3**, 244.
Schneider, K. (1927). Die abnormen seelischen Reaktionen. In Aschaffenburg, G. *Handbuch der Psychiatrie*, ed. G. Aschaffenburg, Spez. Teil, 7. Abt. pp. 1–43. Leipzig & Wien: Deuticke.
Schneider, K. (1950*a*). Letter from Germany: systematic psychiatry. *Am. J. Psychiat.*, **107**, 334.
Schneider, K. (1950*b*). *Klinische Psychopathologie*, 3rd edition. Stuttgart: Thieme. (English translation, 1959, *Clinical psychopathology*, transl. M. W. Hamilton. New York & London: Grune & Stratton.)
Selye, H. (1956). *The stress of life*. New York: McGraw-Hill.
Slater, E. (1964). Book reviews of Faergeman (1963) and Labhardt (1963). *Br. J. Psychiat.*, **110**, 114.
Slater, E., Beard, A. W. & Glithero, E. (1963). The schizophrenia-like psychoses of epilepsy. *Br. J. Psychiat.*, **109**, 95.
Slater, E. & Roth, M. (1969). *Clinical psychiatry*, 3rd edition. London: Baillière.
Sommer, R. (1894). *Diagnostik der Geisteskrankheiten*. Wien & Leipzig: Urban & Schwarzenberg.
Spitzer, R. L., Williams, J. B. W. & Skodol, A. E. (1980). DSM-III: the major achievements and an overview. *Am. J. Psychiat.*, **137**, 151.
Staehelin, J. E. (1947). Zur Frage der Emotionspsychosen. *Bull. Schweiz. Akad. med. Wiss.*, **2**, 121.
Starobinski, J. (1977). The word reaction: from physics to psychiatry. *Psychol. Med.*, **7**, 373.
Stengel, E. (1959). Classification of mental disorders. *Bull. Wld Hlth Org.*, **21**, 601.
Strömgren, E. (1938). *Beiträge zur psychiatrischen Erblehre*. Copenhagen: Munksgaard.
Strömgren, E. (1968). Reactive psychoses. In *Contributions to Psychiatric Epidemiology and Genetics*. Copenhagen: Munksgaard.
Strömgren, E. (1972). Atypische Psychosen. Reaktive (psychogene) Psychosen. In *Psychiatrie der Gegenwart*, vol. 2, 2nd edition, ed. K. P. Kisker *et al.*, pp. 141–52.
Strömgren, E. (1974). Psychogenic psychoses. In *Themes and variations in European psychiatry*, ed. S. Hirsch & M. Shepherd, pp. 79–117. Bristol: J. Wright.
Susser, M. (1973). *Causal thinking in the health sciences*. London: Oxford Univ. Press.
Szasz, T. (1961). *The myth of mental illness*. New York: Harper.
Weizsäcker, V. von (1951). *Der kranke Mensch*. Stuttgart: Thieme.
Wimmer, A. (1916). Psykogene Sindssygdromsformer (Psychogene Geisteskrankheits

formen). In *St Hans Hospital* 1816–1916, *Jubiläumsschrift*, pp. 85–216. Copenhagen: Gad.

Wing, L. (1970). Observations on the psychiatric section of the ICD and the British Glossary of Mental Disorders. *Psychol. Med.*, 1, 79.

World Health Organisation (1978). *Mental disorders: glossary and guide to their classification in accordance with the ninth revision of the International Classification of Diseases*. Geneva: WHO.

Ziehen, T. (1894). *Psychiatrie für Arzte und Studierende*. Berlin: Wreden.

Zilboorg, G. & Henry, G. W. (1941). *A history of medical psychology*. New York: Norton.

2

Life events and mental disorder: biological theories of their mode of action*

G. TURPIN & M. LADER

As suggested by the title of this book, the role of life events in the aetiology of mental illness is controversial. Disagreements abound at a descriptive level concerning the magnitude or even the existence of any association between life events and particular forms of psychiatric disability. Few models have been proposed concerning the nature of mechanisms which might underlie these associations, and little consensus has been reached regarding mediational processes. This applies to both biological and psychological accounts of the deleterious effects of life events on psychological well being. Sadly, the lack of sound biological models to explain these effects is also mirrored by an equally confusing literature concerning the mechanisms responsible for mental illness itself. Thus, it might appear foolhardy even to attempt to integrate these diverse and speculative areas. However, we believe that the lack of theoretical integration within this area reflects the widespread occurrence of methodological and conceptual difficulties which have previously led to confusion and controversy. Accordingly, one purpose of this chapter is to describe critically possible psychobiological models of psychiatric illness which can incorporate the influences of life events, and to outline the implications of these models for future psychiatric research.

Finally, the status of psychobiological models as they relate to individual psychiatric disorders will be reviewed. The purpose of this section is to furnish examples of the application of these models rather than to provide a definitive theoretical account of the mechanisms responsible for the effects of life events on specific psychiatric illness.

Theories of psychiatric disorder

Before specifying a model of the action of life events in relation to psychiatric disorder, relevant theoretical accounts of illness *per se* need

* Preparation of this manuscript was supported by a grant from the Medical Research Council.

considering. An obvious requirement of any model of mental disorder which can accommodate the influence of life events is that it emphasizes environmental agents either as formative or precipitating factors. This immediately precludes traditional biomedical models which have stressed the sole importance of endogenous biological pathogens in the causation of mental illness (see Engel, 1977; Spring & Coons, 1982). Similarly, solely behavioural explanations are likely to be too general to be predictive (Ohman, 1981*a*; Spring & Coons, 1982). This is particularly relevant to life event research since recent studies stress the small proportion of the experimental variance accounted by such episodes (e.g. Andrews & Tennant, 1978). Hence, the occurrence of a life event is neither a necessary nor sufficient condition for the onset of mental disorder. An adequate explanation of the influence of life events, therefore, must predict those conditions under which they produce psychological dysfunction and identify those people at risk. Since behavioural explanations focus on current environmental contingencies, insufficient emphasis is placed upon features in the person's history influencing susceptibility to life events.

Several recently developed models of illness attempt to overcome some of the above difficulties (Engel, 1977; Weiner, 1977). Rather than limiting explanations of disease* to functional descriptions of disorder, Weiner (1977) has addresed the problem of predicting the risk and temporal onset of disease within a population: ultimately, any explanation of disease must also concern the mediational processes responsible for both its predisposition and its initiation in certain individuals. To encompass the breadth of factors influencing the prevalence of illness, so-called 'psychobiological' or 'biopsychosocial' models of disease have been advocated (Engel, 1977; Van Praag, 1981). As well as social and cultural factors, these models also stress the reciprocal nature of the environment–brain–behaviour relationship.

Theoretical models of disease have also incorporated the indisputable contribution of genetic factors to most psychiatric conditions (Rosenthal, 1970; Kety *et al.*, 1983). Of particular importance is the notion of 'vulnerability' or 'diathesis' whereby an inherited predisposition for disease is expressed only under certain environmental conditions of a 'stressful' nature. Two such interactionist model examples are those of Meehl (1962) and Zubin & Spring (1977), both concerning the aetiology of schizophrenia. These models divide the manifestation of illness into predispositional or vulnerability factors and environmental events initiating or precipitating the onset of illness. Such models readily incorporate life

* The term 'disease' is used to describe a theory of mental disorder (Wing, 1979).

Figure 2.1. The role of life events in 'stress-vulnerability' models of psychiatric disorder.

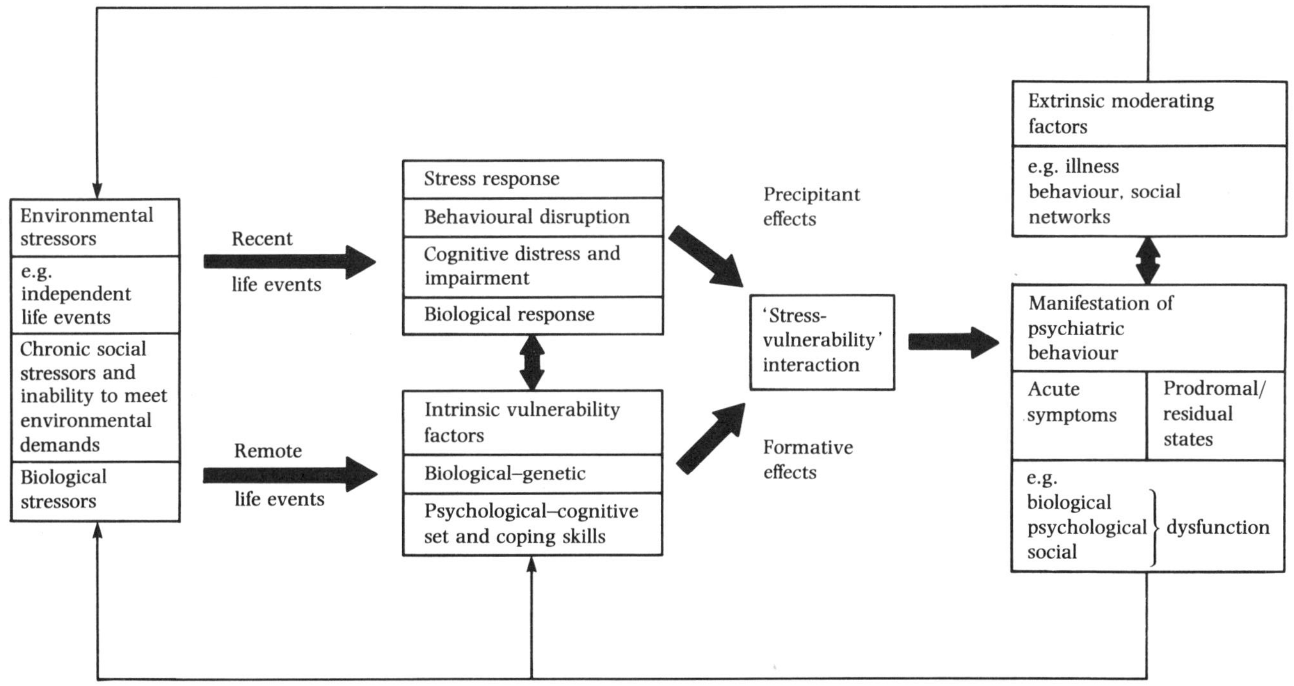

events as initiating environmental factors. Moreover, individual differences in vulnerability might also account for the majority of the population being without serious psychological impairment despite having undergone serious life events.

Although diathesis as described by Meehl (1962) refers primarily to inherited predispositional factors, its companion term 'vulnerability' has been expanded to include predispositional environmental factors (Zubin & Spring, 1977; Spring & Coons, 1982). Indeed, Depue, Monroe & Shackman (1979) stress that predispositional factors may not even be specific to particular diseases but depend on a constellation of factors operating via a final common pathway underlying a particular psychological dysfunction. They characterize biological predisposition as the dysfunction of a specific physiological regulatory system. Psychological predisposition takes the form of particular cognitive biases which operate when a person appraises an environmental event and which, in turn, influences the 'emotional–biologic' response. The inclusion of environmental and psychological factors in determining vulnerability also allows life events to contribute not only to the initiation of disease but to be possible causes predisposing a person to disease. Thus, recent life events may be triggering factors which alter the timing of disease but not its probability of occurrence, whereas remote life events may be formative factors that are usually irreversible and increase the likelihood of disease.

The notion of life events as formative factors causally related to the development of illness is also consistent with the role of 'psychosocial stress' in the aetiology of so-called 'psychosomatic illness'. This emphasis on 'stress'-induced disease has been promoted by Selye's influential writings concerning the effects of environmental challenges upon a generalized, hormonally mediated stress response known as the General Adaptation Syndrome. Selye (1979) suggests that disease results from the inability of the physiological systems subserving the General Adaptation Syndrome to adapt effectively to the challenge imposed by environmental stressors.

In summary, several models of psychiatric disorder exist which might accommodate the deleterious effects of life events. Figure 2.1 outlines a possible 'stress-vulnerability' model and serves as a basis for investigating biological mechanisms underlying the effects of life events on psychiatric disorder. The conceptual problems raised by 'stress-vulnerability' models and the implications of such models for research are examined in the next section.

'Stress-vulnerability' models

Psychobiological models similar to those discussed in the previous section have been employed in the case of psychiatric disorder (Zubin & Spring, 1977; Dohrenwend & Dohrenwend, 1979), 'psychosomatic illness' (Levi, 1972; Weiner, 1977) and cardiovascular disease (Garrity & Marx, 1979). The purpose of this section is to examine critically such models in relation to biological mechanisms underlying the effects of life events and to assess their implication for future research. This will entail both a conceptual and methodological analysis.

At a conceptual level, one strength of psychobiological models is that they embrace many different levels of explanation. Unfortunately, this has also led to the criticism (e.g. Dimsdale, 1982) that they are too general and cannot predict specific effects. The problem of specificity also arises when the exact meaning or usage of the terms employed by these models is examined. This is probably best illustrated by the use of the term 'stress' within the 'stress-vulnerability' model.

Concepts of stress

Lay definitions of stress include both the idea of a constraining or impelling force and that of demand upon the energy of the constrained object. Physics uses the term to mean the constraining force (stimulus), the deformations produced in the object by that force being termed strain (response). The lay confusion has unfortunately persisted in medicine and psychology (Hinkle, 1977). The distinction between 'stress' as stimulus and 'stress' as response is extremely important for psychobiological models. For example, Spring & Coons (1982) suggest that the causal role of 'stress' in schizophrenia cannot be examined using response definitions of 'stress'. This is due to the confounding of psychological impairment, experiential distress, poor social functioning and possible changes in physiological arousal as indicators of a stress response and as possible diagnostic indicators of schizophrenia. Since the stress response may have resulted from the disease process said to underlie schizophrenia, the causal relationship between the two is unclear. Thus, in the remainder of this chapter a distinction will be made between the use of the term 'stressor' as an indication of a stressful stimulus and the term 'stress response' as the organism's reaction to particular stressors.

The definition of a stressor is not without problems. Essentially, there are two approaches: normative models defining stressors objectively and independently of the organism upon which they impinge; and the interactionist perspective that emphasizes the specific context or meaning to the organism associated with the stressor (Spring & Coons, 1982). Examples of the former are using noxious stimuli (e.g. loud noises, shock) in laboratory studies or the construction of normative life event schedules in epidemiological studies. Unfortunately, the lack of agreement between different criterion measures of the stress response (see later) produces difficulties in establishing the validity of these measures (Mason, 1971; Rabkin & Struening, 1976; Tennant, Bebbington & Hurry, 1981). On the other hand, an interactionist approach which attempts to identify stressors idiographically on the basis of the degree of perceived threat (Lazarus, 1966; Rahe, 1978) also raises conceptual problems. The most important of these refers to causality since the appraisal of stress by the individual may already reflect the presence of psychological dysfunction or illness. Similarly, so-called 'dependent life events' which arise as a probable consequence of illness might be regarded as the outcome of stress responses rather than the manifestation of a stressor. Many more problems are associated with the measurement of life events and include issues of reliability, content validity, and the retrospective falsification of life stress (see the chapters by Katschnig; Bebbington; Brown & Harris, this volume; Rabkin & Struening, 1976; Dohrenwend & Dohrenwend, 1978; 1979; Tennant *et al.*, 1981). A further discussion of these crucial methodological issues is beyond the scope of this chapter.

Given the problem of defining psychosocial stressors, the question arises as to whether the term 'stressor' is useful within the context of psychobiological models. Indeed, Hinkle (1977) has argued that 'stress theory' has outlived its usefulness, and that rather than using terms such as 'stress' and 'stressor', more attention should be paid to the objective measurement and definition of each social variable studied. Other researchers have used more descriptive terms such as life change which may be positively or negatively evaluated by the patient (Holmes & Rahe, 1967) or simply threat, upset or distress (Brown & Harris, 1978; Paykel, 1979; Bebbington, Tennant & Hurry, 1981). Although the use of these terms may profitably increase the use of operational definitions, they do not cover environmental changes relevant to psychobiological models. For instance, it would be difficult to subsume under these headings the putative effects of birth complications on later schizophrenic pathology (e.g. Beuhring *et al.*, 1982). Thus, the term 'stressor' may generally but restrictedly describe the many environmental influences which might affect the occurrence of psychiatric disorder but only if subsequent descriptions of individual stressors are objectively defined.

Response definitions of 'stress' pose probably even more insoluble problems than stressors do. First, if stress responses are defined as changes in an organism's functioning following the imposition of a stressor, several different responses are implicated. For example, Serban (1975) has used the term 'stress' to describe the inability of people to meet environmental demands successfully. Clearly, psychological dysfunction, subjective distress and poor social functioning may all be described as stress responses. Perhaps the most generally accepted response measures of 'stress' are physiological changes which may be quantified either psychophysiologically or biochemically (Lader, 1975). Physiological changes which are said to accompany stress responses include increases in heart rate, cardiac output, systolic blood pressure, peripheral vasoconstriction, palmar sweating, muscle tension and desynchrony of the electroencephalogram. These changes are often described as increases in arousal or activation (Lader, 1975; Ursin, 1978). A wide range of biochemical indices has also been examined, especially urinary excretion rates of adrenal cortical and adrenal medullary hormones and their metabolites (Mason, 1971; Levi, 1972; Frankenhaeuser, 1976; Selye, 1979).

If the concept of a general stress response is to have any explanatory value, then these disparate measures should be highly interrelated. Unfortunately, few data relate measures of stressor-induced changes in social performance to physiological indices of stress responding. The sparse extant data suggest that the relationship is complex. For example, Cobb & Kasl (1977) measured repeatedly several different physiological indices in a sample of men facing job loss through factory closure. Different measures were differentially affected depending upon whether the men were anticipating shutdown, experiencing the actual closure or suffering subsequent unemployment. Cardiovascular and endocrine measures were also employed by Rose, Hurst & Herd (1979) in their prospective study of air traffic controllers. Although these measures were reasonably stable across different testing sessions they were unrelated to measures of subjective distress as assessed using the Psychiatric Status Schedule.

Obviously, such field studies are subject to many moderating variables which might explain the low interrelationship between psychosocial and physiological measures of stress responding. Accordingly most research on the non-specificity of stress responses has examined physiological and behavioural responses to laboratory stressors. A central feature of Selye's (1979) classical model of stress is a physiological response pattern, the General Adaptation Syndrome (GAS), mediated by the pituitary–adrenal axis. Since the GAS is claimed to be a stable response pattern and is mediated by stressors in general, it should be an objective index of the stress response. The most ardent critic of this position is Mason (1971; Mason *et al.*, 1976) who has questioned both the non-specificity of the GAS and the use of purely physiological indices to measure 'stress'. In a series of animal studies of the characteristics of the adrenal cortical response to physical stressors, Mason demonstrated different patterns of hormonal activity to different stressors and to the same stressor but under different environmental conditions. Mason therefore rejected the notion of a non-specific GAS and emphasized the role of psychological variables in determining the pattern of physiological response to so-called 'physical stressors'.

Recently, Steptoe (1980) has extended Mason's critique of non-specificity to include a variety of autonomic and neuroendocrine 'stress responses'. He urges the careful analysis of environmental contingencies and response requirements when attempting to identify physiological responses to physical stressors. He also emphasizes the importance of behavioural variables such as predictability and control over the physical stressor and the availability of active coping responses as opposed to passive helplessness in determining the nature of 'stress responses'. Indeed, he suggests that the availability of active avoidance responding leads to increased sympathoadrenal activity whereas adrenal cortical activity actually decreases under conditions of control. Similarly, a unitary concept of arousal is not without its critics (Andrew, 1974; Fahrenberg & Foerster, 1982, but see Lader, 1975) and more recent arousal theories have also stressed the importance of response requirements (Vanderwolf & Robinson, 1981).

Thus, the notion of a general stress response, even at either a psychological or neurochemical level of measurement, is not justified. Researchers wishing to assess the nature of psychological change elicited by environmental stressors cannot rely on the measurement of a single index of neuroendocrine activity. Instead, a range of indices may be needed to obtain a comprehensive profile of neuroendocrine responses to different stressors (Mason *et al.*, 1976). Within the context of psychobiological models, the notion of a stress response must be seen only as a general indication of disturbance after environmental change. The nature of the disturbance must be quantified as broadly as possible and no assumptions made which might lead to the use of a single 'stress index'. We will return to the 'stress' specificity problem when discussing models of 'stress-vulnerability' interaction.

Psychiatric disorder

The use of psychobiological models assumes the existence of an underlying disease process identifiable by the manifestation of psychiatric disorder. However, not all behaviours associated with a particular psychiatric syndrome are necessarily causally related directly to an underlying disease process. For example, Hemsley (1977) has argued in the case of schizophrenia that some patterns of deviant behaviour might represent coping strategies which alleviate distress associated with a core psychological dysfunction. Similarly, the importance of social variables in determining care-seeking behaviour also needs to be recognized (Mechanic, 1978). Finally, acute psychiatric disturbances are generally distinguished from chronic residual states with associated handicaps which are probably unrelated to the processes underlying the acute form of disorder (Zubin & Spring, 1977; Wing, 1978). These issues have important implications for studying psychobiological models, especially when considering the problem of identifying disease onset. The exact time of onset of psychiatric disorders, unlike many physical disorders, may be difficult to date exactly. Ideally, onset would be manifested by signs consistent with reliable diagnostic criteria for the acute condition. However, many forms of psychiatric disorder are not characterized by a sudden appearance of symptoms but by a gradual deterioration of functioning, as in some cases of schizophrenia. The effects of life events must be examined within a longitudinal framework which allows for the episodic nature of acute disorder and the problems of prodromal and residual psychiatric states (Zubin & Steinhauer, 1981; Spring & Coons, 1982). The symptoms of acute psychiatric disorder must be distinguished from the distress of the life events (Bebbington *et al.*, 1981). Finally, for both physical and psychiatric disorders, life events increase the likelihood of illness or care-seeking behaviours independent of the specific disease process (Ingham & Miller, 1976; Mechanic, 1978).

Vulnerability

The question of psychiatric nosology has important implications for the concept of vulnerability. Vulnerability or the predisposition to disease is central to psychobiological models. Moreover, in relation to the effects of life events on psychiatric morbidity, it is a crucial concept which links the effects of environmental stressors to hypothetical disease processes. This raises an important issue concerning the nature of disease itself. Psychiatric disorders may be construed either as qualitatively discrete entities or as extreme examples of psychological impairment on a continuum of universally distributed behavioural traits (Kendell, 1975). These two alternatives have important implications for the relationship between vulnerability factors and the disease process itself. Should vulnerability factors be considered as lying on the same dimension as the disease process or should they be visualized as independent attributes? A continuum model seems more appropriate given the nature of most vulnerability factors. However, this issue has yet to be fully addressed.

In the context of the above discussion, vulnerability factors must be adequately defined and objectively measured. Unfortunately, several definitions of vulnerability need consideration. Vulnerability within the framework of the 'stress vulnerability' model outlined by Zubin & Spring (1977) collectively describes those factors which hazard an individual for developing a particular psychiatric illness. In addition, illness is only shown in those individuals exposed to environmental stressors who are also vulnerable. Thus, vulnerability may be distinguished from acute psychiatric illness by the association of a recent stressor with the latter condition. Vulnerability may also be defined as an intrinsic mediating variable which is related to psychiatric morbidity (Rabkin & Struening, 1976; Spring & Coons, 1982). This needs distinguishing from extrinsic moderating variables which are independent of both the disease process and any precipitant stressor, but which may also modify the risk of illness. An example of this type of factor would be the proposed influence of social support networks in buffering the effect of life events on the risk of depression (Cassel, 1976; but also see Aneshensel & Stone, 1982). It should be noted that the model of depression of Brown & Harris (1978) describes both extrinsic 'vulnerability' factors such as the presence of a confiding relationship and an intrinsic notion of vulnerability as an individual's cognitive appraisal of these factors. Thus, a working definition of vulnerability concerns those stable characteristics of an individual which are related to that individual's risk for developing psychiatric disorder, given the presence of a sufficient level of 'stress' provoked by various different stressors. In this context, Ohman (1981*b*) has suggested that stability in the case of a hypothetical electrodermal vulnerability index might be represented by both test–retest reliability and cross-situational consistency.

Several strategies have been employed in attempts to identify vulnerability factors. An obvious approach seeks to identify behavioural or biochemical indices of genetic diathesis (Rieder & Gershon, 1978; Gershon, 1983). Such an index would be identified if during the course of, say, a twin study, a marker in the patient was also detected in the non-affected proband. Such a marker would also have to be shown to be related to 'stress'-induced psychiatric morbidity in the general population. The intricacies of this approach have been detailed by Erlenmeyer-Kimling (1979) in relation to schizophrenia. A similar approach is to study longitudinally subjects thought to be at high risk for developing a particular disorder and to identify those factors predicting subsequent breakdown. Classic examples of this form of 'high-risk' research are the studies of Mednick and his colleagues (e.g. Beuhring *et al.*, 1982). Finally, vulnerability factors may also be identified by following up patients who have already presented with psychiatric disorder, but who are in remission at the time of study. Vulnerability factors here would predict the occurrence of future relapses.

The above strategies may employ several measures, especially if vulnerability is defined in general terms and not just restricted to genetic diathesis. Zubin & Steinhauer (1981) have attempted to catalogue an almost encyclopaedic range of measures which might be usefully applied. We shall provide only a few examples and restrict these to intrinsic factors since we believe that some of the extrinsic or 'ecological markers' described by Zubin & Steinhauer might best be classified as moderating variables rather than vulnerability factors. At the biological level, markers used previously include measures of enzyme activity such as platelet monoamine oxidase, neurotransmitter metabolites such as homovanillic acid, and neurophysiological and psychophysiological measures. A concise review of potential biological markers in schizophrenia has been undertaken by Melzer (1979) and has also been the topic of a recent symposium (Usdin & Hanin, 1982). Behavioural markers have included measures of autonomic conditioning, eye-tracking performance, reaction times (Spring & Zubin, 1978; Zubin, 1979; Spring & Coons, 1982).

To conclude our discussion of vulnerability measures, we must emphasize some necessary conditions if a measure is to be identified accurately. The 'stress-vulnerability' model defines vulnerability in the context of a provoking agent which is characterized as a precipitating stressor. This definition clearly states, therefore, that vulnerability factors are associated with risk only in the presence of a stressor and, hence, will be identified in any analysis of psychiatric morbidity as an interaction between the marker and stressor present together. Factors associated with either the presence of illness in the absence of a stressor or with the presence of a stressor in the absence of illness cannot be identified as true vulnerability factors (Tennant & Bebbington, 1978; Bebbington, 1980). Thus, measures which characterize the onset of acute illness may not necessarily predict the future course of that illness. Indeed, this lack of association between diagnostic indicators and prognosis has been stressed recently in the case of schizophrenia (Carpenter *et al.*, 1978). Similarly, the dysfunction and distress associated with acute illness might also be unrelated to its future course and thus help to obscure the measurement of underlying vulnerability measures. Furthermore, a variety of provoking agents or moderating variables may be identified which initiate illness but only in the presence of true vulnerability factors and which do not affect the probability of future illness episodes. For these reasons attempts to measure vulnerability must distinguish between the various types of markers assessing different aspects of the illness process. Such studies require prospective designs whereby the variance associated with the presence of stressors, acute illness states, remitted states and the 'stress-vulnerability' interaction can be partitioned and identified. The complexity of identifying these different sources of variance is illustrated by Zubin & Steinhauer's (1981) attempt to classify such markers into eight different types. Therefore, the kinds of statistical approach used in personality research (e.g. Cronbach *et al.*, 1972) may be needed in order to separate these different classes of 'state' and 'trait' variables.

The 'stress-vulnerability' interaction

The purpose of this section is to describe several different ways in which the 'stress-vulnerability' interaction may be formulated. The theories mentioned in this context are, of course, provided as examples of different types of 'stress-vulnerability' models and not as definitive accounts of the aetiology of specific psychiatric illnesses. Also, the different formulations presented here may overlap in terms of different levels of explanation, and as such should not be considered exclusive.

Before discussing these models, the distinction between triggering and formative effects of life events needs reiteration. Formative effects relate to fairly permanent changes in psychiatric morbidity which we have termed vulnerability. Examples of such factors would include the effects of birth complications or perinatal maternal distress on the subsequent development of schizophrenia (Beuhring *et al.*, 1982), the effects of early loss in the aetiology of depression (Lloyd, 1980), and the relevance of early parental separation in the development of neurotic behaviour (Brown & Harris, 1978). Presumably, such effects are mediated by relatively permanent changes in behavioural and cognitive response tendencies which in turn might be associated with underlying neurochemical changes. These effects might also be used as measures of vulnerability. Since the difficulties encountered in investigating these historical effects of life events on vulnerability are immense, we shall not discuss the general nature of this problem any further in this current section. However, such mechanisms will be speculated on later when the role of life events for individual psychiatric conditions is discussed.

Life events are generally conceptualized in terms of their triggering effect on psychiatric illness. We would like to present four schemata which describe generally their possible mode of action as regards the 'stress-vulnerability' model. The first formulation concerns the specific and direct effect of a life event stressor on a brain system subsuming both a particular component of the stress response and also implicated in the dysfunction responsible for a specific impairment. Vulnerability in this model would represent, amongst other things, the original biochemical dysfunction responsible for impairment but activated by the presence of a stressor. This type of approach has frequently been adopted for psychobiological models of depression, especially those that have emphasized the role of brain monoamines (Akiskal, 1979). Since this topic will be discussed at length in the next section, we present here only a concise version of the argument. Essentially, depression is characterized by a dysfunction of so-called diencephalic reinforcement centres which arises as a result of the depletion of monoamines. It is suggested that specific life events may mimic the effect observed in the laboratory of inescapable aversive events in reducing monoamine levels. However, depression is only manifested as a clinical entity in those vulnerable individuals who already demonstrate abnormal monoamine turnover in the brain. Akiskal (1979) cites several possible vulnerability factors which may affect turnover, such as ageing, hypothyroid dysfunction, the puerperium, alcoholism and possible genetic influences.

The second 'stress-vulnerability' model also describes a specific effect of a stressor but relies on an interaction between the brain system implicated in the stress response and a separate system which underlies the psychological dysfunction. Another example from the area of depression is also relevant here. Weiss *et al.*, (1979) have also implicated monoamines in the origins of depression but have conceptualized the behavioural deficit in terms of reduced motor activity. Since dopaminergic systems are more readily identified as subserving motor activity, Weiss *et al.*, have speculated that the association between behavioural deficits and monoamines which is observed under conditions of inescapable aversive events may be mediated by noradrenergic alterations in dopaminergic transmission.

The last two models are concerned with the general effects of 'stress responses' on behaviour and may or may not be subsumed under neurochemical 'stress-vulnerability' models. Both models characterize the effects of stressors in terms of generalized stress responses or increases in arousal. Obviously, the issue of a non-specific stress response is raised by these models. However, as long as this problem is borne in mind when investigating these theories, they may still provide a useful and perhaps less restrictive framework than the two earlier models. The third model relates to the effects of the stress response on psychological function and characterizes dysfunction not as a qualitative breakdown in performance but as an extreme of normal functioning. Vulnerability, therefore, might be represented as poor premorbid functioning which is exacerbated by an acute stressor. The numerous examples of this type of model include drive theories of schizophrenia (Epstein & Coleman, 1970), Lader & Mathew's model of phobic anxiety (1968) and the arousal model of schizophrenic relapse postulated by Leff *et al.*, (1983).

Finally, as Zubin & Spring (1977) point out, stressors may break down coping behaviours and give rise to temporary periods of distress. However, in the vulnerable individual, this breakdown may provide an opportunity 'for more fundamental problems to manifest themselves'. Thus, the stressor results in the breakdown of coping strategies which may have compensated for premorbid dysfunctioning in the highly vulnerable individual.

Implications for research

The different levels of explanation represented by the four models discussed above have important implications for research. Essentially, investigation of the 'stress-vulnerability' model in terms of the biological effects of life events requires information ranging from biochemical functioning to the assessment of psychiatric state and social functioning. Any study which attempts to span these diverse aspects of measurement faces a Sisyphean task. Three strategies can be adopted to simplify such an approach; 'high-risk' studies where risk is defined either genetically, behaviourally or psychiatrically as in the case of remitted patients (Lewine, Watt & Grubb, 1981), extensive single-case studies (Strauss, 1981), or by the use of appropriate animal models (Weiner, 1982). Furthermore, several propositions implicit in the stress-vulnerability model may need to be tested independently. For example, investigation of the biological effects of stressors may be conducted using both human (e.g. Levi, 1972) and animal subjects (Mason *et al.*, 1976). Similarly, the biological effects of life events might be investigated in different patient and control groups. Examples of this approach already include the effects of life events on catecholamines (Theorell *et al.*, 1972) and evoked potentials (von Knorring *et al.*, 1980).

Studies which seek to investigate the relationship between the physiological effects of stressors and psychiatric disorder face numerous problems. Several suggested approaches include investigations of the relationship between stressors such as natural disasters, war or occupational demands and physiological and psychological functioning (Hinkle, 1977). A good example of the latter approach is the study conducted by Rose *et al.*, (1979) which examined prospectively the interrelationship between patterns of psychiatric impairment and physiological and biochemical measures in a group of air traffic controllers. Another approach, advocated by Zubin & Spring (1977), concerns the relationship between physiological and behavioural measures of adaptation and psychiatric symptoms in the day to day experience of psychiatric patients. Examples include Stevens' (1959) study of emotional triggering factors in epilepsy and the work of Leff and his colleagues on the effects of social interaction between schizophrenic patients and their relatives on measures of electrodermal 'arousal' (Sturgeon *et al.*, 1984). Finally, the use of animal models of psychiatric disorder may also be of use but poses immense problems of interpretation. This approach has especially been advocated in the case of both depression (e.g. Akiskal & McKinney, 1975; Weiss *et al.*, 1979) and anxiety (Gray, 1982).

The next section will overview the relevance of these diverse approaches to 'stress-vulnerability' models of specific psychiatric disorders.

Specific models of 'stress-vulnerability' interactions

As we remarked in the introduction to this chapter, attempts to specify the biological mechanisms underlying the effects of life events on psychiatric disorder might be considered speculative and foolhardy, given the current state of knowledge in biological psychiatry. Nevertheless, we shall accept the challenge and outline some possible hypotheses which might be entertained when considering future research in this area. However, a definitive model would require both an understanding of the biological mechanisms implicated in a specific disease theory and a more thorough exposition of the effects of life events on these mechanisms in non-psychiatric populations. Furthermore, the magnitude of the effect of life events on the precipitation of a particular psychiatric disorder would also need to be clearly established. We shall attempt, therefore, to summarize information concerning these prerequisites, as regards specific psychiatric syndromes, and try where possible to integrate this knowledge in relation to a 'stress-vulnerability' model.

Anxiety

Before attempting to disentangle interactions between life events and the neurochemical substrates of anxiety, the effects of life events on psychiatric morbidity *per se* needs to be clearly established. Unfortunately the effects of life events either on the aetiology or precipitation of neurotic disorders are unclear. Retrospective studies of life events or specific stressors related to phobic behaviour suggest that such events may trigger neurotic disorders but only in a few of the patients studied (Myers, Lindenthal & Pepper, 1971; Cooper & Sylph, 1973; Buglass *et al.*, 1977). Andrews & Tennant (1978) in their concise review of the effects of life events on psychiatric morbidity suggest that these do not constitute a major determinant of severe neurotic illness. A further complication in evaluating the effects of life events concerns the distinction between distress responses and abnormal neurotic reactions. Bebbington *et al.* (1981) argue that both the association of life events and disorder, and the pattern of symptoms observed may differ between general population and out-patient samples.

So, the role of life events in neurotic disorders has not been demonstrated unequivocally. This confusion in the literature is also reflected in neurochemical models of the mechanisms responsible for the mediation of anxiety. Current animal models of anxiety have implicated specific noradrenergic systems situated in the locus coeruleus (Redmond & Huang, 1979; but see Mason & Fibiger, 1979), along with interactions between both serotonergic and γ-aminobutyric acid (GABA-ergic) neurotransmitter systems (Hoehn-Saric, 1982). Recently, Gray (1982) has proposed an integrative model of anxiety and septo-hippocampal function which involves noradrenergic, serotonergic and cholinergic pathways.

None of the above theories refers specifically to the role of life events. However, the effects of both short-term and chronic stressors in animal studies have made an important contribution to the empirical basis of the theories. Indeed, Hoehn-Saric (1982) documents stress-induced changes in GABA-ergic, noradrenergic, serotonergic and selective dopaminergic systems. Similarly, Warburton (1979) has argued that the subjective experience of anxiety is associated with increased adrenocortical activity. Furthermore, he speculates that increased cortisol may be associated with increased 'proneness to anxiety' given the presence of an anxiety-provoking stimulus.

Perhaps the most comprehensive attempt to integrate the neurochemical changes induced by stressors and an underlying substrate of anxiety is provided by Gray (1982). He identifies three consequences of a stressor on noradrenergic activity. The first phase constitutes an initial increase in activity which is followed by a second depletion phase due to the prolonged presence of a severe stressor. However, the increase in noradrenergic impulse traffic which results in depletion also gives rise to subsequent increased noradrenaline synthesis which eventually results in a third phase whereby equilibrium between noradrenaline synthesis and release is restored but maintained at a higher level. Gray suggests that these changes in noradrenergic activity produced by stressors are associated with functional changes in both the septo-hippocampal system implicated in his model of anxiety and the hypothalamic mechanisms subserving defensive and aggressive behaviour. In terms of behaviour and Gray's extrapolation of animal models to psychiatric disorder, the functional changes in these two brain systems correspond to both symptoms of anxiety and depression. Hence, the initial increase in noradrenergic activity in these systems is associated with anxiety, whereas the relative depletion of noradrenaline results in anxiety plus depression and eventually depression alone.

The above simplified account of animal models of anxiety may provide a basis for investigating neurochemical changes associated with the acute effects of life events on neurotic disorders. In particular, these models stress the importance of temporal factors underlying both change in noradrenergic activity and the cumulative effects of stressors. These factors may have important implications for the cumulative effects of life events and differences in psychiatric symptoms associated with distress elicited by stressful life events. For example, the pattern of anxious or depressive symptoms may be related to the temporal patterning of life event stressors and individual differences in the relative rates of noradrenaline release and synthesis. This balance between patterns of depressive and anxious symptoms may also have some bearing on pharmacotherapeutic strategies (Gray, 1982).

Finally, it should be recognized that life events may also play a formative role in the aetiology of neurotic disorders. The effects of stressors on long-term neurochemical changes may be implicated in these effects. For instance, chronic repeated exposure to stressors might facilitate the turnover of noradrenaline which results in tolerance to 'stress': a phenomenon known as 'toughening' in the animal literature. Gray *et al.*, (1981) suggest that tolerance may be due to the long-term effects of stressors on the build-up of tyrosine hydroxylase, an enzyme which determines the rate of noradrenaline synthesis. Another area which has also examined long-term effects of stressors concerns the influence of pre- and postnatal trauma on the maturation of brain systems in the infant (Denenberg,

1982; Herrenkohl, 1982). Unfortunately, it would be premature to speculate on the integration of these changes and the effects of life events on vulnerability to neurotic disorders.

Depression

The area of depression has probably generated the earliest and most comprehensive psychobiological models of 'stress-vulnerability'. Some of this impetus was derived from attempts to identify biological distinctions between unipolar and bipolar affective disorders. For example, Goodwin & Bunney (1973) suggested that disruption of brain monoamine systems might be responsible both for unipolar depression and for the switch between mania and depression in bipolar affective disorders. The conditions controlling these transitions were said to result from both genetic vulnerability and the deleterious effects of stressors on monoamine brain systems. A more specific model was proposed in the same year by Akiskal & McKinney (1973) who attempted to integrate findings from animal research relating to early separation experiences in primates, the effects of biogenic amines on animal behaviour and the phenomena of 'learned helplessness' induced by uncontrollable stressors. It was postulated that the vegetative symptoms of depression such as motor retardation, loss of appetite and libido, and sleep disturbances might be explained by a disruption of the 'diencephalic mechanisms of reinforcement'. This dysfunction would be reflected by changes in serotonergic, noradrenergic and cholinergic transmitters and would be brought about by the interaction of diathesis, object loss in childhood and the experience of uncontrollable stressors in the environment. A more explicit formulation of their theory was presented 2 years later (Akiskal & McKinney, 1975) which described in further detail the relationship between different neurophysiological systems and symptoms of depression.

Recent research into 'stress-vulnerability' models of depression have tended to follow two distinct approaches. The first of these has concentrated specifically on 'learned helplessness' models of depression and has focused exclusively on the psychopharmacology of animal behaviour. The second approach has attempted to integrate the life event literature with the findings derived from animal research conducted on the various monoamine theories of depression.

In the interests of brevity only a concise account of the controversies surrounding current animal models of depression can be given. Much of this research involves studies of 'learned helplessness', a phenomenon observed in animals which have experienced uncontrollable and inescapable aversive events. Essentially, exposure to such stressors results in a behavioural deficit in subsequent tasks which require active avoidance responding (Seligman, 1975). In particular, three crucial questions which have arisen from this research may be asked when considering the later application of these findings to 'stress-vulnerability' models. The first question concerns the relative contribution of learning versus non-associative effects of neurochemical changes in explaining the nature of the 'helplessness' deficit. On the one hand, Seligman and his colleagues have proposed a cognitive model of 'helplessness' based on current learnt expectancies and previously acquired attributions (see Abramson, Seligman & Teasdale, 1978). In contrast, researchers such as Weiss and Anisman (Weiss, 1980; Anisman & Lapierre, 1982) have emphasized time-locked, non-associative neurochemical changes as being responsible for the behavioural deficit. Similarly, the effects of such neurochemical changes have been explained either in terms of a motor deficit (Weiss *et al.*, 1979) or disruption of reinforcement systems (Wise, 1978). The second question raised by this research concerns the relationship between the various types of 'helplessness' phenomena and the clinical state of depression (see Gray, 1982). Thirdly, controversy surrounds the nature of the monoamine systems implicated in depression and in particular the relative involvement of either noradrenaline or serotonin as the crucial neurotransmitter (Schildkraut, 1978; Anisman & Zacharko, 1982). Although it is essential that these issues are resolved, it has been argued that they do not pose a serious problem for the larger conceptual framework employed by the 'stress-vulnerability' model of depression itself (Anisman & Zacharko, 1982).

Several authors have recently attempted to integrate life event research with the current neurochemical models of depression described above (Akiskal, 1979; Depue *et al.*, 1979; Anisman & Zacharko, 1982). Essentially, two questions must be posed by this research: the role of life events in precipitating episodes of affective disorder and the nature of vulnerability to depression. Researchers interested in approaching the precipitant effects of life events have tended to rely heavily on the monoamine theories of depression. As has been argued above, changes in brain monoamines are associated with behavioural deficits in animals which are regarded as analogous to symptoms of affective disorders. Moreover, it is argued that uncontrollable aversive events may induce such changes. Several researchers have suggested, therefore, that 'stress-vulnerability' models might be investigated in depressed patients by examining the effects of both acute stressors and life events on peripheral indices of brain monoamine metabolism. For example, Sweeney & Maas (1979) have examined urinary 3-methoxy-4-hydroxy-phenethyleneglycol (MHPG) as an index of noradrenergic activity in depressed patients. These authors demonstrated that changes in MHPG levels were related to changes in state anxiety induced by increasing the demand for physical activity in these patients. Moreover, neither baseline state anxiety nor physical activity *per se* were related to MHPG. Sweeney & Maas suggest that MHPG may prove an index of noradrenergic reactivity to stressors and, thus, could be employed as a vulnerability marker of depression. This study could not be said to support the proposition that stressful life events might mimic the effects of uncontrollable laboratory stressors in bringing about depletion of noradrenaline. However, it does illustrate the direction that research must adopt if this problem is to be tackled. In particular, the prospective study of life events on peripheral measures of monoamine activity in both normal subjects and those predisposed to depression deserves greater attention. In this connection, the problem of predictability and control over the consequences of life events needs to be taken into consideration if the life event–laboratory stress analogue is to be taken seriously.

Stress-vulnerability models of depression are required to explain both the mechanisms involved in the stress–disorder relationship and also the concept of vulnerability. This is particularly important since it has been frequently argued that life events are neither necessary nor sufficient conditions for the occurrence of affective disorder (Bebbington, 1980). With regard to the monoamine theories of depression, vulnerability has been conceptualized in a number of different ways which include the effects of early loss, biological stressors, individual differences in cognitive appraisal and genetic diathesis (Akiskal, 1979; Depue *et al.*, 1979; Anisman & Lapierre, 1982; Anisman & Zacharko, 1982). However, it is argued that these disparate effects operate via common neurochemical mediators resulting in rapid or prolonged monoamine depletion in vulnerable persons. Unfortunately, other than rearing studies in primates (e.g. Kraemer & McKinney, 1979), little evidence exists to demonstrate that developmental factors may affect subsequent monoamine responses to uncontrolled stressors. Moreover, recent stress–depression models (e.g. Anisman & Zacharko, 1982) have been criticized since they focus more on the precipitating effects of life events than on their possible formative effects on vulnerability (Akiskal, 1982). However, given that factors such as early loss and separation may only account for about 10% of the variance (Lloyd, 1980; Tennant, Bebbington & Hurry, 1982), this bias might be justified.

Schizophrenia

The influence of life events on the aetiology and course of schizophrenic disorders has received much recent attention (Rabkin, 1980; Day, 1981; Spring & Coons, 1982). From these comprehensive reviews, it might be concluded that life events may play a role in precipitating acute episodes of disorder, especially in remitted patients with a previous history of illness. However, as Day (1981) has stressed, the problems imposed by the possible heterogeneity of schizophrenia and the diagnostic uncertainty of reactive psychoses or schizophreniform illnesses detracts from any firm conclusions in this area. Similarly, Spring & Coons (1982) suggest that the evidence in support of the formative effects of early trauma such as birth complications, separation or prenatal maternal distress on the later risk of developing schizophrenia is as yet unproven.

The lack of consensus regarding the effects of life events is also mirrored by the absence of an agreed biological mechanism underlying the disease process. Indeed, both genetic and biochemical accounts of schizophrenia now stress the possible heterogeneity of processes thought to underlie the manifestation of schizophrenic symptoms. Although neurotransmitters such as dopamine (e.g. Langer, Brown & Docherty, 1981; Haracz, 1982), noradrenaline (e.g. Mason, 1982), and acetylcholine (e.g. Warburton, 1979) have been currently implicated, firm evidence for the involvement of any one particular brain system is sadly lacking (Oades, 1982). Given this lack of knowledge surrounding both the effects of life events and the biological mechanisms underlying the disorder, it is not surprising that there have been no specific attempts to explain possible 'stress-vulnerability' interactions. In contrast, however, the general concept of 'stress-vulnerability' models of schizophrenia have become increasingly popular (e.g. Zubin & Spring, 1977; Zubin & Steinhauer, 1981; Spring & Coons, 1982) in attempts to reconcile the genetic versus environmental accounts of aetiology. The purpose of this section, therefore, will be to highlight some research conducted into biological mechanisms involved generally in vulnerability as opposed to any specific explanation of 'stress-vulnerability' mechanisms.

Several recent reviews have attempted to detail the numerous vulnerability markers which might be employed in 'high-risk' studies of either the offspring of schizophrenic parents or prospective studies of patients (Klorman, Strauss & Kokes, 1977; Zubin, 1979; Zubin & Steinhauer, 1981). Since these reviews clearly demonstrate the inchoate nature of this area of research we shall not attempt a comprehensive integration of the disparate and frequently equivocal findings. Instead, we will deal with one particular approach which currently has attracted considerable attention and use it to exemplify the kinds of approach adopted in this field.

Psychophysiological measures of autonomic nervous system activity, especially electrodermal measures, have frequently been employed in schizophrenia research (see Spohn & Patterson, 1979). Several researchers have proposed that these measures may reflect both episodic schizophrenic states and, more importantly, trait vulnerability characteristics. Both Zahn (1980) and Frith *et al.* (1979) have reported that electrodermal hyper-responsivity predicts treatment outcome in schizophrenic patients. Patients who responded repeatedly to an habituation series of auditory stimuli improved in a limited way later. Ohman (1981 *b*), in a recent review of the use of electrodermal measures in schizophrenia, also suggested that the 'high-risk' studies have demonstrated to varying degrees hyper-responsivity in the affected probands. Electrodermal overreactivity may therefore provide a vulnerability marker for schizophrenia. However, there is a number of problems with this argument. Perhaps the most important of these concerns the fact that most schizophrenics display a hyporesponsive pattern both in the acute phase (Bernstein *et al.*, 1982) and also in remission (Iacono, 1982). Moreover, hyperresponsivity only appears to predict poor outcome in patients with relatively good prognosis and who display more florid positive symptoms; the reverse is true for socially withdrawn chronic patients (Schneider, 1982).

Support for the notion that electrodermal hyper-responsivity may represent a vulnerability marker in at least some groups of patients has also been adduced from studies concerned with the effects of family and social factors on schizophrenic relapse. Factors such as phenothiazine medication, the presence of a critical or over-involved relative (referred to as high 'expressed emotion'), and high social contact with that relative have been identified as predictors of relapse (Leff, 1978). A mediational model has evolved within this research area whereby these factors are said to bring about relapse via a common pathway of elevated 'arousal' (Brown, Birley & Wing, 1972; Leff & Tarrier, 1981; Leff *et al.*, 1983; Turpin, 1983). Accordingly, several studies have been performed to see whether patients living in high expressed emotion homes differed electrodermally from those residing with low expressed emotion relatives (Tarrier *et al.*, 1979; Sturgeon *et al.*, 1981, 1984). The findings suggest a difference in that patients with high expressed emotion relatives are more 'aroused' electrodermally. More importantly, the frequency of electrodermal responding, recorded from patients when acutely ill, predicts subsequent relapse. Thus, at 9 months following testing, those patients who had relapsed had higher initial response rates than those that remained well (Sturgeon *et al.*, 1984). It may also be possible to implicate the role of life events in bringing about relapse in these patients (see Leff & Vaughn, 1980). The threshold model proposed by Leff *et al.* (1983) predicts that relapse will occur once a critical arousal level has been exceeded. Life events, therefore, may be one of a set of factors which modify a patient's arousal level, since preliminary data by Tarrier *et al.* (1979) suggest that patients who have experienced a recent life event demonstrate higher levels of electrodermal 'arousal'.

Finally, none of the above studies has attempted to identify the possible locus of a 'stress-vulnerability' interaction. However, Dawson, Nuechterlein & Liberman (1984) have argued that electrodermal over-reactivity may be implicated in the attentional dysfunction observed in some schizophrenics and have presented a 'stress-vulnerability' model which incorporates social, behavioural and biological factors. For the sake of completeness, it may be that the speculated effects of life events on noradrenergic systems which have been discussed in relation to depression may also be involved in a noradrenergic/dopaminergic common pathway implicated in the attentional deficit in schizophrenia (Antelman & Caggiula, 1977).

Conclusion

The aim of this chapter has been to present at a conceptual level the contribution of 'stress-vulnerability' models to the understanding of possible biological mechanisms of the effects of life events on psychiatric disorders. Although several theoretical models are clearly established (e.g. Zubin & Steinhauer, 1981; Anisman & Zacharko, 1982), it is apparent that the empirical support for these models is lacking. Hence, in the form of a conclusion, a number of areas which require more extensive research will be identified. Firstly, there is a dearth of empirical findings concerning the biological changes which occur as a consequence of life events in normal populations. Secondly, more prospective studies which can separate out 'state–trait' interactions and, of equal importance, the conditions necessary for identifying vulnerability and episode markers, are clearly required. Thirdly, the measurement of stressors needs to be extended to include other factors such as chronic difficulties, minor life events, and biological environmental stressors which are not currently subsumed under life event methodology. This is particularly important for 'stress-vulnerability' models which emphasize the presence of a precipitant stressor, despite the fact that current epidemiological studies suggest that only a minor proportion of the variance is explained by measurable life events. Fourthly, the mechanisms responsible for the 'stress-vulnerability' interaction require further attention. In particular, the differential time course of the effects of life events on different psychiatric disorders needs to be addressed along with the question of individual differences in vulnerability for specific psychiatric disorders. This level of analysis may require the use of more sophisticated animal models of disorder as advocated by Weiner (1982) in the context of 'psychosomatic disorders'. Finally, studies designed to examine the above problems need also to consider non-biological vulnerability factors which may be psychologically mediated. Similarly, the operation of social moderating factors will also need to be considered if the comprehensive nature of 'stress-vulnerability' models are to be adequately tested.

References

Abramson, L. Y., Seligman, M. E. P. & Teasdale, J. D. (1978). Learned helplessness in humans: critique and reformulation. *Journal of Abnormal Psychology*, **87**, 49–74.

Akiskal, H. S. (1979). A biobehavioral approach to depression. In *The psychobiology of depressive disorders: implications for the effects of stress*, ed. R. A. Depue, pp. 409–37. New York: Academic Press.

Akiskal, H. S. (1982). Is stress a predisposing or precipitating factor in clinical depression? *Behavioural and Brain Sciences*, **5**, 99–100.

Akiskal, H. S. & McKinney, W. T., Jr (1973). Depressive disorders: toward a unified hypothesis. *Science*. **182**, 20–29.

Akiskal, H. S. & McKinney, W. T., Jr (1975). Overview of recent research in depression: an integration of ten conceptual models into a comprehensive clinical frame. *Archives of General Psychiatry*, **32**, 285–301.

Andrew, R. J. (1974). Arousal and the causation of behaviour. *Behaviour*, **51**, 135–65.

Andrews, G. & Tennant, C. (1978). Life event stress and psychiatric illness. *Psychological Medicine*, **8**, 545–49.

Aneshensel, C. S. & Stone, J. D. (1982). Stress and depression: a test of the buffering model of social support. *Archives of General Psychiatry*, **39**, 1392–96.

Anisman, H. & Lapierre, Y. (1982). Neurochemical aspects of stress and depression: formulations and caveats. In *Psychological stress and psychopathology*, ed. R. W. J. Neufeld, pp. 179–217. New York: McGraw-Hill.

Anisman, H. & Zacharko, R. M. (1982). Depression: the predisposing influence of stress. *Behavioral and Brain Sciences*, **5**, 89–137.

Antelman, S. M. & Caggiula, A. R. (1977). Norepinephrine–dopamine interactions and behavior: a new hypothesis of stress-related interaction between brain norepinephrine and dopamine is proposed. *Science*, **195**, 646–53.

Bebbington, P. (1980). Causal models and logical inference in epidemiological psychiatry. *British Journal of Psychiatry*, **136**, 317–25.

Bebbington, P. E., Tennant, C. & Hurry, J. (1981). Adversity and the nature of psychiatric disorder in the community. *Journal of Affective Disorders*, **3**, 345–66.

Bernstein, A. S., Frith, C. D., Gruzelier, J. H., Patterson, T., Straube, E., Venables, P. H. & Zahn, T. P. (1982). An analysis of the skin conductance orienting response in samples of American, British, and German schizophrenics. *Biological Psychology*, **14**, 155–211.

Beuhring, T., Cudek, R., Mednick, S. A., Walker, E. F. & Schulsinger, F. (1982). Vulnerability to environmental stress: high-risk research on the development of schizophrenia. In *Psychological stress and psychopathology*, ed. R. W. J. Neufeld, pp. 67–89. New York: McGraw-Hill.

Brown, G. W., Birley, J. L. T. & Wing, J. K. (1972). Influence of family life on the course of schizophrenic disorders: a replication. *British Journal of Psychiatry*, **121**, 241–58.

Brown, G. W. & Harris, T. (1978). *The social origins of depression*. London: Tavistock.

Buglass, D., Clarke, J., Henderson, A. S., Kreitman, N. & Presley, A. S. (1977). A study of agoraphobic housewives. *Psychological Medicine*, **7**, 73–86.

Carpenter, W. T., Bartko, J. J., Strauss, J. S. & Hawk, A. B. (1978). Signs and symptoms as predictors of outcome: a report from the international pilot study of schizophrenia. *American Journal of Psychiatry*, **135**, 940–5.

Cassel, J. (1976). The contribution of the social environment to host resistance. *American Journal of Epidemiology*, **104**, 107–23.

Cobb, S. & Kasl, S. V. (1977). *Termination: the consequences of job loss*. N.I.O.S.H. Research Report. Washington: DHEW Publications.

Cooper, B. & Sylph, J. (1973). Life events and the onset of neurotic illness: an investigation in general practice. *Psychological Medicine*, **3**, 421–35.

Cronbach, L. J., Gleser, G. C., Nanda, H. & Rajavatnam, N. (1972). *The dependability of behavioral measurements: theory of generalizability for scores and profiles*. New York: Wiley.

Dawson, M. E., Nuechterlein, K. H. & Liberman, R. P. (1984). Relapse in schizophrenic disorders: possible contributing factors and implications for behavior therapy. In *Perspectives on behavior therapy in the eighties*, ed. M. Rosenbaum, C. M. Franks & Y. Jaffe, pp. 265–86. New York: Springer.

Day, R. (1981). Life events and schizophrenia: the 'triggering' hypothesis. *Acta Psychiatrica Scandinavica*, **64**, 97–122.

Denenberg, V. H. (1982). Postnatal stimulation, brain lateralization, and emotional reactivity. In *The biology of anxiety*, ed. R. J. Mathew, pp. 87–103. New York: Brunner/Mazel.

Depue, R. A., Monroe, S. M. & Shackman, S. L. (1979). The psychobiology of human disease: implications for conceptualizing the depressive disorders. In *The psychobiology of the depressive disorders: implications for the effects of stress*, ed. R. A. Depue, pp. 3–20. New York: Academic Press.

Dimsdale, J. E. (1982). Appraising psychobiological approaches to the influence of stress on depression. *Behavioral and Brain Sciences*, **5**, 104–5.

Dohrenwend, B. P. & Dohrenwend, B. S. (1979). The conceptualization of measurement of stressful life events: an overview of the issues. In *The psychobiology of the depressive disorders: implications for the effects of stress*, ed. R. A. Depue, pp. 105–21. New York: Academic Press.

Dohrenwend, B. S. & Dohrenwend, B. P. (1978). Some issues in research on stressful life events. *Journal of Nervous and Mental Disease*, **166**, 7–15.

Engel, G. L. (1977). The need for a new medical model: a challenge for biomedicine. *Science*, **196**, 129–36.

Epstein, S. & Coleman, M. (1970). Drive theories of schizophrenia. *Psychosomatic Medicine*, **32**, 113–40.

Erlenmeyer-Kimling, L. (1979). Advantages of a behavior–genetic approach to investigating stress in the depressive disorders. In *The psychobiology of the depressive disorders: implications for the effects of stress*, ed. R. A. Depue, pp. 391–407. New York: Academic Press.

Fahrenberg, J. & Foerster, F. (1982). Covariation and consistency of activation parameters. *Biological Psychology*, **15**, 151–69.

Frankenhaeuser, M. (1976). The role of peripheral catecholamines in adaptation to understimulation and overstimulation. In *Psychopathology of human adaptation*, ed. G. Serban, pp. 173–89. New York: Plenum Press.

Frith, C. D., Stevens, M., Johnstone, E. C. & Crow, T. J. (1979). Skin conductance responsivity during acute episodes of schizophrenia as a predictor of symptomatic improvement. *Psychological Medicine*, **9**, 101–6.

Garrity, T. F. & Marx, M. B. (1979). Critical life events and coronary disease. In *Psychological aspects of myocardial infarction and coronary care*, ed. W. D. Gentry & R. B. Williams, pp. 31–49. St Louis: Mosby.

Gershon, E. S. (1983). Genetics of the major psychoses. In *Genetics of neurological and psychiatric disorders*, ed. S. S. Kety, L. P. Rowland, R. L. Sidman & S. W. Matthysse, pp. 121–44. New York: Raven Press.

Goodwin, F. & Bunney, W. E., Jr (1973). A psychobiological approach to affective illness. *Psychiatric Annals*, **3**, 19–53.

Gray, J. A. (1982). *The neuropsychology of anxiety: an enquiry into the functions of the septo-hippocampal system*. Oxford: Clarendon.

Gray, J. A., Davis, N., Feldar, J., Owen, S. & Boarder, M. (1981). Stress tolerance: possible neural mechanisms. In *Foundations of Psychosomatics*, ed. M. J. Christie & P. G. Mellet, pp. 153–67. Chichester: Wiley.

Haracz, J. L. (1982). The dopamine hypothesis: an overview of studies with schizophrenic patients. *Schizophrenia Bulletin*, **8**, 438–69.

Hemsley, D. R. (1977). What have cognitive deficits to do with schizophrenic symptoms? *British Journal of Psychiatry*, **130**, 167–73.

Herrenkohl, L. R. (1982). The anxiety-prone personality: effects of prenatal stress on the infant. In *The biology of anxiety*, pp. 51–86. New York: Brunner/Mazel.

Hinkle, L. E. (1977). The concept of 'stress' in the biological and social sciences. In *Psychosomatic medicine: current trends and clinical applications*, ed. Z. J. Zipowski, D. R. Lipsitt & P. C. Whybrow, pp. 27–49. New York: Oxford University Press.

Hoehn-Saric, R. (1982). Neurotransmitters in anxiety. *Archives of General Psychiatry*, **39**, 735–42.

Holmes, Th. H. & Rahe, R. H. (1967). The Social Readjustment Rating Scale. *Journal of Psychosomatic Research*, **11**, 213–18.

Iacono, W. G. (1982). Bilateral electrodermal habituation–dishabituation and resting EEG in remitted schizophrenics. *Journal of Nervous and Mental Disease*, **170**, 91–101.

Ingham, J. G. & Miller, P. M. (1976). The determinants of illness declaration. *Journal of Psychosomatic Research*, **20**, 309–16.

Kendell, R. E. (1975). *The role of diagnosis in psychiatry*. Oxford: Blackwell.

Kety, S. S., Rowland, L. P., Sidman, R. L. & Matthysse, S. W. (1983). *Genetics of neurological and psychiatric disorders*. New York: Raven Press.

Klorman, R. K., Strauss, J. S. & Kokes, R. F. (1977). Premorbid adjustment in schizophrenia. Part IV. Some biological approaches in research on premorbid functioning in schizophrenia. *Schizophrenia Bulletin*, **3**, 226–39.

von Knorring, L., Jacobsson, L., Perris, C. & Perris, H. (1980). Reactivity to incoming stimuli and the experience of life-events. *Neuropsychobiology*, **6**, 297–303.

Kraemer, G. W. & McKinney, W. T. (1979). Interactions of pharmacological agents which alter biogenic amine metabolism and depression: an analysis of contributing factors within a primate model of depression. *Journal of Affective Disorders*, **1**, 33–54.

Lader, M. H. (1975). *The psychophysiology of mental illness*. London: Routledge & Kegan Paul.

Lader, M. H. & Mathews, A. M. (1968). A physiological model of phobic anxiety and desensitization. *Behaviour Research and Therapy*, **6**, 411–21.

Langer, D. H., Brown, G. L. & Docherty, J. P. (1981). Receptor supersensitivity and schizophrenia: a review. *Schizophrenia Bulletin*, **7**, 208–24.

Lazarus, R. S. (1966). *Psychological stress and the coping process*. New York: McGraw-Hill.

Leff, J. (1978). Social and psychological causes of the acute attack. In *Schizophrenia: towards a new synthesis*, ed. J. K. Wing, pp. 139–65. London: Academic Press.

Leff, J., Kuipers, L., Berkowitz, R., Vaughn, C. & Sturgeon, D. (1983). Life events, relatives' expressed emotion and maintenance neuroleptics in schizophrenic relapse. *Psychological Medicine*, **13**, 799–806.

Leff, J. & Tarrier, N. (1981). The home environments of schizophrenic patients, and their response to treatment. In *Foundations of psychosomatics*, ed. M. J. Christie & P. G. Mellet, pp. 407–20. Chichester: Wiley.

Leff, J. & Vaughn, C. (1980). The interaction of life events and relatives' expressed emotion in schizophrenia and depressive neurosis. *British Journal of Psychiatry*, **136**, 146–53.

Levi, L. (1972). Introduction: psychosocial stimuli, psychophysiological reactions, and disease. *Stress and distress in response to psychosocial stimuli*, ed. L. Levi. (Suppl. 528, *Acta Medica Scandinavica*.)

Lewine, R. R. J., Watt, N. F. & Grubb, T. W. (1981). High-risk-for-schizophrenia research. *Schizophrenia Bulletin*, **7**, 273–80.

Lloyd, C. (1980). Life events and depressive disorders reviewed. *Archives of General Psychiatry*, **37**, 529–48.

Mason, J. W. (1971). A re-evaluation of the concept of 'non-specificity' in stress theory. *Journal of Psychiatric Research*, **8**, 323–33.

Mason, J. W., Maher, J. T., Hartley, L. H., Mougey, E. H., Perlow, M. J. & Jones, L. G. (1976). Selectivity of corticosteroid and catecholamine responses to various natural stimuli. In *Psychopathology of human adaptation*, ed. G. Serban, pp. 147–71. New York: Plenum Press.

Mason, S. T. (1982). Schizophrenia, not depression, as a result of depleted brain norepinephrine. *Behavioral and Brain Sciences*, **5**, 113–14.

Mason, S. T. & Fibiger, H. C. (1979). Anxiety: the locus coeruleus disconnection. *Life Sciences*, **25**, 2141–7.

Mechanic, D. (1978). Explanations of mental illness. *Journal of Nervous and Mental Disease*, **166**, 381–6.

Meehl, P. E. (1962). Schizotaxia, schizotypy, schizophrenia. *American Psychologist*, **17**, 827–38.

Melzer, H. (1979). Biology of schizophrenia subtypes: a review and proposal for method of study. *Schizophrenia Bulletin*, **5**, 460–79.

Myers, J. K., Lindenthal, J. J. & Pepper, M. P. (1971). Life events and psychiatric impairment. *Journal of Nervous and Mental Disease*, **153**, 149–57.

Oades, R. D. (1982). *Attention and schizophrenia: neurological bases.* Boston: Pitman.

Ohman, A. (1981*a*). The role of experimental psychology in the scientific analysis of psychopathology. *International Journal of Psychology*, **16**, 299–321.

Ohman, A. (1981*b*). Electrodermal activity and vulnerability to schizophrenia: a review. *Biological Psychology*, **12**, 87–145.

Paykel, E. S. (1979). Recent life events in the development of the depressive disorders. In *The psychobiology of the depressive orders: implications for the effects of stress*, ed. R. A. Depue, pp. 245–62. New York: Academic Press.

Rabkin, J. G. (1980). Stressful life events and schizophrenia: a review of the research literature. *Psychological Bulletin*, **87**, 408–25.

Rabkin, J. G. & Struening, E. L. (1976). Life events, stress and illness. *Science*, **194**, 1013–20.

Rahe, R. H. (1978). Life change measurement clarification. *Psychosomatic Medicine*, **40**, 95–8.

Redmond, D. E., Jr & Huang, Y. H. (1979). New evidence for a locus coeruleus–norepinephrine connection with anxiety. *Life Sciences*, **25**, 2149–62.

Rieder, R. O. & Gershon, E. S. (1978). Genetic strategies in biological psychiatry. *Archives of General Psychiatry*, **35**, 866–73.

Rose, R. M., Hurst, M. W. & Herd, J. A. (1979). Cardiovascular and endocrine responses to work and the risk for psychiatric symptomatology among air traffic controllers. In *Stress and mental disorder*, ed. J. E. Barrett, R. M. Rose & G. L. Klerman, pp. 237–50. New York: Raven Press.

Rosenthal, D. (1970). *Genetic theory and abnormal behavior.* New York: McGraw-Hill.

Schildkraut, J. J. (1978). Current status of the catecholamine hypothesis of affective disorders. In *Psychopharmacology: A generation of progress*, ed. M. A. Lipton, A. Di Mascio & K. F. Killam, pp. 1223–34. New York: Raven Press.

Schneider, S. J. (1982). Electrodermal activity and therapeutic response to neuroleptic treatment in chronic schizophrenic inpatients. *Psychological Medicine*, **12**, 607–14.

Seligman, M. E. P. (1975). *Helplessness: on depression, development and death.* San Francisco: W. H. Freeman.

Selye, H. (1979). The stress concept and some of its implications. In *Human stress and cognition: an information processing approach*, ed. V. Hamilton & D. M. Warburton, pp. 11–32. Chichester: Wiley.

Serban, G. (1975). Stress in schizophrenics and normals. *British Journal of Psychiatry*, **126**, 397–407.

Spohn, H. E. & Patterson, T. (1979). Recent studies of psychophysiology in schizophrenia. *Schizophrenia Bulletin*, **5**, 581–611.

Spring, B. & Coòns, H. (1982). Stress as a precursor of schizophrenia. In *Psychological stress and psychopathology*, ed. R. W. J. Neufeld, pp. 13–54. New York: McGraw-Hill.

Spring, B. & Zubin, J. (1978). Attention and information processing as indicators of vulnerability to schizophrenic episodes. In *Nature of schizophrenia: new findings and future strategies*, ed. L. Wynne, R. Cromwell, & S. Matthysse, pp. 366–75. New York: Wiley.

Steptoe, A. (1980). Stress and medical disorders. In *Contributions to medical psychology*, vol. II, ed. S. J. Rachman, pp. 55–77. Oxford: Pergamon Press.

Stevens, J. R. (1959). Emotional activation of the electroencephalogram in patients with convulsive disorders. *Journal of Nervous and Mental Disease*, **123**, 339–51.

Strauss, J. S. (1981). Comment on 'How to break the logjam in schizophrenia'. *Journal of Nervous and Mental Disease*, **169**, 493–4.

Sturgeon, D., Kuipers, L., Berkowitz, R., Turpin, G. & Leff, J. (1981). Psychophysiological responses of schizophrenic patients to high and low expressed emotion relatives. *British Journal of Psychiatry*, **138**, 40–5.

Sturgeon, D., Turpin, G., Kuipers, L., Berkowitz, R. & Leff, J. (1984). Psychophysiological responses of schizophrenic patients to high and low expressed emotion relatives: a follow up study. *British Journal of Psychiatry*, **145**, 62–9.

Sweeney, D. R. & Mass, J. W. (1979). Stress and non-adrenergic function in depression. In *The Psychobiology of the depressive disorders: implications for the effects of stress*, ed. R. A. Depue, pp. 161–76. New York: Academic Press.

Tarrier, N., Vaughn, C. E., Lader, M. H. & Leff, J. P. (1979). Bodily reactions to people and events in schizophrenics. *Archives of General Psychiatry*, **36**, 311–15.

Tennant, B. & Bebbington, P. (1978). The social causation of depression: a critique of the work of Brown and his colleagues. *Psychological Medicine*, **8**, 565–75.

Tennant, C., Bebbington, P. & Hurry, J. (1981). The role of life events in depressive illness: is there a substantial causal relation? *Psychological Medicine*, **11**, 379–89.

Tennant, C., Bebbington, P. & Hurry, J. (1982). Social experiences in childhood and adult psychiatric morbidity: a multiple regression analysis. *Psychological Medicine*, **12**, 321–7.

Theorell, T., Lind, E., Fröberg, J., Karlsson, C.-G. & Levi, L. (1972). A longitudinal study of 21 subjects with coronary heart disease: life changes, catecholamine excretion and related biochemical reactions. *Psychosomatic Medicine*, **34**, 505–15.

Turpin, G. (1983). Psychophysiology, psychopathology and the social environment. In *Physiological correlates of human behaviour*, vol. 3. *Individual differences and psychopathology*, ed. A. Gale & J. Edwards, pp. 265–80. London: Academic Press.

Ursin, H. (1978). Activation, coping and psychosomatics. In *Psychobiology of stress: a study of coping men*, ed. H. Ursin, E. Baade & S. Levine, pp. 202–28. New York: Academic Press.

Usdin, E. & Hanin, I. (1982). *Biological markers in psychiatry and neurology*. Oxford: Pergamon Press.

Vanderwolf, C. H. & Robinson, T. E. (1981). Reticulo-cortical activity and behavior: a critique of the arousal theory and a new synthesis. *Behavioral and Brain Sciences*, **3**, 459–76.

Van Praag, H. M. (1981). Socio-biological psychiatry. *Comprehensive Psychiatry*, **22**, 441–9.

Warburton, D. M. (1979). Physiological aspects of anxiety and schizophrenia. In *Human stress and cognition: an information processing approach*, ed. V. Hamilton & D. M. Warburton, pp. 431–65. Chichester: Wiley.

Weiner, H. (1977). *Psychobiology and human disease*. New York: Elsevier.

Weiner, H. (1982). The prospects for psychosomatic medicine: selected topics. *Psychosomatic Medicine*, **44**, 491–517.

Weiss, J. M. (1980). Learned helplessness, physiological change and learned inactivity. Part V. Explaining behavioral depression following controllable stressful events. *Behaviour Research and Therapy*, **18**, 485–504.

Weiss, J. M., Glazer, H. I., Pohorecky, L. A., Bailey, W. H. & Schnider, L. H. (1979). Coping behavior and stress-induced behavioral depression: studies of the role of brain catecholamines. In *The psychobiology of depressive disorders: implications for the effects of stress*, ed. R. A. Depue, pp. 125–60. New York: Academic Press.

Wing, J. K. (1978). Clinical concepts of schizophrenia. In *Schizophrenia: towards a new synthesis*, ed. J. K. Wing, pp. 1–30. London: Academic Press.

Wing, J. K. (1979). The concept of disease in psychiatry. *Journal of the Royal Society of Medicine*, **72**, 316–21.

Wise, R. A. (1978). Catecholamine theories of reward: a critical review. *Brain Research*, **152**, 215–47.

Zahn, T. P. (1980). Predicting outcome from measures of attention and autonomic functioning. In *Perspectives in schizophrenic research*, ed. C. Baxter & T. Melnechuk, pp. 81–104. New York: Raven Press.

Zubin, J. (1979). Markers of vulnerability to mental disorders. *Psychopharmacology Bulletin*, **15**, 7–49.

Zubin, J. & Spring, B. (1977). Vulnerability: a new view of schizophrenia. *Journal of Abnormal Psychology*, **86**, 103–26.

Zubin, J. & Steinhauer, S. (1981). How to break the logjam in schizophrenia: a look beyond genetics. *Journal of Nervous and Mental Disease*, **169**, 477–92.

3

Life events as predisposing and precipitating factors for mental disorders: some psychological considerations

A. BECKER

Introduction

No definite model of how life events may contribute to the development of psychiatric disorders is available today. The model presented by Brown & Harris (page 107, this volume) together with the work of Dohrenwend & Dohrenwend (1979) provide an abstract framework for the possible processes involved in the pathogenic effects of life events. I will present some more unsystematic considerations from the perspective of psychological and psychotherapeutic thinking in order to complement the more abstract models.

The following reflections focus on psychological mechanisms. However, it is my conviction that such mechanisms do correspond to biological processes of high complexity (see the chapter by Turpin & Lader, page 33, this volume), i.e. that their existence does not constitute a separate class of psychogenic disorders. On the other hand, I would also like to warn those who believe in the existence of a purely biological class of psychiatric diseases. Since psychiatry is a subdiscipline of medicine it is dominated by a 'general concept of disease' in one way or another. Even if such a general concept of disease is not explicitly formulated, it nevertheless dominates – through prejudice based on it being taken for granted – the ways of nosological systematization of forms of illnesses both in research and clinical practice. One should not forget the trivial fact that definitions of terms are basically normative and arbitrary and cannot be empirically confirmed or refuted. For this reason they can neither be 'true' nor 'false' but can only serve given purposes to either greater or lesser degrees (Sadegh-zadeh, 1977, 1981; see also Cooper, this volume).

With these caveats in mind I will first examine some psychoanalytic ideas about how life events create vulnerabilities to develop specific diseases or act as triggering factors, and then discuss some concepts from the realm of behavioural and cognitive psychology. Finally, an attempt at providing an integrative view will be presented.

Psychoanalysis, behavioural and cognitive psychology

Freud & Breuer (1895) were the first to approach the effects of life events systematically by means of a new method of treatment (hypnocatharsis) by which not only apparent but also hidden biographical data were worked through, where 'hidden' implies that the meaning for the patient is on a 'subconscious' level. In the short account of the life history and suffering of Elisabeth v. R., the death of the father and a sister is mentioned as preceding the onset of a functional gait disorder. However, problems of guilt and self-esteem proved to be of 'traumatic' aetiological significance for the patient's symptom and for her chronic despair (which was hidden behind the hysteric 'belle indifference'). These problems of guilt and self-esteem were connected with the forbidden, and therefore unadmitted, love for the deceased sister's spouse. Accordingly, a strong resistance to the process of non-hypnotic uncovering of the 'defences' and 'repressions' emerged; these processes in fact amount to a re-traumatization which is justified by its therapeutic purpose. The authors assumed a sequence of 'several partial traumas' which only become effective as a group of events by their accumulation; in the case of Elisabeth v. R. these led to a 'conversion' for the purpose of 'defence', blocking certain motor functions in a manner similar to posthypnotic tasks. The paralysis could not be dismissed as being a form of simulation.

Without relying on extensive 'metapsychological' constructs, psychoanalysis has shown by this early example that after-effects of the most personal and intensely emotional events of the not too distant past do exist, whose full meaning for an individual need not be conscious at all, or becomes conscious only in a distorted way or to a partial degree. This assumption was extended to the occurrence of 'traumatic' events of early childhood which are much more difficult to ascertain. This highlights the limitations of enquiring into the idiosyncratic meanings of 'secret' traumas with regard to the feasibility of life event research. One need only consider the costs which would arise in such biographical research as a result of such unavoidable resistance.

One of the physiological metaphors used by Freud is the concept of a 'stimulus barrier' from which the concept of 'inner' defence processes is derived (see Sulloway, 1979). The process of becoming ill is explicitly attributed to the unsuccessful attempts to maintain a tolerable equilibrium through subconscious regulatory defence mechanisms. Consequently, the various so-called 'defence mechanisms' described by Anna Freud (1936) and others are in no way simply pathogenic; they may also have protective effects, depending on their type and intensity and on time factors. This is exemplified by Horowitz (1983) with regard to 'denial' in relation to serious life events. According to Lazarus (1983), 'denial' not only entails 'costs', but also brings 'benefits'. Furthermore the concept of 'stimulus barrier' had to be modified in order to take into consideration not only that overstimulation may be harmful, but also that effects of understimulation through sensory or social isolation may be traumatic. In this perspective it is conceivable that specific stimulus configurations of optimal intensity and optimal duration have to exist for each individual at a given point in time. If attempts at achieving this optimum fail, pathology might ensue.

As a result of psychoanalytic experiences with depressive patients, Bibring (1953) stressed the effects of subjective conditions of helplessness and powerlessness which develop when self-esteem is diminished owing to the unattainability of exaggerated super-ego ideals.

Since 1958 Bowlby has developed his 'attachment theory' from empirical data by using elements of psychoanalytic thought, ethology, control theory and cognitive psychology (Bowlby, 1969, 1973, 1977). 'Attachment theory' is concerned with the propensity of human beings to make strong, emotional bonds to significant others. The secure basis of parental attachment encourages the child to explore and to extend its relationships, and thereby enables it to become self-reliant. On the other hand, undesired separations and other negative influences lead to the development of 'anxious attachment', which gives rise to the susceptibility of reacting to death or separation with pathological forms of mourning (Parkes, 1972). Bowlby postulates that those representational models of the attachment figure and of the self that a person has built up during his development from early childhood onwards tend to persist relatively unchanged into and throughout adulthood and influence the manner in which emotional bonds are made and broken. It is assumed that such attachment is not of 'oral' origin, dependent on food supply, but is a behaviour system of its own. Early disturbances in this behaviour system would have severe and long-lasting after-effects. Two psychoanalytically orientated empirical studies can serve to illustrate how vulnerating experiences earlier in life and later experiences and abilities to cope with stress situations are interconnected.

Keilson (1979) has very thoroughly studied the 'sequential traumatization of children' experienced by 204 Jewish war orphans in the Netherlands from 1940–45 and followed up their fate approximately 25 years after the end of the war. Like many other authors he is of the opinion that the suffering which people have been through cannot be stated in terms of numbers. The author therefore decided to be content with eliciting only the external factors of extreme stress sequences and not to attempt to 'measure' the psychic reality. Only what happened to the child in question was recorded and not the manner in which the child experienced and assimilated it. The author distinguished three traumatic phases: (1) the occupation of the country and the beginning of the terror against the Jewish population; (2) direct persecution, e.g. the deportation of parents and children to concentration camps, or the separation of children from their parents and their going into hiding with impromptu foster families; (3) the post-war period during which the main issue was that of appointing guardians and finding new homes. The follow-up study, approximately 25 years after the end of the war, showed that not only the two phases of persecution, but also the third phase – initially assumed to be unproblematic – was of considerable significance for the resultant impairment of psychological functioning during adulthood. The degree of impairment was determined by the quality of the post-war environment whereby its capacity to break the chain of traumatizing factors could mitigate the entire process. The example shows that once the traumas of separation and life threat had been overcome, the child's further development depended on whether or not the resultant conflicts of ethnic–religious identity and emotional loyalty could be mastered with adequate social help. Social and intrapsychic conflicts are therefore intimately linked to each other in this example.

Matussek (1971, 1975), in his studies on the late effects of the concentration camp situation on prisoners, attempted to define as adequately as possible the specific stress factors and to identify their pathogenic character. For this purpose, the constituents of the complex stressor concept were differentiated according to different levels of intensity. It could be shown that the 'work situation' in the concentration camps was the most important factor for the development of later impairments. Low social status, which was connected with heavy manual work, determined the intensity of hunger, sickness, torture and humiliations, and also the chances of survival and the later impairments. Along with a 'psychophysical syndrome', which can be interpreted as a long-lasting general state of exhaustion, enduring disturbances of social-communicative functions were found in many cases, amongst which the most serious were called 'resignation and desperation', resembling the 'deep depression' described in the clinical literature. Individuals who already had a high 'capacity for interpersonal contact', characterized by initiative and cooperative activities, were able to escape stressing work situations and had fewer such later impairments. A lack of such positive personality characteristics was found to be connected with a disturbed mother–child relationship, showing that early psychological experiences and later stress situations and the ability and possibility to cope with them are intimately connected.

In the primate experiments of the school of Harlow (1958), both extreme and long-lasting after-effects of early social deprivation were described. The possible relevance of these results for human behaviour – they seem to give support to the theory of Bowlby (1969) – can be deducted from the phylogenetic proximity between primates and humans (Harlow & Harlow, 1966; Harlow, Harlow & Suomi, 1971; McKinney, Suomi & Harlow, 1971; Suomi & Harlow, 1972; Young *et al.*, 1973; Kaufman, 1977).

Although classical psychoanalysis and behaviourism (including Pavlov's reflexology) obviously have a common basis in the idea of an association between stimulus and reaction, a crucial difference resides in the fact that psychoanalysis departed from verbal productions whereas behaviourism ignored them (at least at the beginning). Certainly no one would maintain that laboratory animals experience no feelings; however, dogs, rats or pigeons do not have a verbal medium to reflect upon these inner qualities and to express them directly. The growing self-restriction of psychoanalysis to 'intrapsychic' processes was partly the unavoidable consequence of a form of therapy which centred around biographical aspects of human beings. The turn to cognitive psychology in behaviourism shows that therapy is obviously impossible without taking 'private' events and intrapsychic functions into consideration. This development confirms the fruitfulness of the original psychoanalytic approach. Differences between different psychological schools are becoming more and more restricted to terminology and to some practical clinical rituals, and are no longer as substantial as they seemed to be in the past.

The clinical interest of the behavioural schools of psychology was mainly centred around the problem of the development of depression. Their general stance is that loss of a significant source of positive 'reinforcement' leads to conditions which may range from a 'transient blue mood' to 'sustained melancholia' (Liberman & Ruskin, 1971). What constitutes a 'reinforcer' for a specific person can only be deduced from the biography of the individual (i.e. by an idiographic approach) and cannot be stated as a general rule. This so-called 'reinforcement hypothesis' includes the occurrence of adverse events, the absence of supportive systems, lack of social skills, and the amount of anxiety level as antecedent conditions. The main assumption is that a low rate of reinforcement leads to depression. A second causal hypothesis considers depression as related to a decreased reinforcement *potential* leading to a search for biochemical antecedents. It is important to note that these two hypotheses are by no means regarded as mutually exclusive. In fact, both mechanisms could operate as a vicious circle whereby a low rate of reinforcement leads to depression, which in turn alters the biochemical substrates of reinforcement potential and so forth (Lewinsohn, Youngren & Grosscup, 1979).

If psychoanalysis and behavioural psychology are compared one could say that the hedonistic principle of the pleasure–aversion regulation of psychoanalysis, which is related to the psychic apparatus, is analogous to the hedonistic scheme of behavioural psychology implying the withdrawal or presentation of positive or negative 'reinforcers'. These reinforcement mechanisms are represented in the reinforcement apparatus of the central nervous system with its 'rewarding' (medial forebrain bundle) and 'punishing' areas (periventricular system).

The concept of 'learned helplessness' (Seligman, 1975) refers to the after-effects of experiences of uncontrollability of a traumatic situation leading to an apathy in animals which resembles states of depression. In applying this hypothesis to humans, it was modified in the sense that the expectation of a lack of control over stressful events was regarded as the main causal factor for those deficits which are similar to depression (Abramson, Seligman & Teasdale, 1978; Garber, Miller & Seaman, 1979).

Finally, Bandura's concept of 'self-efficacy' (1977) deserves mentioning here. It refers to the process of learning of expectations in relation to a lack of coping abilities; in this concept the role of learning from a model is important.

R. S. Lazarus can be taken as the spokesman for the 'Berkeley School' with its 'cognitive phenomenological analysis' of psychological stress. This relational or transactional concept describes certain kinds of adaptive interplay between any (kind of) systems; in our case, between a subjective personal and an ecological environmental system with the assumption of a reciprocal causation. The concept of 'stress' in its wider meaning embraces any event in which environmental or internal demands (or both) tax or exceed the adaptive resources of an individual, a social system, or an organismic system. The distinction between a physiological, psychological and sociological level may be adequate for research. For medicine, however, as I understand it, the continuous relationship of the subject system to the variables of the ecological and organismic systems (and its dependence upon them) should remain in the foreground.

'Cognitive appraisal' is one of the basic concepts of this specific theory of emotion (Lazarus, Averill & Opton, 1970). The evaluation of reality implied here is essentially personal, i.e. actually emotional. According to this school, the individual attempts, first of all, to extract the meaning, which is relevant for immediate survival, from the perceived actual circumstances, which to me suggests an analogy to the 'orientation reaction', which can either lead to habituation or an alarm reaction. In the next step so-called 'secondary appraisals', which work on a medium-term basis, shape the mentioned emotional cognitive processes by feedback and assess the available coping resources. Such 'reappraisals' reconsider again and again all information about the environment, the self, and their interaction, in order to change, if necessary, preconceived notions in such a way that the individual's activities correspond better to the problems he encounters.

The word 'coping' tends to become an all-purpose word, the meaning of which ranges from 'adjustment' (as person–environment fit, see French, Rodgers & Cobb, 1974), to 'mastery', to 'accuracy of self or reality assessment', and finally, to 'defence'. Lazarus & Launier (1978) have recommended the constriction of its meaning to specific problem-solving and emotion-regulating efforts, which may be both action orientated and intrapsychic; namely, those which can maintain the 'balance of power' between demands (environmental and internal, including conflicts) and resources (supplies, abilities) or re-establish it when disturbed. This involves the mobilization of various activities which may be conscious or subconscious, organismic, psychic and interpersonal. A distinction between problem-solving instrumental skills on the one hand and emotion-regulating 'palliative' measures on the other hand seems rather artificial. After all, keeping cool is a prerequisite for a rational approach to coping with difficulties.

An integrative view

Both the onset and the course of any disease, including emotional diseases, depend on the balance between facilitating (i.e. noxious), and protective factors. These factors may be of a hereditary, environmental, or biographical, i.e. information-processing, nature. With regard to the aforementioned mechanisms of 'appraisal', which are of central importance for coping with life events, it seems important not to conceive of them as if they were merely taking cognizance of abstractly interesting facts, but to regard them also as emotional-orientating reactions which may imply different degrees of threat. In the process of evaluation of perceptions, so-called 'collateral models of transduction' (Weiner, 1977) handle different components on different central nervous pathways: partly on the experiential level of knowledge and feeling, partly in motor behavioural preparations for action, and partly on an autonomic and endocrine level. The latter two overlap to different degrees with functions which have traditionally been termed motivational and emotional.

Life events have to be differentiated from gradually developing life difficulties without apparent alarming occurrences, which nevertheless exert a stressing influence. In such life difficulties the cognitive part of the appraisal process becomes blurred and difficult to analyse, while the accumulation of emotional uneasiness may have considerable effects, both on corresponding physiological regulations and on sets of expectancies which are implicit and not easy to grasp verbally. Such complex processes probably have considerable negative effects on the development of self-esteem and self-efficacy, with all its consequences. However, they are difficult to describe and evaluate for research purposes.

For any 'appraisal' of internal or external events, a frame of reference is required. The way in which the available information is put into an evaluative order of priorities depends on this frame of reference. It seems desirable to me, along with Dörner (1976), to attach the area of subconscious cognitive and evaluative processes (in the sense of Freud's primary processes) to this epistemic data base. Averill (1979) uses the term 'meaning' in a transactional way when stating that 'in order for a person to impose meaning on events, he must possess some model or cognitive structure which represents the environment and his place within it. A person informs or structures his environment, as well as vice versa.'

Piaget's concept of assimilation refers to building up this cognitive data base, upon which both reproductive thinking and routine actions are based (Piaget, 1971). However, owing to its primary-process character, this data base contains contradictions which constitute a psychological threat for the person concerned when they become excessive. The assimilation of negative critical life events into this data base may be impeded by emotional resistance. Adverse events which cannot be assimilated, or only with difficulty, place a demand on the individual concerned to cope with them by accommodation, i.e. by changing his own cognitive emotional schemes.

According to Horowitz (1983) models based on the past must interpret the present and be revised to meet the future. The difficulty in revising or giving up such fundamental accustomed patterns is illustrated by the phantom sensations after amputation. Further examples are Freud's 'grief work' (1917) which refers to various processes of mastery which are related to a factual loss, and the concept of the 'work of worrying' (Janis, 1958) which refers to anticipatory coping if a misfortune is imminent.

There is little doubt that most critical life events require accommodative, problem-solving and assimilative evaluation processes, which operate both on a cognitive and on an emotional level. These regulative activities, which include all processes usually referred to as 'coping' and 'defence', in many cases seriously overtax the existing abilities and resources of the person concerned. The persistence of unrevised early patterns of person-to-person relationships into adulthood (called 'transference' in psychoanalysis) is an example of how problems, which could be unimportant at a later life stage, are perpetuated. Postponing the revision of fundamental emotional epistemic structures diminishes the chance of coping adequately and constructively with future life problems. Unresolved problems resulting from various conflicts may accumulate to such a degree that a point is reached where resources are exhausted and decompensation begins.

In brief, a hypothetical model of how life events and the failure to cope with them may lead to psychiatric disorders could be formulated as such: if the formation and constant revision of an epistemic representation of the self and of the environment is impeded by various unfavourable conditions, the prerequisites for solving current problems are insufficient and unresolved problems accumulate. Specific predispositions for suffering pathogenic effects from life events, i.e. vulnerabilities, may subsequently develop if certain other factors (e.g. hereditary ones) are present. As a result, the risk of developing certain types of illness may increase.

These specific vulnerabilities may, for example, refer to the importance attached to one's social prestige, to the possible harm and threat experienced by close persons, or to a relatively low tolerance of emotional closeness or emotional distance. Once a person has become vulnerable to specific life events, these may trigger pathological conditions which, in accordance with the prevalent concept of disease, are defined as illnesses.

In coming back to the introductory remarks, it must be stated that regulatory mechanisms of the central nervous system are obviously responsible for the onset and termination, cure, or relapse of the various forms of diseases called endogenic, albeit to different degrees. These mechanisms determine, for example, different degrees of arousal, hedonistic equilibrium, emotional qualities, cognitive abilities and so on. It would indeed be surprising if the aforementioned acquired psychological vulnerabilities were not also based on these and similar nervous functions. An example of such an integrative view is the hypothesis of the diencephalic final common pathway for the development of depression (Akiskal & McKinney, 1975; Akiskal, 1979). In this model the chain of antecedent factors includes physiological and psychological stressors, and genetic and developmental predispositions, which 'relate to the diencephalic centres of mood, reward, and arousal through interoceptive and exteroceptive circuits' (Akiskal, 1979). It is not only conceivable but also the hope that similar integrative aetiological models will be constructed for other psychiatric illnesses.

References

Abramson, L. Y., Seligman, M. E. P. & Teasdale, J. (1978). Learned helplessness in humans: critique and reformulation. *Journal of Abnormal Psychology*, **87**, 49–74.

Akiskal, H. S. (1979). A biobehavioral approach to depression. In *The psychobiology of the depressive disorders, implications for the effects of stress*, ed. R. A. Depue, pp. 409–37. New York: Academic Press.

Akiskal, H. S. & McKinney, W. T., Jr (1975). Overview of recent research in depression. Integration of ten conceptual models into a comprehensive clinical frame. *Archives of General Psychiatry*, **32**, 285–305.

Averill, J. R. (1979). A selective review of cognitive and behavioral factors involved in the regulation of stress. In *The psychobiology of depressive disorders: implications for the effects of stress*, ed. R. A. Depue, pp. 365–87. New York: Academic Press.

Bandura, A. (1977). Self-efficacy: toward a unifying theory of behavioral change. *Psychological Review*, **84**, 191–216.

Bibring, E. (1953). The mechanism of depression. In *Affective disorders*, ed. Ph. Greenacre, pp. 13–48. New York: International Universities Press.

Bowlby, J. (1958). The nature of the child's tie to his mother. *International Journal of Psychoanalysis*, **39**, 350–73.

Bowlby, J. (1969). *Attachment and loss*, vol. I, *Attachment*. London: Hogarth Press.

Bowlby, J. (1973). *Attachment and loss*, vol. II, *Separation*. London: Hogarth Press.

Bowlby, J. (1977). The making and breaking of affectional bonds. I. Aetiology and psychopathology in the light of attachment theory. *British Journal of Psychiatry*, **130**, 201–10.

Dohrenwend, B. P. & Dohrenwend, B. S. (1979). The conceptualization of measurement of stressful life events: an overview of the issues. In *The psychobiology of the depressive disorders: implications for the effects of stress*, ed. R. A. Depue, pp. 105–21. New York: Academic Press.

Dörner, D. (1976). *Problemlösen als Informationsverarbeitung*. Stuttgart: Kohlhammer.

French, J. R. P., Jr, Rodgers, W. & Cobb, S. (1974). Adjustment as person–environment fit. In *Coping and adaptation*, ed. G. V. Coelho, D. A. Hamburg & J. E. Adams, pp. 316–33. New York: Basic Books.

Freud, A. (1936). *The ego and the mechanisms of defence*. London: Hogarth Press, 1937.

Freud, S. (1917). *Mourning and melancholia. Standard edition of the complete psychological works of Sigmund Freud*, vol. 14. London: Hogarth Press.

Freud, S. & Breuer, J. (1895). *Studies on hysteria. Standard edition of the complete psychological works of Sigmund Freud*, vol. 2. London: Hogarth Press.

Garber, J., Miller, W. R. & Seaman, S. F. (1979). Learned helplessness, stress and the depressive disorders. In *The psychology of depressive disorders: implications for the effects of stress*, ed. R. A. Depue, pp. 335–63. New York: Academic Press.

Harlow, H. F. (1958). The nature of love. *American Journal of Psychology*, **13**, 673–83.

Harlow, H. F. & Harlow, M. K. (1966). Learning to love. *American Science*, **54**, 244–72.

Harlow, H. F., Harlow, M. K. & Suomi, S. J. (1971). From thought to therapy: lessons from a primate laboratory. *American Scientist*, **59**, 538–49.
Horowitz, M. J. (1983). Psychological response to serious life events. In *The denial of stress*, ed. S. Breznitz, pp. 129–59. International Universities Press. Reprinted from *Human stress and cognition*, ed. V. Hamilton & D. Warburton. Chichester: Interscience (1979).
Janis, I. L. (1958). *Psychological stress: psychoanalytic and behavioural studies of surgical patients*. London: Chapman & Hall.
Kaufman, I. C. (1977). Developmental considerations of anxiety and depression: psychobiological studies in monkeys. In *Psychoanalysis and contemporary science*, ed. T. Shapiro, pp. 317–63. New York: International Universities Press.
Keilson, H. (1979). *Sequentielle Traumatisierung bei Kindern*. Stuttgart: Enke Verlag.
Lazarus, R. S. (1983). The costs and benefits of denial. In *The denial of stress*, ed. S. Breznitz, pp. 1–30. New York: International Universities Press.
Lazarus, R. S., Averill, J. R. & Opton, E. M., Jr (1970). Toward a cognitive theory of emotion. In *Feelings and emotions*, ed. M. Arnold, pp. 207–31. New York: Academic Press.
Lazarus, R. S. & Launier, R. (1978). Transactions between person and environment. In *Perspectives in interactional psychology*, ed. L. A. Pervin & M. Lewis, pp. 287–327. New York: Plenum Press.
Lewinsohn, P. M., Youngren, M. A. & Grosscup, S. J. (1979). Reinforcement and depression. In *The psychobiology of the depressive disorders: implications for the effects of stress*, ed. R. A. Depue, pp. 291–316. New York: Academic Press.
Liberman, R. P. & Ruskin, D. E. (1971). Depression: a behavioral formulation. *Archives of General Psychiatry*, **24**, 515–23.
McKinney, W. T., Jr, Suomi, S. J. & Harlow, H. F. (1971). Depression in primates. *American Journal of Psychiatry*, **127**, 1313–20.
Matussek, P. (1971). *Die Konzentrationslagerhaft und ihre Folgen*. Berlin: Springer.
Matussek, P. (1975). Psychische Schäden bei Konzentrationslagerhäftlingen. In *Psychiatrie der Gegenwart. Soziale und angewandte Psychiatrie*, 2nd edition, vol. 3, ed. K. P. Kisker, J. E. Meyer, C. Müller & E. Strömgren, pp. 387–427. Berlin: Springer.
Parkes, C. M. (1972). *Bereavement. Studies of grief in adult life*. London: Tavistock Publications.
Piaget, J. (1971). *Biology and knowledge*. Chicago: University of Chicago Press.
Sadegh-zadeh, K. (1977). Krankheitsbegriffe und nosologische System. *Metamedicine*, **1**, 4–41.
Sadegh-zadeh, K. (1981). Foundations of clinical praxicology. Part 1. The relativity of medical diagnosis. *Metamedicine*, **2**, 183–96.
Seligman, M. E. P. (1975). *Helplessness: on depression, development and death*. San Francisco: W. H. Freeman.
Sulloway, F. J. (1979). *Freud, biologist of the mind. Beyond the psychoanalytic legend*. London: Burnett.
Suomi, S. J. & Harlow, H. F. (1972). Depressive behavior in young monkeys subjected to vertical chamber confinement. *Journal of Comparative and Physiological Psychology*, **80**, 11–18.
Weiner, H. (1977). *Psychobiology and human disease*. New York: Elsevier.
Young, L., Suomi, S. J., Harlow, H. F. & McKinney, W. T., Jr (1973). Early stress and later response to separation in rhesus monkeys. *American Journal of Psychiatry*, **130**, 400–5.

4

Measuring life stress – a comparison of the checklist and the panel technique

H. KATSCHNIG

Introduction

Since the publication of Lindemann's (1944) seminal paper on grief, studies on the relationship between life stress and the development of physical and mental diseases have, at least up to the early sixties, relied mainly on investigating the health consequences of single events such as bereavement, divorce, expatriation, or retirement. The design of these studies was either prospective, i.e. the study population was chosen at the time of the event and then followed up regularly in order to find out about health consequences, or retrospective, i.e. both the selection of probands, who had experienced a specific life event in the past, and the gathering of data about health consequences were carried out retrospectively (Figure 4.1).

The publication of the 'Schedule of Recent Experience', a 42-item self-rating list for life changes with predetermined adjustment scores (Holmes & Rahe, 1967), signalled the advent of a completely new methodological approach to establishing links between life stress and

Figure 4.1. Types of life event studies I: studying the various health consequences of a single type of life event.

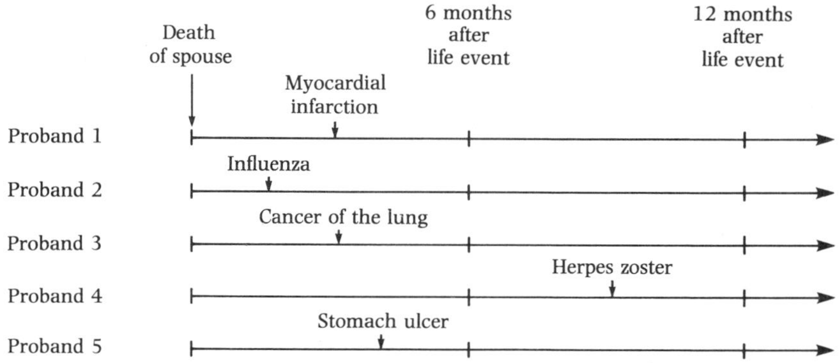

illness. Whereas in the traditional research design the various health consequences of a single (often catastrophic) type of life event are studied (e.g. Kasl, Gore & Cobb, 1975, on health changes after losing a job), the new research strategy involves the study of individuals suffering from a single specific disease such as myocardial infarction or depression, whose various (catastrophic and non-catastrophic) life stresses over a given period before disease onset are elicited retrospectively and assessed with regard to their cumulative stress effect (e.g. Brown & Harris, 1978, on life events preceding the onset of depression). By its very nature this design can only be retrospective (Figure 4.2).

This latter approach implies the necessity of using a quantitative stress measure representing the total amount of life stress experienced by a person over a specified time period. Studies employing this design are numerous. There is, however, no uniformity in such retrospective quantification of life stress as can be seen in the examples of results of life event and illness studies presented in Figures 4.3 to 4.5. Nevertheless the results are very similar for such different conditions as depression, schizophrenia, attempted suicide and coronary heart disease, all showing an increase of life stress before illness onset.

Some differences in methodology are obvious from inspecting the graphs: the time intervals chosen differ in the three studies, ranging from four 3-week periods over six 1-month periods to twelve 3-month periods; the stress measures constructed for each of these intervals imply either a *threshold* model ('at least one life event in a given time period'; Figure 4.3) or an *additive* model, in which life events are simply counted (Figure 4.4) or predetermined weights of single life events are added up (Figure 4.5). Other differences, such as in the methodology of data collection and the

Figure 4.2. Types of life event studies II: studying the various life events preceding the onset of a single type of disease.

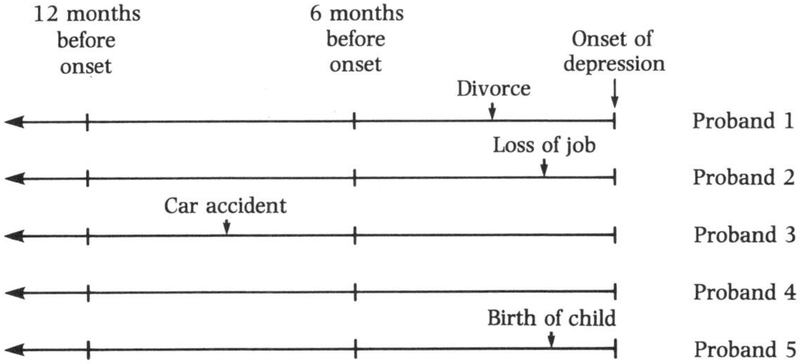

Figure 4.3. Percentage of persons with at least one event in the four 3-week periods before onset (patients) or interview (general population) (from Brown & Birley, 1970).

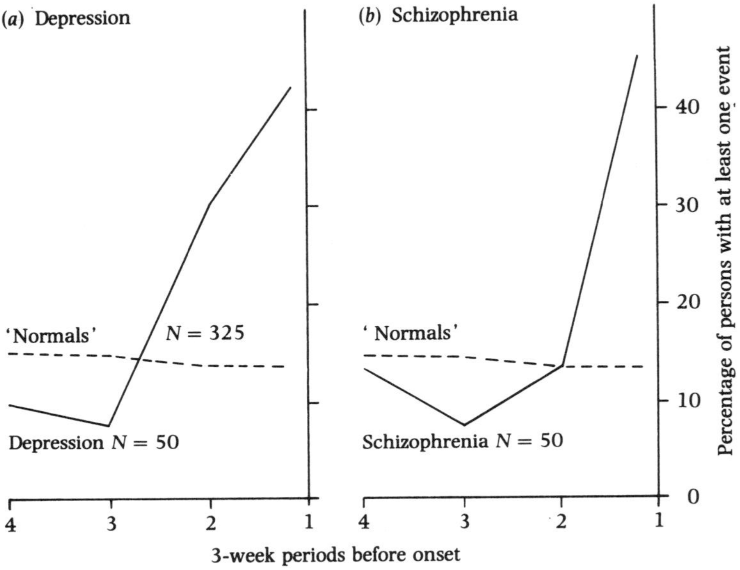

Figure 4.4. Mean number of events reported during each one-month period prior to attempted suicide, onset of illness, or interview (from Paykel *et al.*, 1975). Key: triangles, suicide attempts; squares, depressives; circles, general population controls.

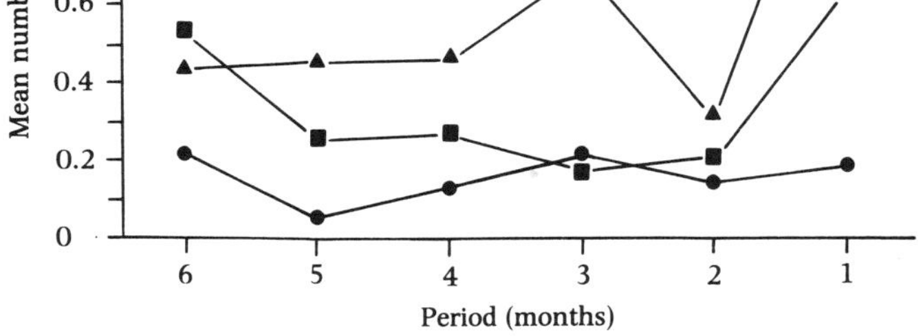

evaluation of the stressfulness of single life events, are not obvious unless one knows the distinct traditions in which the authors have carried out their studies. In fact, Brown & Birley (1970), Paykel, Prusoff & Myers (1975) and Theorell & Rahe (1971) all employ different methodologies.

Among the many methods used for collecting data about life events and quantifying life stress retrospectively, two approaches have, over the past 15 years, obtained a kind of paradigmatic status. It is the aim of this chapter to analyse the problems inherent in the measurement of life stress by comparing these two approaches, which are usually referred to as the *checklist* (or *inventory*) and the *panel* approach. The 'Schedule of Recent Experience' (SRE) by Holmes & Rahe (1967) will serve to illustrate the checklist approach, while the London 'Life Event and Difficulty Schedule' (LEDS) will be used as an example for the panel technique. These two instruments will first be briefly characterized. Data about a cross-validation study will then be presented before a more thorough description of the differences between the two approaches is given. Finally a taxonomy of life stress measures is proposed.

Figure 4.5. Quarter-year mean life change unit (LCU) totals, over the 3 years prior to hospitalization for 27 coronary heart disease in-patients with no previous signs and/or symptoms of coronary heart disease (from Theorell & Rahe, 1971).

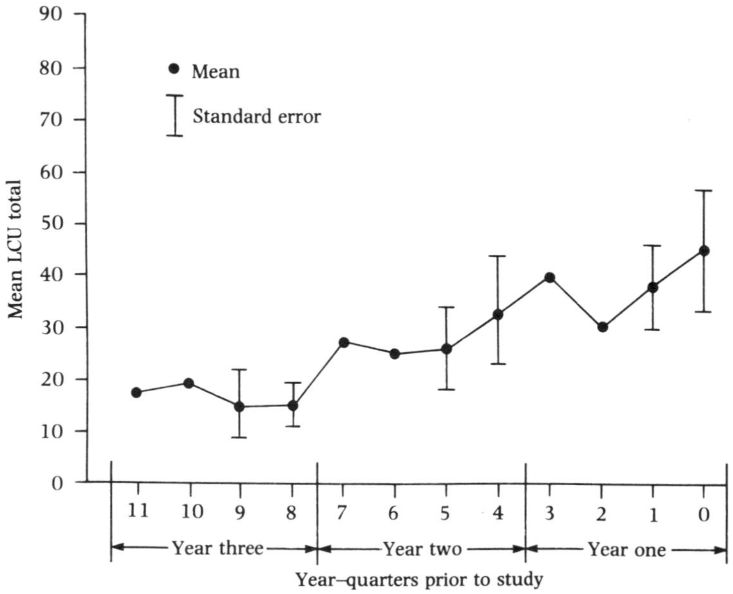

Two techniques for quantifying life stress

The fact that the SRE is both simple to apply (being basically a self-rating list) and yields a seemingly clearcut quantitative measure for life stress may explain its popularity with students of life stress and illness throughout the world, as documented by the translation of the SRE into numerous languages (Rahe, 1969). The SRE and derivative instruments (e.g. Paykel, Prusoff & Uhlenhuth, 1971; Cochrane & Robertson, 1973; Tennant & Andrews, 1976; Dohrenwend *et al.*, 1978) use a standard checklist of a fixed number of life changes with predetermined weighted scores. For the SRE the list of these stress scores – called 'Life Change Units' (LCUs) – has been named the 'Social Readjustment Rating Scale' (SRRS) (Holmes & Rahe, 1967). For illustrative purposes the first and the last few items of the SRRS are presented here together with their LCUs.

Rank	Life change	LCU
1	Death of spouse	100
2	Divorce	73
3	Separation	65
4	Jail term	63
5	Death of a close family member	63
.	.	
.	.	
.	.	
40	Change in eating habits	15
41	Vacation	12
42	Minor violations of the law	11

Such stress scores are usually obtained by asking samples of the general population to rate the stressfulness of each event on the list (conceptualized, in the case of the SRE, as the amount of 'readjustment' required by the average person to cope with a specific life change) and calculating mean values. This procedure has led Tennant *et al.* (1979) to call this approach the 'consensus a priori' technique. The SRE and similar checklists are nearly always (although not necessarily) employed as self-rating instruments. Attention has been drawn repeatedly to the serious drawbacks of the SRE, in particular its inaccuracy in defining life changes and its low reliability (e.g. Mendels & Weinstein, 1972; Brown, 1974; Katschnig, 1980*a*, *b*; Steele, Henderson & Duncan-Jones, 1980). However, little notice seems to have been taken of this criticism and the SRE and similar checklists continue to be widely employed.

The London LEDS developed by Brown (1974, see also Brown & Harris, this volume, p. 113) is an alternative to the checklist approach to measuring life stress. It consists of a lengthy, semi-standardized interview for eliciting information on life events and the subject's social background, and makes use of an extensive glossary of definitions and of elaborate scoring rules. The amount of stress involved for the individual under study is determined – after all relevant information has been gathered by an interviewer – by a team of raters (a 'panel') who have all the information about each life event of the proband and about the specific social context of its occurrence, but have no information about the subject's psychiatric state or emotional reactions. The degree of 'threat' of each event is first assessed independently by each rater on a four-point scale; then judgments are pooled in order to reach a consensus. Consequently, Tennant *et al.* (1979) have called this technique the 'consensus a posteriori' approach. The LEDS is a carefully designed method with a high reliability (Tennant *et al.*, 1979; Parry, Shapiro & Davies, 1981); it has, however, not gained as equally wide an acceptance as the SRE, mainly because of its more complex structure, which makes it both laborious and difficult to apply.

It is astonishing that despite the existence of a vast literature on both the checklist and the panel approach (see, e.g., the papers contained in Dohrenwend & Dohrenwend, 1981), only exceptionally are cross-references made between the two (e.g. Katschnig, 1980*a*, *b*; Bebbington *et al.*, 1984; Brugha *et al.*, 1985). It is the specific purpose of this paper to compare and contrast these two techniques both on an analytical and – by using data of two cross-validation studies – on an empirical level. In this way, not only will the relative advantages and disadvantages of the two techniques become apparent but also some principal limitations of the quantitative methods used in research on stressful life events will emerge.

A cross-validation study of the SRE and the London LEDS

A cross-validation study of the SRE and the London LEDS, carried out at the Royal Infirmary in Edinburgh on 42 patients who had attempted suicide, demonstrated that congruency between these two principal methods for measuring life stress was very low (Katschnig, 1980*a*, *b*). It could be shown that such cross-validation studies can be heuristically helpful for analysing differences between various research methods.

The possibility of making more extensive analyses was limited in that study because of the small number of cases. The Edinburgh study was therefore repeated on a larger number of cases involving 147 depressed patients admitted either to the Psychiatric Clinic of the University of Vienna or to a large psychiatric hospital near Vienna (Katschnig & Fuchs-Robetin, 1984). Depressed patients were chosen for this study, since it is well documented that they experience an increase in the frequency of life events prior to the onset of their illness (Paykel *et al.*, 1975; Brown & Harris, 1978). The two research instruments were applied only after the depressive episode had remitted, thus excluding the possibility of the depressed mood influencing recall (Schless *et al.*, 1974).

Patients first received the SRE as a self-rating list, which enquired about the occurrence of each of 42 life changes in four consecutive 6-month periods prior to admission. Since for the purpose of this methodological study either the date of admission or that of illness onset could have been chosen, the former was used as being the more reliable one. The LEDS interview was carried out immediately after the patient had completed the SRE, and also covered the two-year period before admission. The expected effect of applying one technique immediately after the other would be to increase congruency between the two measurements obtained, since a respondent is unlikely to give completely different answers to the same question within a matter of one or two hours. Any incongruencies between the resulting stress measures would therefore have to be regarded as a serious indicator that the two methods do not correspond.

Life stress prior to admission as measured separately by the SRE and the LEDS

The two usual ways of analysing life event data obtained by the use of checklists such as the SRE consist of either simply counting the number of life events which have occurred in specified time periods and calculating the respective means for the whole group under study (see, e.g., Figure 4.4) or adding up the predetermined LCUs and calculating their mean values for the group (see, e.g., Figure 4.5). In our study, both when simply counting the number of life changes and when calculating the total LCU scores for each of the four 6-month periods separately, a clearcut rise in the amount of life stress experienced by our patients was found (Figures 4.6 and 4.7). The rise between the first and the second 6-month periods before onset is statistically highly significant. Furthermore, a close correlation was found between the number of life events and the total LCU score for individual patients (Spearman's rank correlation coefficient was 0·94 for the first 6-month period and 0·97 for the second period). This finding suggests that one could dispense with the LCU scores (for a more detailed analysis of this problem see Shrout, 1981).

Figure 4.6. Schedule of Recent Experience: mean numbers of life changes reported by 147 depressed patients for each of the four 6-month periods preceding admission. Rise 7–12 months → 0–6 months: $P < 0{\cdot}0001$.

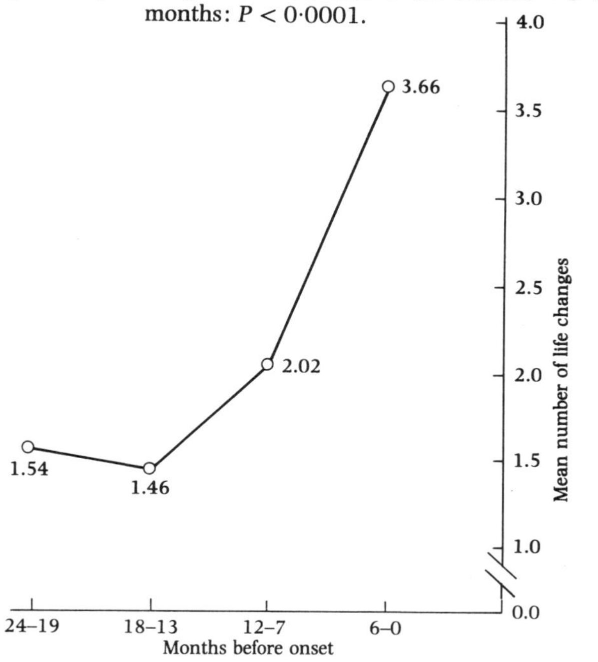

Figure 4.7. Schedule of Recent Experience: means of total life change unit (LCU) scores (for life changes reported by 147 depressed patients) for each of the four 6-month periods preceding admission. Rise 7–12 months → 0–6 months: $P < 0.0001$.

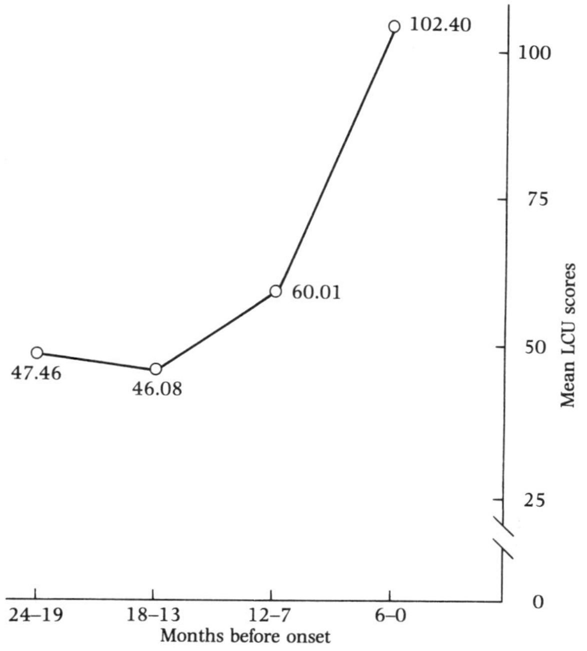

Figure 4.8. London Life Event and Difficulty Schedule: mean numbers of life events reported by 147 depressed patients for each of the four 6-month periods preceding admission. Rise 7–12 months → 0–6 months: $P < 0.05$.

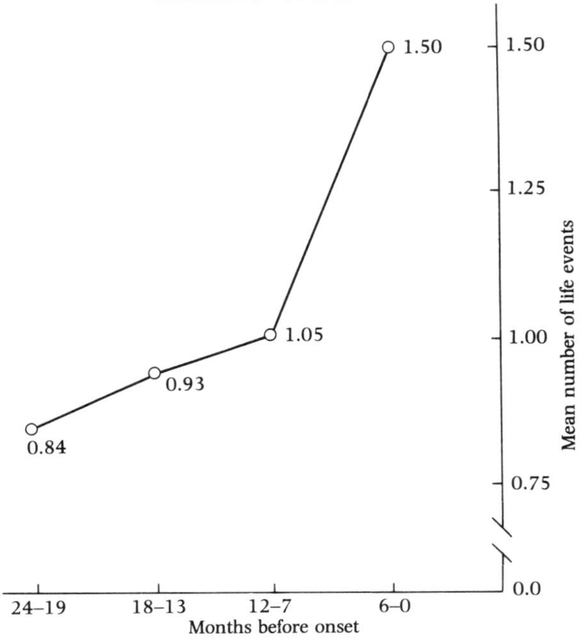

Figure 4.9. London Life Event and Difficulty Schedule: percentage of patients reporting the occurrence of at least one life event for each of the four 6-month periods preceding admission.

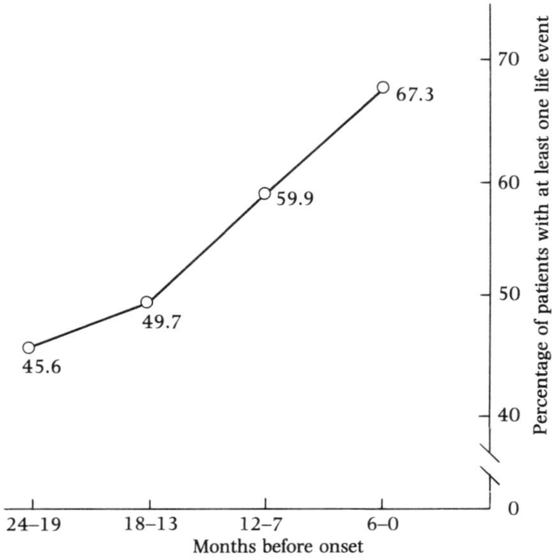

When turning to the LEDS and calculating the mean number of life events picked up by the LEDS for the four 6-month periods, the results obtained are practically identical to those found with the SRE. There is a clearcut rise from the distant to the proximal 6-month period, whereby the difference between the first and second 6-month period before onset is statistically significant (see Figure 4.8). A similar picture emerges when using the threshold model, more frequently applied with the LEDS. The percentage of patients experiencing at least one life event in each time period increases towards the admission date, although this rise is not statistically significant (see Figure 4.9).

One can thus conclude that applying the SRE and the LEDS to groups of depressed patients yields identical results. This replicates the earlier findings for attempted suicide patients (Katschnig, 1980*a*, *b*) and at first sight suggests that it would be sensible to use the more economical SRE rather than its more complicated and expensive counterpart, the LEDS. However, this conclusion cannot be accepted without first comparing the SRE and the LEDS in relation to individual patients.

Comparing the global stress measures of the SRE and the LEDS in individual patients

In order to find out whether there is a correspondence between the stress measures provided by each of the two methods also on the level of the individual patient, analyses are restricted to the 6-month period immediately preceding admission.

Applying the SRE to our sample of 147 depressed patients yielded 538 life changes during this period, whereas the number of life events recorded by the LEDS for the same time period was substantially lower, numbering only 220. LEDS life events are obviously more narrowly defined than SRE life changes. Calculating Spearman's rank correlation coefficient for the total number of SRE life changes and LEDS life events recorded for each patient yields a moderately high value (0.31, $P < 0.001$). It seems that LEDS life events carry with them a 'cloud' of less strictly defined SRE life changes. No judgment can, however, be made at this stage as to whether individual SRE life changes in the 'cloud' do in fact correspond to the LEDS life events of a given patient.

The total number of life events is not usually used as a stress measure when employing the LEDS. Instead, a frequent stress measure applied in LEDS studies is the proportion of persons experiencing at least one life event in a given time period (see, e.g., Figure 4.3). For both SRE life changes and LEDS life events this measure is used in the comparison presented in Table

4.1. While 87·5% of patients have experienced at least one SRE life change in the 6 months before admission, 67·3% reported at least one LEDS life event (which is not significantly different). For 95 (64·6%) of the 147 depressed patients the result was identical with both methods, whereas in the remaining 52 (35·4%) there was disagreement about this stress indicator. The value of the Kappa agreement coefficient, which, unlike the Spearman's coefficient takes chance agreement into consideration, yields a value of 0·04 which corresponds to virtually no correlation.

In a series of further cross-tabulations (Katschnig & Fuchs-Robetin, 1984) the agreement between the two methods was either low or practically non-existent. Only two further examples (both involving LCU totals) are given here. In tables 4.2 and 4.3 patients were divided into those above ($N = 59$) and those below ($N = 88$) the LCU group mean (102), representing patients with 'high' and 'low' life stress during the 6 months before admission. In a cross-tabulation with the LEDS, using as stress indicator the index of 'at least one LEDS life event', the Kappa coefficient was 0·24 (Table 4.2), and still lower (though still significant) if only 'severe LEDS life events' were taken into consideration (Table 4.3; for the definition of a 'severe' life event see the chapter by Brown & Harris, p. 107, this volume).

Thus, when comparing the global stress scores of the SRE and the LEDS on the level of the individual patient, we find a sharp contrast to the seemingly identical results when group mean values are compared. On the level of the individual patient the two methods produce stress measures which correlate only moderately or not at all. Obviously, the uniform picture of an increase in life stress obtained by plotting group mean values

Table 4.1. *Cross-tabulation of patients having at least one life event according to the LEDS or at least one life change according to the SRE during the 6 months before admission*

		LEDS: Number of persons with at least one life event	no life event	Total
SRE: number of persons with	at least one life change	88	41	129 (87·5%)
	no life change	11	7	18 (12·5%)
	Total	99 (67·3%)	48 (32·7%)	147 (100%)

Kappa = 0·04; n.s.

of these stress measures (Figures 4.6 to 4.9) is produced by different patients when different methods are used, i.e. a patient having a high SRE score in the proximal 6 months and a low one in the distal 6-month period may show the inverse pattern when the LEDS is applied. We may suspect that this could also be the case in other studies, for example in those presented in Figures 4.3 to 4.5.

'Group pictures' such as those shown in Figures 4.3 to 4.9 are abstractions from the pictures of the individual patients in each group. This is illustrated in Figure 4.10, where the 'course' of life stress (measured in LCUs of the SRE) is shown both for the whole group and for each individual

Table 4.2. *Cross-tabulation of patients having LCU scores above and below the group mean (SRE) and patients having at least one life event (LEDS)*

		LEDS: Number of persons with at least one life event	no life event	Total
SRE: number of persons with	LCU score above mean	49	10	59
	LCU score below mean	50	38	88
	Total	99	48	147

Kappa = 0·24; $P \leqslant 0{\cdot}01$.

Table 4.3. *Cross-tabulation of patients having LCU scores above and below the group mean (SRE) and patients having at least one severe life event (LEDS)*

		LEDS: Number of persons with at least one severe life event	no severe life event	Total
SRE: number of persons with	LCU score above mean	25	34	59
	LCU score below mean	21	67	88
	Total	46	101	147

Kappa = 0·19; $P \leqslant 0{\cdot}05$.

of the 42 attempted suicides of the Edinburgh cross-validation study (Katschnig, 1980*a, b*). While there was a general rise in the total LCU mean score for the total group from 106.4 LCUs in the distant 6-month period to 182·8 LCUs in the proximal 6-month period (heavy line in Figure 4.10), only 28 patients corresponded to this 'group picture', whereas 12 patients showed an inverse pattern, i.e. a fall in life stress, and two patients had experienced the same amount of life stress during the two periods. Thus,

Figure 4.10. Individual life change unit (LCU) totals for 42 attempted suicides 12–7 and 6–0 months before the attempt (from Katschnig, 1980*a*).

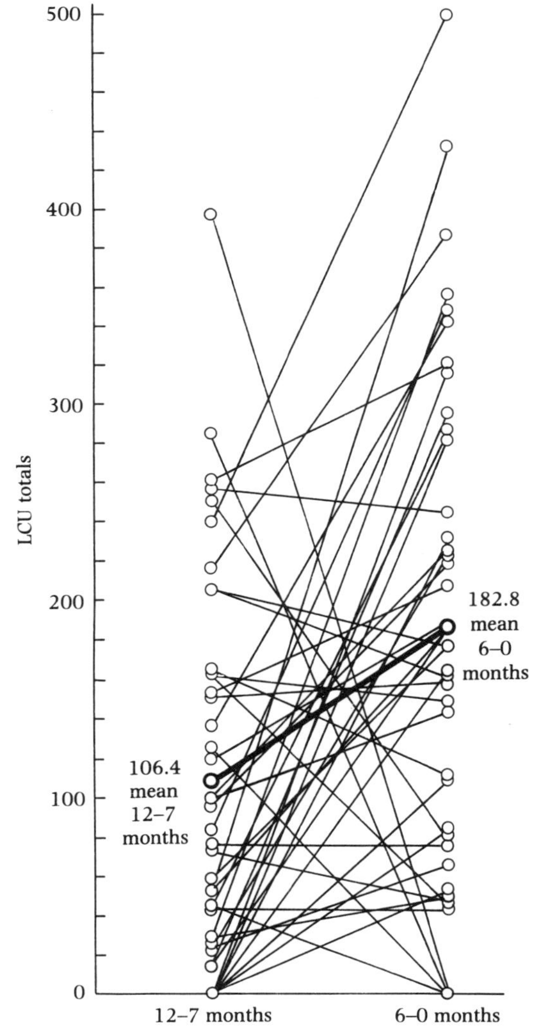

while on a group level there is a consistent correlation across different studies using different life event methodologies (i.e. a low group stress value goes together with a distant time period, a high group stress value is associated with the more proximal time period), individual patients need not necessarily show the identical picture of the course of stress when examined by different life event methods. Table 4.4 shows that only 73 of our 147 depressed patients, or less than 50%, follow an identical 'course' of stress over both methods and that more than 50% show discrepant patterns. Concordance as measured by the Kappa coefficient is therefore rather low (0·19).

These discrepancies between correlations on a group level and correlations on an individual level resemble the so-called 'ecological fallacy' first described by Robinson (1950) in research on voting behaviour: while on the level of the geographical district a correlation may exist between the percentage of votes a specific party obtains and a specific ecological characteristic of a constituency (e.g. the higher the proportion of blacks in a constituency the higher the number of votes for party A) it does not necessarily follow that individuals characterized by the variable used to describe the constituency are in fact responsible for the low or the high percentage of votes for a given party (in our example, if party A receives a higher number of votes in constituencies with high proportions of blacks it does not necessarily follow that the blacks have voted for this party). This

Table 4.4. *Comparison of individual 'course' of stress for 147 depressed patients for the two 6-month periods before admission*

	LEDS			
	More life events in proximal 6 months period	Same number of life events in both periods	More life events in distant 6 months period	Total
SRE				
More life changes in proximal 6 months period	48	27	23	98
Same number of life changes in both periods	10	9	5	24
More life changes in distant 6 months period	4	5	16	25
Total	62	41	44	147

Kappa = 0.19; $P < 0.01$

'ecological fallacy' can be generalized to include our example of a discrepancy between 'group correlations' and 'individual correlations'. Scheuch (1966) has coined the term 'group fallacy' for this phenomenon. A 'group correlation' does not exclude the possibility of an 'individual correlation', but by no means does the latter necessarily follow from the former. In fact, in our example the 'group correlation' does not correspond to a correlation on the level of the individual patient, i.e. while the total life event stress is low for the whole group in the distant time period and high in the proximal one, regardless of whether the LEDS or the SRE is applied, this is not true for the individual patients, who can have experienced an increase in life stress when one method is applied but a fall in life stress according to the other method. Thus the assumption that, regardless of which measurement procedure is applied, life stress increases before the outbreak of a disease is only true on an aggregate level. However, in studying the association between life stress and illness onset in individual patients the results obviously depend on the method chosen.

Comparing individual life events as elicited by the SRE and the LEDS

With this qualification in mind and given the increasing concern with studying the mechanisms of coping with life events (Parker & Brown, 1982; Ray, Lindop & Gibson, 1982), a concentration on single types of life events, in addition to using global scores, seems appropriate. It is,

Table 4.5. *Comparable SRE life changes and LEDS life events picked up by one of the methods or by both 6–0 months before admission (147 patients)*

	Picked up by			
	SRE	LEDS	Either SRE or LEDS	Both SRE and LEDS
Divorce/marital separation	9	9	17	1
Personal injury or illness	40	18	45	13
Marriage	1	3	3	1
Fired at work	11	12	17	6
Retirement	3	1	4	—
Pregnancy	3	5	6	2
Son or daugher leaving home	6	3	6	3
Outstanding personal achievement	3	1	4	—
Begin or end of school	2	—	2	—
Change in residence	10	5	12	3

Figure 4.11. Reliability study – Schedule of Recent Experience (SRE) (first trial). Mean numbers of life changes reported by 26 attempted suicides for the two 6-month periods preceding the attempt (SRE filled out immediately after attempt).

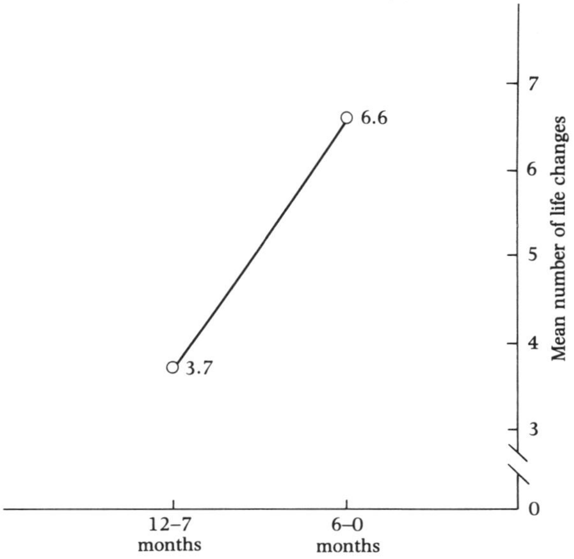

Figure 4.12. Reliability study – Schedule of Recent Experience (SRE) (second trial). Mean numbers of life changes reported by 26 attempted suicides for the two 6-month periods preceding the attempt (SRE filled out two weeks after attempt).

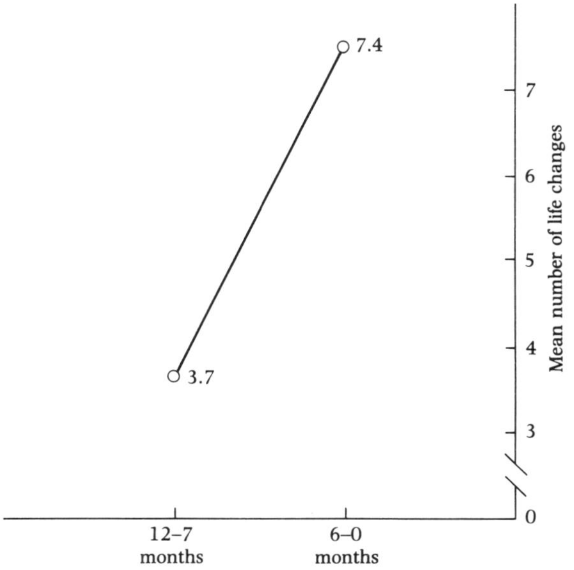

therefore, of some interest to analyse the cross-validity of the SRE and the LEDS not only on the level of the usual global stress measurement but also on the single life event level, i.e. to find out whether the SRE and the LEDS do in fact pick up the same individual life events for a given patient.

Such an exercise cannot be carried out easily because the differences between the two methods already extend to the types of life events included in each of them. When starting from the SRE, 10 life changes can be identified, for which it is easy to find clearcut corresponding life events in the LEDS. These events include the more stressful ones, such as divorce, pregnancy and retirement, which are also easier to define. The selection of these items has been based on their identical formulation in both instruments. Other life changes/life events may be more frequent but no precise correspondence can be established.

The results of this comparison are rather disappointing (Table 4.5): the proportions of identical life changes/life events picked up by both methods are very low, ranging from one in 17 for 'divorce/marital separation' to 3 in 6 for 'son or daughter leaving home'. The possible reason for these astonishing discrepancies (e.g. inexact dating of events in the SRE) will be discussed below.

The point about the 'group fallacy' made in the last section can be even more strikingly illustrated by data from the Edinburgh study (Katschnig, 1980*a*, *b*), which included a reliability study of the SRE. Two weeks after the SRE had been filled out, 26 of the 42 patients filled it out again for the same two 6-month periods preceding the attempted suicide. In Figures 4.11 and 4.12 the results for the two trials are presented, using as stress index the mean number of life events in each of the two 6-month periods.

Table 4.6. *Reliability study of the SRE. Life changes identified in the first and the second trial and those identified in both trials*

	Number of life changes in first trial (in parentheses: life changes identified in first trial only)	Number of life changes in second trial (in parentheses: life changes identified in second trial only)	Number of life changes identical in both trials
6–0 months before onset	173 (42)	193 (62)	131 (55.7% of 235)
7–12 months before onset	95 (41)	95 (41)	54 (39.7% of 136)

Again, the pictures are very similar to one another and to that for the whole group of 42 patients (Figure 4.10), showing an increase in life stress for the whole group. When the number of life changes elicited on both occasions was counted, the correlation coefficient amounted to 0·89 for the proximal and to 0·74 for the distant 6-month period, indicating that the same patient had made a roughly equal number of responses in the first and in the second trial. When, however, the data on individual life changes were analysed, it was found that for the proximal 6-month period only 131 of a total of 235 life changes elicited in both trials (55.7%) were identically reported on the first and the second occasion; for the distant 6-month period only 39.7% of all life changes were identical in both trials (Table 4.6). Thus, while the 'group picture' of an increase of life stress from the distant to the proximal 6-month period is identical on both occasions, it is obvious that *differently reported single life changes* are responsible for this rise on the two occasions of data collection in the reliability study. These results are in agreement with the postulation of a certain 'effort after meaning' in individuals suffering from psychological or somatic disorders (Brown, 1974), which implies a tendency for either 'over-reporting' or 'lowering the threshold of remembrance' for *any* life event. Retrospective data collection by self-rating questionnaires is obviously especially susceptible to mirroring this tendency of the individual, which may 'produce' an increase in life stress before the outbreak of a disease, or at least make such an increase more pronounced. The results of studies using such checklists become thus very questionable, especially if the analysis is also to be carried out on the single life event level.

Concluding remarks to the cross-validation study

We can conclude that the congruence of the two best-known instruments in life event research, the SRE and the LEDS, which appears so promising when aggregate data are used, becomes doubtful when global stress scores are compared for individual patients, and disappears completely when individual life events are examined by each method, or by one and the same method (the SRE) on different occasions in a reliability study. The two most plausible interpretations of this discrepancy are that the methods either measure different phenomena (which would have different implications for interpreting the data) or that the SRE – given its lower reliability on the level of the specific life change – simply produces random results.

Thus a serious obstacle stands in the way of replacing the more laborious, time-consuming technique of the LEDS, with the more economic one of the SRE. If life event stress in general does indeed cause or trigger a large number of diseases (Tennant & Andrews, 1976; Rahe & Arthur, 1978), and if it is accepted that we have to find out under which particular circumstances which types of life events act by which individual pathways to cause which specific diseases (Mechanic, 1974), the identification of concrete life events experienced by an individual will be of paramount importance in future research. Consequently, any discrepancy on the level of eliciting single life events constitutes serious grounds for hesitating before replacing one method with the other. In the following section a step by step comparison of the many differences between the SRE and the LEDS will be carried out in order to give some guidelines for a possible compromise between economical applicability and methodological accuracy.

A description of the differences between the SRE and the LEDS

The cross-validation study described above has not addressed itself to the question of which specific differences in the instruments themselves account for the incongruency, but has only demonstrated that findings based on the two methods do not agree, which in itself is a result which must be taken very seriously. Following the brief description of the SRE and the LEDS in the second part of this chapter and assuming that the reader can make himself better acquainted with the LEDS in the chapter by Brown & Harris (p. 107, this volume) the SRE and the LEDS methodology will now be contrasted in those aspects which may be relevant to the observed discrepancies (Tables 4.7 and 4.8).

Conceptual differences

A very basic difference between the two methods resides on the conceptual level. Whereas the authors of the SRE claim to measure the amount of 'readjustment' (Holmes & Rahe, 1967) necessary after a specific life event has occurred (and therefore not only include events which are commonly regarded as unpleasant, but also pleasant ones, which nevertheless require 'adjustment'), the authors of the LEDS explicitly aim at measuring the 'threat' which ensues after a more or less unpleasant life event has occurred (Brown, 1974). To what extent these different concepts influence the measurement procedure is difficult to judge. For the SRE this influence is confined to the realm of data analysis and interpretation, since the concept of 'readjustment' was only used for arriving at the 'predetermined' LCUs and the person who completes the SRE questionnaire is unaware of this. In the LEDS both the data-gathering procedure and the assignment of a score are directly influenced by the concept of 'threat'. Other methods use still other concepts for measuring life stress, such as the 'upsettingness' of an event (Paykel *et al.*, 1971).

Differences in the method of data collection

There are some important differences between the two methods in the process of data collection (Table 4.7). One of the most salient is that the SRE is usually used as a self-rating questionnaire, whereas the LEDS consists of a rather lengthy, semi-structured interview. This is a substantial difference, for it is very difficult in a self-rating questionnaire to reach uniformity without specific guidelines, whereas a trained interviewer can keep to the rules which have been laid down. The combination of a checklist and a self-rating method implies that it is left completely to the respondent to define a life event. While it is usually quite clear what 'marriage' or 'death of a spouse' means, events such as 'change in eating habits' or 'illness of a family member' may encompass a range of different experiences and one and the same event may be recorded by one patient and not by the other. The reverse may also occur: very different experiences of different patients may be entered in the same SRE rubric. In the LEDS it is the interviewer, who, after having acquired a thorough knowledge of the glossary and its definitions and after having collected the necessary information decides whether a specific occurrence should be counted as a life event or not.

A further difference is that, while data recording with the SRE consists of asking the proband to tick a box in the appropriate column, information

Table 4.7. *Differences between the SRE and the LEDS concerning the data collection procedure*

Aspects of data collection	SRE	LEDS
Method of data collection	Self-rating questionnaire	Interview
Who decides whether or not to include an event?	Respondent alone	Respondent and interviewer
Additional information necessary for stress rating?	No (predetermined value in life change unit list = 'consensus a priori')	Yes (for contextual threat rating, which is done by a team of raters = 'consensus a posteriori')
Data recording	In writing (usually a box is ticked)	In writing and by tape recording
Duration of data collection	Minutes	Hours
Is training of research worker necessary?	No	Yes
Costs of data collection	Low	High

elicited by the LEDS is both recorded in writing during the interview and on tape, the latter usually serving as a basis for later discussions with other experts about the ratings to be made. The LEDS interviewer can, therefore, always go back to the details of a specific life event while the SRE researcher only has a ticked box at his disposal. With the LEDS the information necessary to make the appropriate threat ratings (which largely depend on the circumstances of the life event) must be specifically collected by the interviewer for each life event (for the purpose of a 'consensus a posteriori' rating by the panel of raters); with the SRE, on the other hand, no extra effort is necessary in the data collection process to arrive at a threat rating, because predetermined standardized 'LCU' are used ('consensus a priori').

A number of differences touch on the economical applicability of the two methods. It is self-evident after what has been said that using the LEDS implies a training procedure as a necessary prerequisite, whereas the SRE can be used by any researcher who wishes to do so. Furthermore, whereas it takes only a few minutes to complete the SRE (which can even be used in a postal survey), the time needed to arrive at a reliable stress rating based on the LEDS is considerable: the interview itself may last several hours (depending on the number of life events reported by the subject), and the rating session which ensues requires the presence of several trained raters and may also be quite lengthy.

Of the differences discussed here, the self-rating procedure used with the SRE, in conjunction with the unclear definitions of life changes, is probably most important for the low reliability of this instrument on the level of the individual life change; it is also very probable that these methodological properties constitute an important source for the discrepancies between the SRE and the LEDS found in the cross-validation study. The amount of work necessary to collect *in detail* specific information characterizing the life event itself and the circumstances under which it has occurred, and the training necessary for collecting this information in a reliable way, make the LEDS an expensive technique as compared with the SRE. But complex phenomena must not be oversimplified in the measuring process and expensive data-collection procedures are indispensible in life event research.

Differences in precision/standardization of the measurement of life stress

Under this heading a number of important differences can be listed (Table 4.8) which may well also be at the root of the disappointing result of the cross-validation study (see also Brown, 1974; Hudgens, 1974). To begin with, the two methods cover different populations of life events. The SRE provides a fixed list of 42 life change events (some lists contain 'Christmas' as the 43rd life event which, according to Rahe (1978), had been put into a publication by mistake), whereas the LEDS has an extensive 'life event dictionary'; the typical life events therein, however, serve only as 'anchor' examples. In the LEDS it is thus possible to include life events which are not included in the dictionary but which, according to the general rules, qualify for inclusion. Our attempt at comparing the two methods on the level of individual life events (p. 88) was seriously hindered by the fact that few events qualified for a comparison at all, since they were regarded as an event in only one of the two methods or were so vaguely defined in the SRE that no corresponding event could be found in the LEDS. When

Table 4.8. *Differences between the SRE and the LEDS concerning the precision/standardization of measurement*

Aspects of the precision/ standardization of measurement	SRE	LEDS
Number of possible types of life events	Fixed	Open
Standardization of wording of question	Fully standardized (in writing)	Flexible
Are precise criteria formulated as to whether an event has to be included or excluded?	Not at all	Yes, precise criteria
Are the 'close' persons, whose life events have to be included, precisely defined?	No	Yes (focus rating)
Are acute events distinguished from chronic difficulties?	No	Yes
Are life events separated from symptoms?	No	Yes
Is it possible to make a rating about whether a life event is independent of the person concerned?	No	Yes
To which aspect of the life events do the rules of which stress measure to apply refer?	Only to type of life event	To type of life event plus context
Are subjectively experienced and objective stress separated?	No	Yes
Are immediate stress effects separated from long-term effects?	No	Yes
Are life events dated?	Only in broad time intervals	Precise date

analysing such differences and congruencies in life event coverage between different methods (e.g. Brugha *et al.*, 1985) it is important to take into consideration that verbal identity (e.g. 'serious illness or injury to a close relative') does not guarantee the identification of identical life events by different methods (see p. 95).

Many misunderstandings have arisen concerning the 'standardization' of data collection in the two instruments. Usually the SRE is regarded as a standardized instrument not only as far as the predetermined LCUs are concerned, but also with respect to data collection, since the life change list of the SRE can be seen as a standardized 'stimulus' for a respondent. Every respondent is confronted with the same written words (e.g. 'Did you experience a change in sleeping habits?'). The LEDS, on the other hand, provides only an interview guideline and leaves it more or less to the interviewer to formulate his questions. Thus in the LEDS the verbal 'stimulus' itself is not standardized. When considering the definitions of single life events, however, it has to be restated that the meaning of many of the 'standard' formulations of the SRE is completely open, and it is left to the respondent to decide which kind of experience he subsumes under a specific item in the SRE. The LEDS, on the other hand, provides full definitions and elaborate rules for deciding which event has to be included and which not. In fact, therefore, it is the LEDS which has a standardized data collection procedure, and not the SRE.

The rules for inclusion or exclusion of events in the LEDS contain definitions of the 'close' persons whose life events qualify for inclusion. The LEDS provides, e.g., clear rules as to which persons have to be regarded as 'family or household members' and which do not. In the SRE, on the other hand, one is simply required to remember the 'illness of a family member', which leaves it completely to the respondent to include or exclude a myocardial infarction of, say, a distant cousin or an uncle.

The LEDS makes a number of differentiations bearing on the problem of precision of measurement which are neglected in the SRE. The first concerns the 'event' or 'change' character of the occurrence. In the SRE it is difficult to decide for some so-called life 'changes' whether they represent acute events or long-standing difficulties (e.g. 'difficulties with parents-in-law' may have developed recently or may have existed for many years). In contrast, the LEDS separates acute events from chronic difficulties and provides lengthy rules and a separate 'difficulty dictionary' for correctly identifying such chronic difficulties. Secondly, the SRE includes a number of items which may really mirror psychiatric symptomatology rather than an objective change in the person's life (e.g. 'change in sleeping habits', 'change in eating habits'). In contrast, the LEDS makes a clearcut distinction between life events and possible symptoms. Furthermore, the LEDS provides the possibility to distinguish between those life events which may already be a consequence of an ongoing but subclinical disease or which might have been brought about by the person himself, and those life events which are in fact independent of the person and his disease. If the research aim is aetiological, this distinction is, of course, crucial. The SRE does not provide this possibility.

As far as the standardization of the process of assigning a stress measure to a single life event is concerned, both methods – the SRE and the LEDS – provide standardized procedures. The predetermined stress measure of the SRE can simply be taken from the SRRS which contains the LCUs established by Holmes & Rahe (1967) from the judgments of a 'sample of convenience'. In the SRE 'death of spouse' always receives an LCU value of 100, 'change to different line of work' always has 36 LCUs. In the LEDS the procedure of assigning a stress value (which is called 'contextual threat rating') to life events is also standardized. The rules are laid down in a manual which the interviewer must have in mind when he asks for additional information in order to clarify the circumstances under which the life event has occurred. The threat rating of the LEDS is not only dependent on the type of life event, as in the SRE, but also on the context in which a person finds himself when the life event occurs. This contextual threat rating has a high reliability (Tennant *et al.*, 1979; Katschnig *et al.*, 1981; Parry *et al.*, 1981).

In addition to giving this objective 'contextual threat rating' according to rules laid down in the glossary, the LEDS allows for a separate rating of the subjectively experienced stress as the respondent recalls it ('subjective threat'). While there is, therefore, a neat separation between 'objectivity' and 'subjectivity' in the LEDS, the SRE in fact confounds both aspects: relying on the predetermined standardized LCUs does not guarantee that subjectivity is excluded, as it is left entirely to the respondent to decide which events to tick on the self-rating questionnaire. Thus, given the 'effort after meaning' in sick persons, the patient's subjective retrospective view of the causes of his illness goes into the final stress score without any control. It is probable that for sick persons the SRE just serves as a stimulus to tick more numbers of boxes than healthy persons would do.

A further difference between the SRE and the LEDS concerns the distinction between 'short-term' and 'long-term' threat, (i.e. the probable short-term or long-term consequences of the event), which is made by the LEDS but not by the SRE. Katschnig (1980*a*) could demonstrate that events which, according to the rules of the LEDS, have only short-term threat effects do not show an increase before an attempted suicide, while long-term threat events do.

The two final characteristics distinguishing the SRE from the LEDS refer to the ways that indices of stressfulness are related to time intervals (see also the next section of this paper). While the LEDS asks for the exact dating of an event, the SRE – mainly because it is a self-rating procedure – can only provide broad time intervals within which the occurrence of an event can be recorded. Take, for example, two life events which occurred in the 12 months before data collection: these two events may have occurred shortly after one another in the middle of the 12-month period (i.e. the first at the end of the distant 6-month period and the second at the beginning of the proximal 6-month period) or nearly one year from each other (i.e. the first at the beginning of the distant 6-month period, and the second at the end of the proximal 6-month period). The SRE, providing just two 6-month periods would give the same stress indices for both examples and no detailed analysis would be possible. The exact time relationship between life stress and illness onset can therefore only be analysed by using the LEDS with its possibility of exactly dating the occurrence of events.

Differences in the methods of data analysis

Here two issues have to be distinguished: first, the way in which global stress indices for a time interval are calculated once all information about the individual life events has been collected, and secondly, the way in which the magnitude of the effects that life events may have on the probability of an illness onset is determined.

Concerning the calculation of a 'stress index' for a given time interval two principal models have been used: the additive and the threshold model. In the additive model (usually used in conjunction with the SRE) a quantitative measure is calculated for each patient which is dependent in one way or another on the number of life events in the time interval; it usually consists of either a total count of life events in a given time interval or of the sum of stress values assigned to each life event (such as the LCUs). For the whole group of probands under study a mean value of these total counts or sums is calculated and then used for further analyses.

The second model, the threshold model, implies a yes/no approach. For each person it is determined whether or not, according to rules laid down, this person has to be regarded as 'under stress', usually using a formulation such as 'experienced at least one life event (of a certain severity) in a given time interval'. This approach is frequently used in conjunction with the LEDS.

However, neither of these approaches is obligatory for either the LEDS or the SRE. In the cross-validation study presented above, both approaches were used with both methods, and on a group level the results were very similar regardless of which method of data analysis was used (see Figures 4.6 to 4.9). Correlations on the level of the individual patient, while being on the whole rather modest, depended on the type of model used for data analysis, with the additive model showing higher correlations than the threshold model. One must conclude, therefore, that it does in fact matter which type of stress index is calculated for a time interval, since additive and threshold analyses do not necessarily identify the same individuals as being under stress. This means that, although in a given group of persons – regardless of which model of data analysis is chosen – a similar proportion may prove to have experienced life stress, it will be different persons who contribute to the group picture, depending on which model of data analysis is employed. If more detailed analyses are carried out on subpopulations of the persons under stress, quite different variables may therefore prove to be associated with the outbreak of a disease according to which data analysis model is used.

In calculating the *magnitude* of the effect of life stress in triggering an illness onset, many different approaches have been used. At the simplest level are graphs showing a rise in life stress in the sick population and a lack of such a rise in the control group (see, e.g., Brown & Birley, 1970; Figure 4.3 in this chapter). Comparing rates and calculating probabilities in order to exclude chance differences represents an advance over this first approach (e.g. Paykel *et al.*, 1969; Bebbington, Tennant & Hurry, 1981). More sophisticated techniques include the calculation of the so-called 'brought forward time' (Brown, Harris & Peto, 1973), or of 'relative risk' (Paykel, 1974), and the application of log-linear techniques of analysis (Tennant & Bebbington, 1978). The latter group of authors have demonstrated that applying different techniques of analysis to the same set of data yields different results, and Everitt & Smith (1979), who have further elaborated on this issue, conclude that at this stage of development of data analysis techniques and their theory, no rational basis is available for regarding one data analysis technique as superior to the other.

Concluding remarks concerning differences between the SRE and the LEDS

Probably most of the differences described here share responsibility for the lack of agreement found between the two methods, although the magnitude of their relative contribution to the discrepancies found cannot easily be estimated. Some of these features are intrinsic to each of the two approaches (such as the predetermined stress values for the checklist approach and the 'consensus a posteriori' threat ratings of the LEDS). Others, such as the presentation of a checklist as a self-rating scale, are optional, although it is inherent in the 'cheap' checklist approach not to carry out an interview. Nevertheless, the 'checklist' may also be read out to the proband and it is also possible to collect some additional information at an interview on the circumstances of life events included in a standard checklist. Such a compromise method has been developed by Paykel (1983). Finally, it has to be stressed that specific data analysis techniques are not necessarily restricted to either the LEDS or the SRE, although data analysis techniques should be kept in mind as a possible source of discrepancy when different studies are compared.

A taxonomy of measuring the life stress of a single life event

Regardless of how information is elicited and how it is finally processed, the underlying concept of how the stressfulness of a single life event should be assessed constitutes a fundamental difference between different life event methods. I would like to propose a taxonomy putting four different levels of measurement of the stressfulness of a single life event into a hierarchical relationship, relating these four levels with four basic assumptions about the stressfulness of life events (see Figure 4.13).

Level 1: All life events are regarded as being equally stressful

Life event methods which use the total number of life events experienced by a person over a given time period as a stress measure obviously assume that all life events are equally stressful. The first studies employing the SRE (Rahe *et al.*, 1964), the early studies of the London group (Brown & Birley, 1970) and some studies by Paykel *et al.* (1969, 1975; see Figure 4.4) have used this approach.

Level 2: Different weights are given to different types of life events

The introduction of LCUs by Holmes & Rahe (1967) marks the beginning of a new approach whereby different weights are given to life events according to the assumed differences in their stressfulness. Such life event scales have been published by Paykel *et al.* (1971), Cochrane & Robertson (1973), Tennant & Andrews (1976), Dohrenwend *et al.* (1978) and others.

Level 3: Taking the context into account

While it obviously makes sense to regard 'death of spouse' and 'change in eating habits' as being different in stressfulness, it also makes sense to regard the same kind of life event as variably stressful according to the circumstances in which it occurs. The birth of a child to a happily married woman in good financial circumstances can obviously be regarded as being less stressful than the birth of a child to an unmarried and unemployed woman who is solely responsible for bringing up the child. The LEDS works on this more differentiated level of measurement, i.e. it provides rules for assessing the level of stressfulness of the same type of life event depending on the different contexts in which it has occurred.

Level 4: Subjectively experienced life stress

To measure the amount of stress which is actually experienced by a person at a time when a life event occurs would be the most appropriate way of

Figure 4.13. Measuring the stressfulness of a single event on different levels of differentiation for 'birth of a child' and 'divorce' (Size of column corresponds to amount of stress)

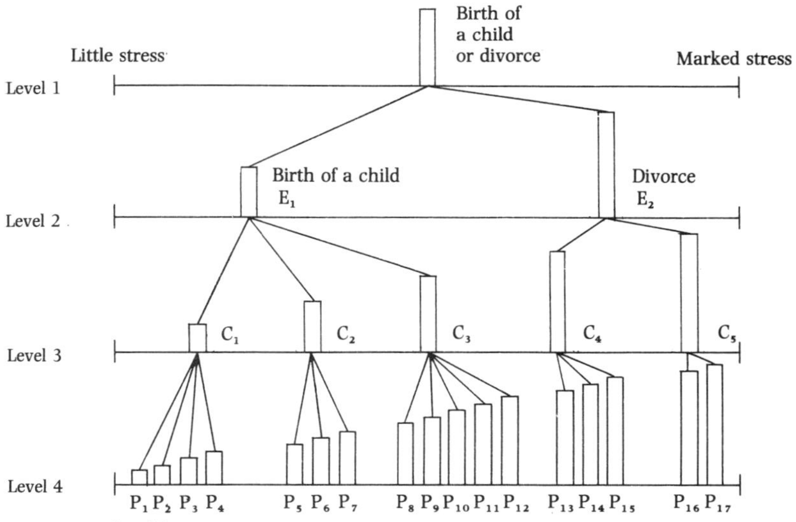

Level 1
Undifferentiated: stress measure corresponds to mean over types of events (E_1, E_2), contexts (C_1–C_5) and subjective experiences of stress (P_1–P_{17})

Level 2
Differentiated according to type of event (E_1, E_2): stress measure corresponds to mean over contexts and subjective experiences of stress (e.g. E_1 = mean over contexts C_1–C_3 and subjective experiences of stress P_1–P_{12})

Level 3
Differentiated according to context (C_1–C_5): stress measure corresponds to mean over subjective experiences of stress (e.g. C_1 = mean over subjective experiences of stress P_1–P_4)

Level 4
Differentiated according to subjective experiences of stress of each person (P_1–P_{17})

studying the possible causal role played by stressful life events in the development of diseases. However, whether or not life stress experienced at a specific time in the past can be reliably reported retrospectively is a highly controversial issue (Brown, 1974). Desirable as such a 'subjective' stress measure may be, it is subject to all kinds of retrospective distortions, and can therefore not be regarded as useful.

The hypothesis behind this 'four-level model' is that measurements on a less differentiated level constitute 'mean values' of the measurements on a more differentiated level. It is clear that a level 1 measurement is the result of averaging out all level 2 measurements. The hypothesis also implies that level 2 measurements (i.e. regarding different *types* of life events as being different in their stressfulness) can be regarded as being averages of level 3 contextual stress ratings which can be different for the same life event if it occurs in different contexts. For example, while 'gain of a new family member' has a predetermined LCU score of 39 in the SRE, 'birth of a child' may, according to the LEDS, receive stress ratings ranging from 1 (highest) to 4 (lowest). It can therefore be hypothesized that those life changes having high predetermined LCU scores in the SRE also have high average contextual threat ratings in the LEDS, while those life events which have low predetermined LCU scores in the SRE have low average contextual threat ratings in the LEDS. The general hypothesis also refers

Table 4.9. *Average short-term threat rating for specific life events (LEDS) and corresponding LCUs (SRE) (number of life events/life changes in parentheses)*

	LEDS Mean short-term threat rating[a]	SRE LCUs[b]
Divorce/marital separation (19)	1.90	73
Personal injury or illness (64)	1.75	53
Marriage (6)	3.50	50
Fired at work (26)	2.42	47
Retirement (8)	3.38	45
Pregnancy (10)	2.30	40
Son or daughter leaving home (6)	3.00	29
Outstanding personal achievement (2)	4.00	28
Begin or end school (1)	4.00	26
Change of residence (21)	3.38	20

[a] Low value = marked threat; high value = little threat.
[b] Low value = little stress; high value = marked stress.
Spearman rank correlation coefficient = -0.71; $P < 0.05$

to the relationship between levels 3 and 4, i.e. to subjectively experienced life stress. It implies that the contextual threat rating for a given life event under given circumstances is the average of the amount of subjective stress experienced by different subjects in the same situation.

In the cross-validation study of the SRE and the LEDS described above data are available for testing this hypothesis for the relationship between levels 2 and 3. For this purpose the 10 life changes/life events which are comparable in the two methods were chosen (see Table 4.5). For these life changes/life events two series of values were obtained. First, the predetermined LCUs of the SRRS (Holmes & Rahe, 1967); secondly, medium threat ratings of the LEDS for events picked up with the LEDS. Divorce/marital separation has thus a mean threat value of 1.90 in the 19 cases where this event was recorded. The corresponding LCU score is 73 (Table 4.9). In both instances this means a rather high stress value. The calculation of the Spearman rank correlation coefficient shows a high concordance between these two series of measurements ($r = -0.71$, $P < 0.05$; the negative value of r is simply a consequence of the different scoring systems). These data obviously support the hypothesis of the stress values on level 2 being average values of contextual threat ratings on level 3. This result implies that the rules of the LEDS, laid down by Brown and his colleagues on the basis of 'commonsense', are in fact anchored in a general 'commonsense' which is mirrored in the average LCUs derived by Holmes & Rahe (1967) for their SRRS.

Conclusion

The starting point for the reflections and analyses presented in this chapter on life event methodology was an unusual one: the striking similarities of results of different life event studies (see, e.g., Figures 4.3 to 4.5), most of which arrive at the conclusion that life event stress does contribute, though to a variable degree, to the onset of such different diseases as myocardial infarction, inguinal hernia, depression or schizophrenia. This is in contrast with the usual starting point for methodological considerations, which is normally the incongruity between such studies rather than a uniformity between results obtained in different studies addressing themselves to the same problem.

In comparing and contrasting the two main types of life event methods, the SRE and the LEDS, it has become apparent that life event methods do in fact differ from one another in many respects and that 'similar' results obtained with different methods are deceptive. It was shown that it is not possible to dispense with the detailed collection of information on life events and their context. It would therefore be wise to refrain from continuing to use self-rating checklists with predetermined life stress values. If nothing else, the differences and incongruencies between the two main life event methods described in this chapter should, at least, make future research workers more cautious when interpreting their life event data and trying to arrive at generalizations.

References

Bebbington, P. E., Tennant, C. & Hurry, J. (1981). Adversity and the nature of psychiatric disorder in the community. *Journal of Affective Disorders*, **3**, 345–66.

Bebbington, P. E., Tennant, C., Sturt, E. & Hurry, J. (1984). The domain of life events: a comparison of two techniques of description. *Psychological Medicine*, **14**, 219–22.

Brown, G. W. (1974). Meaning, measurement and stress of life events. In *Stressful life events: their nature and effects*, ed. B. S. Dohrenwend & B. P. Dohrenwend, pp. 217–43. New York: John Wiley.

Brown, G. W. & Birley, J. L. T. (1970). Social precipitants of severe psychiatric disorders. In *Psychiatric epidemiology*, ed. E. H. Hare & J. K. Wing, pp. 321–5. London: Oxford University Press.

Brown, G. W. & Harris, T. (1978). *Social origins of depression*. London: Tavistock Publications.

Brown, G. W., Harris, T. O. & Peto, J. (1973). Life events and psychiatric disorders. Part 2. Nature of causal link. *Psychological Medicine*, **2**, 159–76.

Brugha, T., Bebbington, P., Tennant, C. & Hurry, J. (1985). The list of threatening experiences: a subset of 12 life event categories with considerable long-term contextual threat. *Psychological Medicine*, **15**, 189–94.

Cochrane, R. & Robertson, A. (1973). The life events inventory: a measure of the relative severity of psycho-social stressors. *Journal of Psychosomatic Research*, **17**, 135–9.

Dohrenwend, B. S. & Dohrenwend, B. P. (1981). *Stressful life events and their contexts*. New York: Prodist.

Dohrenwend, B. S., Krasnoff, L., Askenasy, A. R. & Dohrenwend, B. P. (1978). Exemplification of a method for scaling life events: the PERI life events scale. *Journal of Health and Social Behavior*, **19**, 205–29.

Everitt, B. S. & Smith, A. M. R. (1979). Interactions in contingency tables: a brief discussion of alternative definitions. *Psychological Medicine*, **9**, 581–3.

Holmes, Th. H. & Rahe, R. H. (1967). The Social Readjustment Rating Scale. *Journal of Psychosomatic Research*, **11**, 213–18.

Hudgens, R. W. (1974). Personal catastrophe and depression: a consideration of the subject with respect to medically ill adolescents, and a requiem for retrospective life-event studies. In *Stressful life events: their nature and effects*, ed. B. S. Dohrenwend & B. P. Dohrenwend, pp. 119–34. New York: John Wiley.

Kasl, S. V., Gore, S. & Cobb, S. (1975). The experience of losing a job: reported changes in health symptoms and illness behaviour. *Psychosomatic Medicine*, **37**, 106–22.

Katschnig, H. (1980*a*). Lebensverändernde Ereignisse als Ursache psychischer Krankheiten – Eine Kritik des globalen Ansatzes in der Life-Event-Forschung. In *Sozialer*

Streß und psychische Erkrankung – Lebensverändernde Ereignisse als Ursache seelischer Störungen?, ed. H. Katschnig, pp. 3–93. München, Wien & Baltimore: Urban & Schwarzenberg.

Katschnig, H. (1980*b*). Measuring life stress: a comparison of two methods. In *The suicide syndrome*, ed. R. Farmer & S. Hirsch, pp. 116–23. London: Croom Helm.

Katschnig, H., Brandl-Nebehay, A., Fuchs-Robetin, G., Seelig, P., Eichberger, G., Strobl, R. & Sint, P. P. (1981). *Lebensverändernde Ereignisse, psychosoziale Dispositionen und depressive Verstimmungszustände*. Wien: Psychiatrische Universitätsklinik.

Katschnig, H. & Fuchs-Robetin, G. (1984). *Methodenkritische Untersuchung zur Erfassung von krankheitsrelevantem sozialem Stress*. Wien: Psychiatrische Universitätsklinik.

Lindemann, E. (1944). The symptomatology and management of acute grief. *American Journal of Psychiatry*, **101**, 141–8.

Mechanic, D. (1974). Discussion of research programs on relations between stressful life events and episodes of physical illness. In *Stressful life events: their nature and effects*, ed. B. S. Dohrenwend & B. P. Dohrenwend, pp. 87–97. New York: John Wiley.

Mendels, J. & Weinstein, N. (1972). The schedule of recent experiences: a reliability study. *Psychosomatic Medicine*, **34**, 527–31.

Parker, G. B. & Brown, L. B. (1982). Coping behaviors that mediate between life events and depression. *Archives of General Psychiatry*, **39**, 1386–91.

Parry, G., Shapiro, D. A. & Davies, L. (1981). Reliability of life-event ratings: an independent replication. *British Journal of Clinical Psychology*, **20**, 133–4.

Paykel, E. S. (1974). Recent life events and clinical depression. In *Life stress and illness*, ed. E. K. Gunderson & R. H. Rahe, pp. 134–63. Springfield, Illinois: Charles Thomas.

Paykel, E. S. (1983). Methodological aspects of life event research. *Journal of Psychosomatic Research*, **27**, 341–52.

Paykel, E. S., Myers, J. K., Dienelt, M. N., Klerman, G. L., Lindenthal, J. J. & Pepper, M. P. (1969). Life events and depression. A controlled study. *Archives of General Psychiatry*, **21**, 753–60.

Paykel, E. S., Prusoff, B. A. & Myers, J. K. (1975). Suicide attempts and recent life events. *Archives of General Psychiatry*, **32**, 327–33.

Paykel, E. S., Prusoff, B. A. & Uhlenhuth, E. H. (1971). Scaling of life events. *Archives of General Psychiatry*, **25**, 340–7.

Rahe, R. H. (1969). Multi-cultural correlations of life change scaling: America, Japan, Denmark and Sweden. *Journal of Psychosomatic Research*, **13**, 191–5.

Rahe, R. H. (1978). Life change measurement clarification. *Psychosomatic Medicine*, **40**, 95–7.

Rahe, R. H. & Arthur, J. (1978). Life change and illness studies: past history and future. *Journal of Human Stress*, **4**, 3–15.

Rahe, R. H., Meyer, M., Smith, M., Kjaer, G. & Holmes, T. H. (1964). Social stress and illness onset. *Journal of Psychosomatic Research*, **8**, 35–44.

Ray, C., Lindop, J. & Gibson, S. (1982). The concept of coping. *Psychological Medicine*, **12**,385–95.

Robinson, W. S. (1950). Ecological correlation and behaviour of individuals. *American Social Review*, **14**, 351–7.

Scheuch, E. K. (1966). Cross-national comparisons using aggregate data. In *Comparing nations: the use of quantitative data in cross-national research*, ed. S. Rokkan & R. Merritt, pp. 131–67. New Haven: Yale University Press.

Schless, A., Schwartz, L., Goetz, Ch. & Mendels, J.(1974). How depressives view the significance of life events. *British Journal of Psychiatry*, **125**, 406–10.

Shrout, P. E. (1981). Scaling of stressful life events. In *Stressful life events and their contents*, ed. B. S. Dohrenwend & B. P. Dohrenwend, pp. 29–47. New York: John Wiley.

Steele, G. P., Henderson, S. & Duncan-Jones, P. (1980). The reliability of reporting adverse experiences. *Psychological Medicine*, **10**, 301–6.

Tennant, C. & Andrews, G. (1976). A scale to measure the stress of life events. *Australian and New Zealand Journal of Psychiatry*, **10**, 27–32.

Tennant, C. & Bebbington, P. (1978). The social causation of depression: a critique of the work of Brown and his colleagues. *Psychological Medicine*, **8**, 565–75.

Tennant, C., Smith, A., Bebbington, P. & Hurry, J. (1979). The contextual threat of life events: the concept and its reliability. *Psychological Medicine*, **9**, 525–8.

Theorell, T. & Rahe, R. H. (1971). Psychological factors and myocardial infarction – I. An inpatient study in Sweden. *Journal of Psychosomatic Research*, **15**, 25–31.

5

Establishing causal links: the Bedford College studies of depression

G. W. BROWN & T. HARRIS

Introduction

We have restricted this review to only part of the literature on life events and depression in the hope that this would enable us to review present knowledge in some depth and to convey certain principles by which it can be judged. We have limited ourselves to issues that have arisen following the publication of the first report of the Camberwell study of depression in 1975 (Brown, Ní Bhrolcháin & Harris, 1975) and the full account of the patient and the two community studies in 1978 (Brown & Harris, 1978*a*). Many of the issues arose out of a series of papers stemming from an enquiry carried out in 1979 of the same Camberwell population by members of the Medical Research Council (MRC) Social Psychiatry Unit. If the somewhat emotive term 'controversy' is to be used, it is most relevant for the work of this team as we differ markedly from it on many points of substance, theory and method. (For an introduction, see Bebbington, Tennant & Hurry, 1981*b*).

We are fortunate that over the last decade we have trained members of many research centres in our original measures – both in the United Kingdom and abroad and it is now possible to begin to draw upon the results of their research. On a number of key issues there are already six or more independent replications of the original research. We believe that this increasing use of the London Life Event and Difficulty Schedule (LEDS) has resulted not only from the potential importance of the original findings but also from the widespread frustration with the persistent and apparently irredeemable shortcomings of the main alternative approach based on the use of questionnaires – that is, in essence, asking the respondent rather than the investigator to carry out the job of measurement. As realisation grew that the sums of money saved by the use of easily completed questionnaires rather than the complex and more time-consuming interviewer-based measures was more than outweighed by conflicting and non-cumulative findings, some reaction was inevitable.

Fortunately the investment in interviewer-based measures has led to cumulative results. So much so that certain findings already appear reasonably secure. None-the-less, difficulties have arisen, albeit of a different kind: this in itself should not be surprising as the successive discovery and mastery of problems is at the heart of effective scientific activity – one might say its driving force. Even the most ill-judged controversy may lead to new insights, perhaps about issues neither 'side' had in mind at the start. But even given the possible bonus of serendipitous insights there are certain lessons to be learnt from recent disputes. In particular it would have been helpful to have had greater recognition of two points. First, even with large population samples it is inevitable that relatively few persons will be found to develop an onset of a definite affective disorder within a period of, say, one year. Given also that the causal processes reflected in the aetiology of affective disorders are of considerable subtlety, quite discrepant results may emerge with only small changes in research practice. If there is a wish to see whether work can be replicated, the original procedures need to be closely followed – which in no way rules out doing something different as well, although this is often overlooked. For example, Bebbington and his colleagues claim that, in spite of using the same, LEDS, instrument, they obtained quite different results concerning the role of life events in the onset of depression among *patients* (Bebbington *et al.*, 1981*b*). Yet they conclude this despite changing the original approach in certain critical ways (such as taking a shorter period before onset and excluding certain types of event) which, in terms of the results of the original enquiry, would be bound greatly to reduce the size of the aetiological effect (Brown & Harris, 1982*b*). Such practice is bound to create confusion. We do not argue here for slavish repetition: only that innovation should go with a close regard to past practice so that at every stage of research the new can be related to the old. While if a quite disparate approach should *repeat* a finding then this would tend to add to our confidence about the original result; failure to replicate is more ambiguous. It is essential to be able to argue that the original procedures have been closely followed or, if changes have been made, that these are carefully documented and a case made why they should not have influenced chances of repeating the original result. (The logic of this kind of procedure has been developed in discussions of 'triangulation' and construct validity (Cook & Campbell, 1979)). Moreover, it should always be borne in mind that if changes in sampling or design have resulted in changes in the presence of the factors of underlying causal importance the failure to replicate may actually provide *support* for the original results.

But replication requires an initial set of results to be replicated and it may be useful to begin by summarizing the core results of the original enquiry. The aetiological model of depression developed in Camberwell suggests that certain *provoking agents* occurring currently determine when an episode of depression takes place. Most significant are *severe* events involving an important loss or disappointment, if this is understood to encompass not only loss of a person but loss of a role or even an idea (Brown & Harris, 1978*a*). (Loss in the sense of bereavement formed only a small minority of events associated with onset of depression – at least among women in urban settings.) A second, somewhat less important, provoking agent concerns ongoing major difficulties such as might be brought about by overcrowded and poor housing or by a husband who drinks heavily.

At a conservative estimate the original study in 1975 concluded that such provoking agents probably bring about 60% of all episodes of depression among psychiatric patients (excluding certain groups such as those with bipolar disorder and depression secondary to other conditions) and about 80 to 90% of episodes among women developing depression in the general population (Brown & Harris, 1978*a*). However, the chance of such experience bringing about depression is greatly influenced by the presence of *vulnerability factors*, such as lack of social support. The middle arrow in the diagram represents the fact that these factors increase risk only in the presence of the provoking agent, but have little or no impact without them.

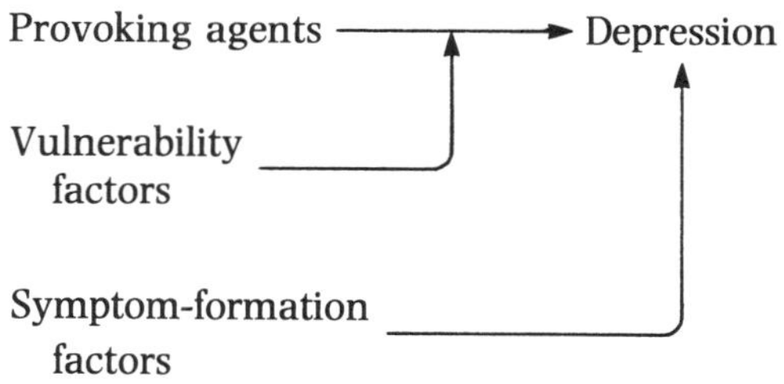

We concluded that lack of an intimate tie with a husband, having three or more children under the age of 14 living at home, and loss of a mother before the age of 11 act as vulnerability factors for women – that is, that risk of depression is increased in their presence once a provoking agent occurs (Brown & Harris, 1978*a*: 181). There was also some suggestion that lack of employment may also play this role under certain circumstances.

The third, symptom-formation, factor in the model is different from the others in that rather than increasing the risk of depression, it influences the form once it occurs – in terms, for instance, of the degree to which it is 'psychotic' rather than 'neurotic', more anxious or without anxiety. The relevant experience leading to such an effect apparently may occur at any point in a person's life – but so far early experience of loss and type of loss have been heavily implicated.

Causal model and theory

Our approach has been predicated on certain assumptions about the most profitable way to proceed in aetiological research and it may be helpful to discuss these. There are two tasks: the development of a model that reflects causal processes, and the building of theory to understand the model. Neither can possibly be accomplished in the short term and the two must go hand in hand and influence each other. However, at any one point in time it is possible to distinguish model and theory and it is highly desirable that this is done. The initial task must be to reflect possible causal processes in a model that has some broadly recognised claim to validity. For this to be done much initial work must be devoted to the development of reliable and valid measures so that a good case can be made for the presence of causal links. Measures should be as reliable as possible because it is extremely difficult to obtain replicable results, or indeed results worthy of attempts to replicate, without this. The measures, however, have only to be valid in one sense: measurement artefacts that may create causal links where none in fact exist must be ruled out. But since the main task is to establish the presence of causal processes that are worth pursuing in a series of enquiries, measures do not have to be totally valid in the other sense of reflecting *exactly* those theoretical processes which they name; it is quite possible that once a causal process has been established as worth pursuing, subsequent refinement of understanding will show that what was being measured was rather different from what was originally thought to have been measured, but the causal link is none-the-less still confirmed. Indeed a factor can be included in a model without the investigator having much idea of what it is reflecting in a theoretical sense: it is enough that he can rule out that the apparent causal link involved is not due to some measurement artefact. This is not to say that the use of crude atheoretical measures in a model is desirable – simply that it may be inevitable and in time can lead to better things. Much will depend on the insights of the investigator, what has already been done in the field, the resources available for the time-consuming business of developing new measures and the degree of experience and skill so far developed as a research worker. However, no matter how sensitive the measures, it will be wise to assume that in all likelihood they are somewhat distant indicators of what is really of significance. There is in any case bound to be a 'gap' between indicator and theoretical concept in the sense that few indicators can be expected to reflect exactly what the investigator thinks is of importance in a theoretical sense. There will therefore be two kinds of slippage between the indicators, the model and, if we may use the term, reality. At one extreme the investigator may have little confidence in his idea of what the indicator represents and at the other, even if he feels reasonably clear, he should never readily assume that what he considers to be theoretically relevant is what is really producing changes in the dependent variable.

There are two ways forward. The investigator can assume the indicator has a certain theoretical significance and seek to gain support for this view *within* the analysis of the data set incorporating the indicator. The second option is to seek to improve measures in the light of empirical findings and theoretical insights. The latter is likely to prove a long road involving much approximation and trial and error; and it is possible that at any one point in time in a programme of research, impressive results may be obtained, in the sense of predictive power and control, without fully settling what the theoretical significance of the indicators may be.

The research on life events and depression is still at quite an early point in this second process: we are only beginning to emerge from the stage where there was fundamental disagreement about whether or not events play a core role in the aetiology of serious depressive illness. Much of this controversy originally centred on shortcomings in the measurement of events. One of the most well-known sceptical articles came from the St Louis group of research workers (Hudgens, Morrison & Barchaa, 1967; Hudgens, Robins & Delong, 1970). A detailed recent review concludes that even in the instance of this flawed research that 'the hypothesis that severely unpleasant life events, particularly events involving loss, are a cause of depression has not been refuted' (Finlay-Jones, 1981). By and large we assume in this review a good case has now been made for the presence of such a causal link and most of our concern will be with problems arising from the model and associated theory once this basic link is accepted. Throughout what follows it is essential to distinguish issues concerning the model itself (whether certain indicators of lack of support act as vulnerability factors) from issues concerning the theoretical significance of particular links (whether the impact of lack of support is through, say, lack of opportunity to work because of the grief consequent upon a loss, or because of feelings of low self-worth which derive from unsuccessful ongoing relationships).

Since the development of the original model of depressive disorder, members of our team have not only undertaken investigations which can provide replications but have also pushed the model into new areas, both conceptually and geographically. We shall refer to some of these new departures in the course of this review since they confer certain new insights: for example, we have become sharply aware of how geography and history seem to change the model without necessarily changing the theory. It may be helpful here to briefly outline what these new departures have been. First, geographically we now have experience of two different islands in the Outer Hebrides, of an outer London borough (Walthamstow) and two further inner London boroughs, Islington and the Regents Park section of Camden. (We do not touch here on influences from research by others whom we have trained and who have sent us feedback from places as far afield as Kenya and Italy.) This has made us aware of the differences not only in the quantity but also the quality of provoking agents in different places. In terms of history we have witnessed changes even within the same borough, not only in provoking agents (housing is better, unemployment is worse than when we started research) but also in terms of social provisions affecting our vulnerability factors (by and large there are more nursery school places than in the late 1960s and a greater availability of easy forms of contraception, both of which would have bearing on the prevalence and implications of having three or more children under 14 at home).

Even more enlightening have been new conceptual developments. First, we have embarked on a prospective study which allows us greater confidence that measures of vulnerability factors such as intimacy are not contaminated by the subsequent development of depression. For this we have developed a range of new measures of social support including some for our pivotal intervening variable 'self-esteem'. Second, in a study specifically focusing upon differences in the dependent variable, between anxiety and depression without anxiety, we have been led to develop new dimensions to categorise life events (e.g. loss and danger). Third, by extending our range of dependent variables to include certain physical disorders we have devised yet further dimensions for events ('goal frustration' and 'potential to produce symptoms for secondary gain'); we have also extended the model so that affective symptoms can be seen as crucial *intervening variables* between provoking agent, vulnerability factor and dependent variable (in this case the physical illness). Fourth, in a study designed to explore the mode of impact of one of the vulnerability factors (early loss of mother) we have developed new measures of yet other intervening variables, such as *childhood*, rather than adult, social vulnerability factors (e.g. lack of adequate parental care) and psychological adult vulnerability factors, such as situational personality measures (e.g. situational helplessness). While detailed discussion of some of these new variables (under all four headings) is out of order in a review of life event research, it may not be irrelevant for the reader to know the general context in which we have come to espouse the positions we shall outline.

Basic concepts and measures

The contextual measurement of life events

In the typical life event instrument based on a questionnaire, each broad type of event is given a simple definition and 'weighted' in terms of its propensity to produce change and disruption, with the implicit assumption that events such as births of babies can be treated as comparable in the sense that they are all likely to involve much the same amount of change and make broadly similar demands on adjustment (Holmes & Rahe, 1967). However, it is clear that the extent of disruption in activities is likely to be influenced by an individual's situation: for example, in the case of a birth, whether the original pregnancy was planned, whether the woman is still in touch with the father, or how far the birth interferes with plans for a career.

There is growing agreement about the importance of meaning and this has lead to a number of interesting attempts to reflect qualities of events other than amount of change in usual activity – say, in terms of their unpleasantness – and this has meant dealing with various characteristics of *particular* classes of event rather than summing events to obtain an overall score of change in a particular period of time for each individual. But despite this concern with meaning, measurement is still in terms of classes of event – for instance, an investigator still has to make up his mind to characterise births as, say, 'pleasant' or 'unpleasant'. At best only *general* meaning is dealt with, and the variety of circumstances that might surround particular births which would give different *specific* meanings are ignored.

The shortcomings of such a 'dictionary approach' have now been thoroughly reviewed (see Wershow & Reinhart, 1974; Sarason, de Monchaux & Hunt, 1975; Brown & Harris, 1978*a*; Jenkins, Hurst & Rose, 1979; Brown, 1981; Paykel, 1983).

A second approach to measurement attempts to deal with meaning for the particular individual. We will refer to it as *contextual*, in recognition of the fact that specific meaning is dealt with by taking into account the circumstances surrounding particular events. The Bedford College London LEDS, using a semi-structured interview, gathers as coherent and as full an account as possible of any incident from a list of events defined as relevant, (the criteria of such relevance having already been established in exploratory research). It is at this stage no more than a dictionary-type instrument. However, unlike other instruments, it covers the occurrence of ongoing difficulties as well as discrete life events (Brown & Harris, 1978*a*: Chapter 8). It is the *investigator*, by the use of a set of previously developed rules and detailed questioning, who decides whether or not an event is to be included. There is, therefore, no question of including, say, the death of a distant uncle if not already covered by rules about what can and cannot be defined as an 'event'. Once the occurrence of 'events' has been established, a second level of interviewing allows the investigator to specify various aspects of meaning by the use of ratings based on the notion of *Verstehen*, or understanding (Brown, 1984). Ratings take into account a person's biography and current circumstances in assessing, say, the threat of having a third child in an overcrowded flat, while ignoring what a woman said she felt about the birth. Raters make an estimate of what most persons in such circumstances would be likely to feel, by taking into account what is known of the person's plans and purposes, particularly insofar as these are reflected in biographical circumstances. By ignoring self-reports about reactions, various potential sources of bias stemming from the respondent can be ruled out; and by using consensus decisions of raters who are ignorant of such self-reports, potential bias stemming from the investigator is brought under control. It is important to note that the approach avoids altogether any judgment about the likely causal link between event and disorder – indeed, it is essential to keep from the raters making such contextual ratings not only anything about what the subject said he or she felt in response, but also whether or not the event was followed by the onset of illness or disorder (Brown & Harris, 1978*a*: 63–99).

A crucial advantage of this approach is its ability to measure the 'severity' of a particular event. Given differences in biographical and social context, some losses will be more 'severe' than others, some 'exits' will be a greater emotional blow than others and so on. 'Severity' in the LEDS is assessed in terms of the immediate impact of stressful events (short-term threat) and their more protracted effects (long-term threat), some 7 to 10 days after their first occurrence. The approach can also be utilised to measure a range of other qualities such as loss, danger, and chances of resolving the consequences of the event. It is important to emphasise that this contextual approach has a great deal of room to account for the individual's likely subjective meaning because what it is ruling out is not consideration of *all* feelings but only of those at the time of the event and subsequent to it. By considering the subjects' prior plans and purposes avowed or implicit in their activity, the interviewer is deliberately taking account of *previous* feelings which form part of the context from which the event derives its meaning.

Those emphasising the theoretical importance of change and disruption have usually followed a respondent-based approach and utilised questionnaires, and those emphasising the importance of specific meaning, an interview and investigator-based approach. However, as already indicated, some, dissatisfied with the former approach, have amended instruments such as the Schedule of Recent Experience (SRE) in important ways, particularly to take some account of *general meaning*. While these have usually continued to use a respondent-based approach, they have tended to move towards a more flexible mode of interviewing. The life event interview developed by Paykel and his colleagues in New Haven has been one of the most important of these, and, although it dealt in its initial form only with *general meaning* (in terms of a general notion of undesirability), it was sufficient to establish a case for there being an important aetiological link between life events and onset of depression (Paykel *et al.*, 1969; Paykel, 1974). A later version deals with more specific meaning in terms of negative impact (Paykel *et al.*, 1980). Research into many psychiatric and physical disorders has now reached a point where it is essential to deal with such *specific* meaning, if more effective theory is to be developed – for instance, in exploring the role of social support in buffering the impact of events. For this, the predictive superiority of the LEDS, in comparison with instruments reflecting general meaning, may well be critical.*

Reliability and fall-off in the reporting of life events

The fall-off in the reporting of life events has been a popular way of judging the accuracy of life event instruments. We have recently discussed this issue at length (Brown & Harris, 1982*a*) and we will summarise certain of our general conclusions. When a period of a year is considered, there

* Attributable risk per cent, a measure of the impact of a causal agent for depressed psychiatric patients, is 33% for undesirable events in the New Haven research using Paykel's original version (Paykel, 1974: 141), and for the Camberwell research, 49% for 'severe' events and 61% if 'major' long-term difficulties are also included – improvements on 'predictive power' of 48% and 85% respectively (Brown & Harris, 1978*a*: Chapter 7).

is little or no evidence for a fall-off in reporting using LEDS with trained interviewers. Given the critical role of severe events in the aetiology of a range of psychiatric and physical conditions this is a result of considerable importance. There is, however, a fall-off in the reporting of events of lesser severity (Figure 5.1). It is not entirely clear when this begins but it seems that significant error can be expected to occur when the gap between interview and event is 5 months or more. It is the salience of the event that appears to be critical for recall.

A group in Zurich using a checklist approach based on our published list of events obtained quite different results (Schmid, Scharfetter & Binder, 1981). Whereas we found a decline of only 8% for the 21 weeks before interview, it was 62% for the Zurich samples. This went with a much higher rate of events in Zurich – more than five times greater. We have argued that this extraordinary difference must be very largely due to the way the two centres conducted and rated the interviews (Brown & Harris, 1982*a*: 25).

The LEDS, like other instruments, is based on a standard list of 'events'; however, the questions are more detailed and only a specified range of circumscribed individuals are covered. The interviewer has also to collect a good deal of material about each reported incident to make sure it meets detailed criteria (e.g. a hospital admission of a close relative is only included as an event if it is serious or lasts more than 7 days). While the main impetus for developing these procedures was to avoid certain kinds of

Figure 5.1. Rate of events over 12 months for 17 3-week periods before interview for Camberwell and Lewis by severity of threat of events. (The final period covers 4 weeks but the rate is readjusted as for a 3-week period.)

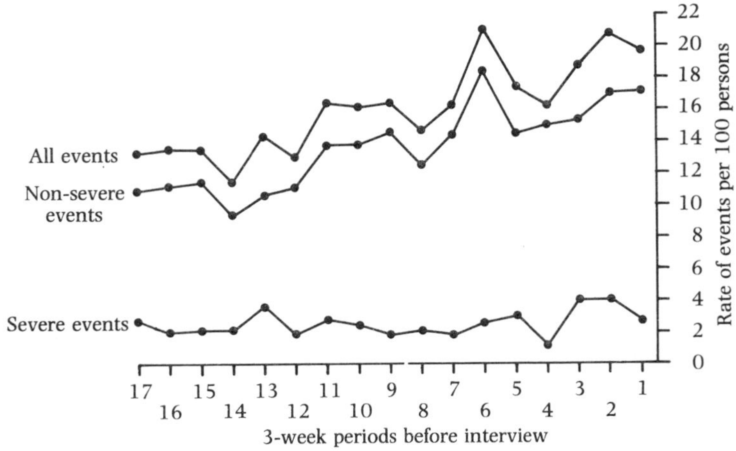

reporting and rating *bias* (for example, 'effort after meaning' on the part of the respondent), they undoubtedly add to the overall accuracy of the instrument. However, training in the use of the instrument, and also access to the extensive notes defining types of events, is essential. The training programme lasts 2 to 3 weeks and includes an opportunity to listen to tape-recorded interviews, discuss interview methods and to receive criticism of interviews carried out by the trainee. As already emphasised, what is to count as an event, and also its severity, is settled by the investigator and the consensus of her or his team within the strict limits provided by the background definitions and by procedural rules for collecting and rating material (Brown, 1981). We are confident about the ability of trainees to reach the necessary level of skill and accuracy (e.g. Tennant *et al.*, 1979; Parry, Shapiro & Davies, 1981). Unfortunately, the Zurich group did not receive this training or have access to the manuals providing criteria for inclusion or exclusion of incidents as 'events', and therefore cannot be said to have employed the LEDS. The published list of events is only a relatively minor part of the total instrument. Without, for example, the extensive list of definitions, it is impossible to settle what incidents should be included as events. It is also, we believe, desirable to follow a certain set of general rules when interviewing. For example, to pursue by further questions any hint on the respondent's part that an incident may have occurred; and also in the course of the interview to 'link' events to each other and to any background difficulties – in short to obtain a coherent 'story' about a particular incident. Once we know, for example, that a person has been rehoused, the interviewer should go back to explore what led to it: were there any important decisions or disappointments; did any crisis initiate the rehousing, and so on? (See Brown & Harris, 1982*a*, for further points along these lines.)

We believe that the much greater overall rate of events in the Zurich sample must be due to the fact that the investigators included almost every incident mentioned in response to one of the standard questions. Thus, to take an example, they have probably accepted *any* illness rather than one reaching defined standards of severity. It is also possible that they have been far more inclusive in the persons covered – we only included close relatives (parents, siblings, spouse and children), persons defined as close confidants, any fiancé, and all household members. In our experience respondents frequently mention events occurring to others such as cousins or aunts whom they rarely see, even though the persons the interviewer wishes to cover have been outlined. This interpretation is supported by the very low reliability reported for checklist instruments such as the SRE of Holmes &

Rahe (1967) – e.g. Yager *et al.* (1981). Paykel (1983) has recently carried out a comprehensive review of this for various life event instruments and since he arrives at very similar conclusions to our own we will not pursue the issue further.

Event dimensions

There are many, perhaps infinite, ways in which life events may be characterised (Hultsch & Plemons, 1979; Brim & Ryff, 1980). The full LEDS, indeed, deals with some 40 dimensions and new ones emerge (Finlay-Jones & Brown, 1981; Miller & Ingham, 1983). However, only a few have so far proved critical for aetiological enquiries and these fortunately have been based on the contextual approach to measurement. The success of this approach to life events has probably stemmed from its restriction of concern with meaning to judgments of likely emotional response (that is, by the 'average' person in such circumstances) rather than trying to deal with possible motives for action. The range of possible emotional responses are certainly highly restricted when compared with possible underlying motives. None-the-less we have already made clear that the approach does involve taking into account background plans in the evaluation of the likely emotional response of the average person with such prior purposes. Thus in assessing the threat of the birth of a second child to a woman living in grossly inadequate accommodation we would take into account that she had been trying for several years by a variety of means to acquire better accommodation; we would probably take some note of the fact that the pregnancy was unplanned and that there was some use of contraceptives, but we would not try to assess the possible motives of husband and wife underlying the pregnancy and birth. Indeed, given the context and desire to move it would make little difference to our rating of threat whether the birth was planned or unplanned. (In recently developed measures of *coping*, however, we would be interested in, say, the fact that the woman in those circumstances had deliberately become pregnant in order to become eligible for local authority housing because of 'overcrowding').

The importance of long-term threat (as opposed to short-term, see previous section) in bringing about depressive conditions has now been amply documented and it is unnecessary to review the evidence in any detail. We repeat the original Camberwell results in Table 5.1 as these have been fairly closely replicated in subsequent studies. (We will deal with the issue of onset of depression among psychiatric patients in a subsequent section.)

At this point it is perhaps important to note that the contextual approach does not necessarily rule out concern at some other point in the analysis with the respondent's subjective experience of threat. This needs to be emphasised as there has been a good deal of confusion about the lack of concern of the contextual approach with such material. A good deal of material about actual response to events is collected by the LEDS and rated on a set of parallel scales – reported short-term and reported long-term threat. The scales, however, have been somewhat neglected probably because of their suspect methodological status and because when used they give results not greatly different from the contextual ratings. Perhaps the point to emphasise is that it is possible to do better. It is also worth noting that such reports have in some cases had an important influence on the contextual ratings in the sense that in the course of rating the threat of thousands of events, any obvious discrepancy between the contextual and the self-report ratings are noted and this might well be taken into account in fixing standards of future contextual ratings. For example, the fact that so many women in our more recent research in North London (Regents Park, Walthamstow, Islington) have sailed through experiences of termination with relief (in marked contrast to the marked or moderate threat they reported feeling some weeks earlier on discovering an unwanted pregnancy) led us to change our rating standards on the contextual threat of an early induced abortion sought for unwanted pregnancy, putting it down one

Table 5.1. *Proportion with at least one provoking agent in the period before onset for patients and onset cases, or interview for 'normal' and 'borderline case' women*[a]

	Psychiatric patients (%) (N = 114)		Onset cases (%) (N = 37)		'Normal' and 'borderline case' women (%) (N = 382)	
1. Severe event alone	30	76	41	89	13	30
2. Severe event and major difficulty	32		24		6	
3. Major difficulty alone	14		24		11	
4. No severe event or major difficulty	25		11		70	

[a] The average period before onset for the patient group was 38 weeks so for normal and borderline case women the period taken is 38 weeks before interview.

point on contextual threat. We sent out instructions to this effect to all the raters we had trained in our methods.*

Subsequent developments of the ratings have concentrated less on the severity of emotional response than on aspects of the events that could be expected to lead to characteristic emotional responses. The two most important of these concern *loss* and *danger* (Finlay-Jones & Brown, 1981). Only events previously rated at least moderate on long-term threat are rated. Loss is a reasonably straightforward category although the inclusion of loss of a cherished idea (say, unexpectedly learning of a husband's infidelity) is worth noting. The idea of danger breaks newer ground and relates to the degree of unpleasantness of a specific future crisis which might occur as a result of the event. The most salient future specific crisis stemming from the news that a woman's father has cancer is his possible death. Severity of danger depends on judgment of how unpleasant it would be to the woman (not her father) given the context. For a rating of danger the specific future crisis that might occur (i.e. death) is assessed not the present associated difficulties that might stem from the news of the cancer such as the need for nursing. The future crisis has to have some probability of occurring but not be inevitable. If clearly inevitable, it is argued, such an experience is more like a loss since the future crisis could reasonably be assumed to be going to occur. (In the most recent version we have tidied up our approach somewhat to rate inevitability of danger and reversibility of losses.) Inter-rater agreement, as with all the contextual ratings so far developed, is high (Finlay-Jones & Brown, 1981: 808).

The importance of the distinction has been demonstrated in a study of the onset of depressive disorders and anxiety states. Loss was clearly related to onset of depression and danger to anxiety, but perhaps the most revealing result was the link of both loss and danger events with the onset of mixed conditions judged to reach a caseness level of severity on both depression and anxiety (Finlay-Jones & Brown, 1981).

Miller & Ingham (1983, 1986) have recently developed an interesting series of dimensions which, although less global, appear broadly to parallel the notions of loss and danger. Preliminary results suggest that somewhat similar findings might emerge in terms of symptoms of depression and anxiety.

* It is important to realise that such 'rules' only provide a general guidance: the rater can rate otherwise if she feels that there are particular biographical and current circumstances that justify it.

Diagnosis and specificity of response

Consideration of dimensions leads naturally to the question of how far particular domains of meaning and emotional response relate to the aetiology of specific psychiatric and physical disorders. It is now evident that important specific links occur. It remains to settle how general these are. We have already noted the clearcut results for depressive and anxiety disorders once the measure of general long-term threat is expanded to take account of loss and danger.

	Threat of event	
Onset period	Short-term	Long-term
Short	1	2
Long	3	4

An important step is to distinguish short- and long-term threat and short- and long-term response in the sense of the maximum length of time between event and onset of the disorder. For instance, in these terms schizophrenia probably falls within box 1 (short-term threat; short period) and depression straddles boxes 2 and 4 (long-term threat; and both short and long periods). A number of studies have now documented that a florid onset or relapse in schizophrenia occurs within a few weeks of an event (e.g. Brown & Birley, 1968; Leff & Vaughn, 1980; Day, Nielsen & Korten, 1982). A more recent paper by Leff & Vaughn (1983) is particularly interesting as it suggests that *some* threat needs to be present however minor (as reflected in the LEDS) whereas Brown & Harris (1978*a*) had suggested that *any* event reflected by the LEDS may play a role (i.e. even one without minor threat). We are happy to concede that in general some threat is probably required, but given the small size of the schizophrenic series so far studied the matter needs further enquiry. However, in more theoretical terms we do believe that events rated without threat can at times play a role. Since a raised risk of onset of schizophrenia has only been shown to occur within 3 weeks of an event the issue of long-term versus short-term threat is bound to be somewhat confused. However, in the sense that many develop florid symptoms within 7 to 10 days of the event, short-term threat, in the technical sense of the LEDS system of measurement, is obviously often critical. But we would not wish to rule out altogether the possibility of a longer-term impact of particularly threatening events.

(One patient in our 1968 series developed an acute schizophrenic episode 11 weeks after her mother with whom she lived committed suicide.) However, this again needs much larger series and would in any case be difficult to disentangle from the effect of important changes in the 'expressed emotion 'level of the home (Brown, Birley & Wing, 1972; Vaughn & Leff, 1976).

The possible importance of the short- and long-term threat distinction, however, may well prove a far more important issue as research is extended to other conditions. Creed (1981) has shown that the proportion of patients with severe events occurring before appendicectomy of normal or only mildly inflamed appendices was remarkably similar to the proportion of depressive patients in Camberwell with such an event. However, for those with acutely inflamed appendices the proportion with a severe event was no different from the general population comparison group. Such patients, however, did have in the 13 weeks before the operation a raised rate of events showing at least *some* short- or long-term threat. Connolly, using an early version of the LEDS, has shown an increased rate of such events in the 6 weeks before an infarct (Connolly, 1976; Craig & Brown, 1984*a*: table 1). The result is, in fact, reasonably comparable to that obtained in the work on schizophrenic patients and a classic study of streptococcal infections of the throat in children (Meyer & Haggerty, 1962). Such results do raise the possibility that for a number of organic disorders insofar as life events are involved aetiologically it is in terms of short-term threat and a short onset period (box 1, p. 121) and that they play a 'triggering' rather than a 'formative' causal role, 'triggering' implying that they provoke a disorder that would have been likely to occur before long in any case (see Brown, Harris & Peto, 1973; Brown & Harris, 1978*a*).

An additional complexity that possibly arises in the study of physical disorder should be noted. It is illustrated by a study of women in the general population selected because they reported on a screening questionnaire the recent development of new physical symptoms of moderate or severe intensity (Murphy & Brown, 1980). The relationship of severely threatening events to physical symptoms appeared to be mediated by an intervening psychiatric disorder of an affective nature, the mean length of time between the onset of the psychiatric disorder and onset of 'organic' disorder being 7 weeks. (The possible importance of affective disturbance as a mediating factor is also raised by the study of those admitted for an emergency appendicectomy (Creed, 1981), and by two studies still undergoing analysis in our unit concerned with gastrointestinal disorder and menorrhagia.) While long-term threat is clearly of importance the issue of onset period is complicated by the apparently intervening role of affective disorder. Given the preliminary nature of the findings it is inappropriate to deal with the issue in any detail and in any case much larger series are essential in order to establish more securely the length of the periods involved. One final point should be made about the diagram on p. 121. For certain physical conditions such as coronary heart disease it may prove necessary to add another row representing an onset period of more than one year. (We have been developing an approach with some success that collects events and difficulties over a 5 to 10 year period for this purpose – Neilson & Brown, 1984.)

In general a great deal more research remains to be done concerning specificity of response and particularly the link between physical and psychiatric disorder (Craig & Brown, 1984*a*). It should be added that there is almost certainly a need to take account of other dimensions of 'events'. For example, an impressive recent study by Kasl, Evans & Neiderman (1979) of officer cadets relates development of infectious mononucleosis to the importance placed by the individual cadets on success in their training course and to frustrations and challenges to such success. This suggests a need to supplement our notions of danger and threatened loss by the experience of special 'challenge' situations. In our own unit we have evidence of the importance of another dimension in the onset of gastro-intestinal disorder (Craig & Brown, 1984*b*) 'goal frustration', which seeks to take account of the degree to which an event interferes with the subject's prior plans and goals. A second dimension, 'potential to produce symptoms for secondary gain', seeks to explore the hypothesis that certain types of events which regularly precede symptoms of acute physical pain have aspects reliably categorisable by blind raters as imposing a need to claim care and attention from significant others upon those who experience them. (The hypothesis of 'secondary gain' in the traditional psychiatric literature rests upon the not unreasonable assumption that relatives and significant others do tend to respond to dramatic physical symptoms by giving more care and attention to the sufferer.) So, for example, a fiancée intimating that she may rethink the engagement because she is not sure whether she wishes to marry the subject would have marked 'Potential to Produce Symptoms for Secondary Gain' (PPSSG), whereas a fiancée dying would not, though both would be events of marked threat. In the first instance the continued existence of the fiancée would mean that she could be appealed to by the physical symptoms of pain to restore the care and attention she was threatening to withdraw. In the second, although pain symptoms developed after her death might gain him care and attention from other relatives they could never restore her care and attention which he lost through her death. The classic example of a marked PPSSG event is the case of someone awaiting compensation after an industrial accident: the notably long continuation of symptoms in such instances has often been attributed to the expectation of a greater gain in compensation accruing to those with greater 'damage' from the accident. This PPSSG dimension has now been piloted and developed; among a consecutive sample of women with an onset of gastrointestinal disorder the proportion with one of these PPSSG events among events rated severe was significantly higher than among severe events occurring to a comparison group from the general population.

The independence dimension

Consideration of dimensions would not be complete without a discussion of 'independence'. This was one of the earliest dimensions used in an attempt to safeguard against the possibility that a life event might be the result of an onset of disorder before symptoms became really obvious, rather than a cause. By distinguishing events which on logical grounds could not be the result of such an 'onset' (because their source was so 'independent' of the subject's agency), possible contamination is avoided. Events which because of the subject's agency could not be clearly rated 'independent' were relegated to the category 'possibly independent'. (Compare a house move forced upon a family by the decision of the local council to demolish a whole terrace with a move decided upon quite voluntarily.) The use of this dimension originally represented a considerable advance but in the hands of purists it has recently threatened to confuse the understanding of aetiology. Presenting a separate aetiological 'analysis' of 'independent' events should be a preliminary methodological exercise to convince readers that any apparent causal link obtained cannot simply be the result of bias in measurement. But once having done this it is essential to move on to analyse events which are possibly independent along with those which are independent. Those rare 'illness-related' events which are likely to be the result of disorder such as a suicide attempt or dismissal from a job would be excluded from all analyses of onset, though they might be included in studies of recovery. It is important to emphasise that the logic behind the concept of 'possibly independent' events is not that such events are no longer part of the social stressors in a person's environment; it hardly makes sense that any measure of adversity should ignore a bankruptcy or a marital separation just because the subject has played a part in bringing them about. Yet such is the hold of our culture's moral influence that time and time again trainees in the LEDS have been tempted to see the aetiological contribution of events such as these as stemming entirely from within the person and thus as not part of the social environment. In a similar way they will try to rate them lower on contextual threat on the grounds that the subject has somehow been responsible for the event's occurrence and thus, perhaps, deserves less sympathy. The distinction from each other of the contextual threat and the independence dimensions cannot be too heavily emphasised; and its logical corollary, that severe threat is severe whatever its source, requires that 'possibly independent' events are given much the same weight in analyses as 'independent' ones if the impact of severely threatening events is to be fairly assessed (Brown & Harris, 1982*b*).

On the other hand it is reasonable to suggest that so far not enough has been done to exploit this dimension in analysis (Bebbington *et al.*, 1981*b*). Perhaps the ratio of independent to possibly independent events varies with different groups of depressives, say, referred psychiatric patients as compared with those treated by general practitioners only, neurotic as compared with psychotic patients and so on. Perhaps too it might be useful to conceive of varying degrees of independence rather than the present fairly crude three categories. If differences did emerge, they might suggest further avenues of exploration particularly in terms of the personality predispositions that might partly account for them. For example, a proneness to disrupted relationships after rows might distinguish certain groups of depressives, as might carelessness or a tendency to suffer physical illnesses. In order to investigate these possibilities we have refined the scale and reanalysed our Camberwell data.

The new scale has 12 points. The first four deal with 'independent' events. Point 1, or the most 'independent', describes events whose immediate origin is unconnected with the subject and whose more distant origin it is difficult to attribute to him or her with any plausibility. The second describes events whose immediate origin is unconnected with the subject but it is impossible to rule out entirely that some aspect of his or her behaviour might have influenced it – say, the subject's friend deciding to move to a distant part of the country. Point 3, 'negligence not obvious but not impossible', covers events where influence of the subject's behaviour upon the other person's actions has a certain outside plausibility but where there is nothing whatever to suggest that it did occur. Certain accidents to children are included here, though others where the subject's neglect or carelessness might more clearly be implicated would fall in a later less 'independent' category. It is necessary to emphasise here that our usage is very conservative: that is, erring against the hypothesis that events totally external to the subject are producing her depression. Events like a child falling over at school and becoming concussed, would not in the normal course of affairs be thought to have any relationship to an insidious onset of depression in the mother. However, in the Camberwell data an association had emerged between accidents to children and recent previous onset of depression in the mother (Brown & Davidson, 1978). Following the theory that it is withdrawal of the mother's care and concern after her symptoms develop which acts as the intervening variable between maternal depression and accidents to children, we argue that accidents may not be as completely independent as they seem even when occurring to husbands and lovers. (Even before revision of the scale, the rules had specified that it was inappropriate to rate certain types of accidents as 'independent', for example if a hot kettle had been left too close to the edge of a table and fell off onto the child.)

Point 4 includes all illnesses to the subject: this is seen as the least independent of the four 'independent' categories and allows for the possibility that somatic complaints of a person may just be harbingers of their impending psychiatric breakdown. Against this it may be thought curious that physical illnesses to the subject had at any stage been seen as independent, since they are so clearly located within the person and not in the outside environment. The rationale for this originally derived from an unwillingness to assume the truth of the psychosomatic perspective before it was clearly independently established. A separate category for these events involving illness means that analyses can now be carried out in both ways, once making the psychosomatic assumption and once without it.

Point 5 is the most independent of the 'possibly independent' categories: called 'consent' it copes with events where an incident from an external source forces the subject to make a decision, for example a fall by an elderly mother and the decision of a woman to have her come to live with her although she would never have decided on such a course without the fall. Point 6 is for 'intentional actions', the classic examples of possibly independent events, such as moving house, pregnancies, engagements. Point 7 describes events which have clearly occurred as a result of the subject's probable negligence. Thus since point 3 ('negligence not obvious but not impossible') is treated conservatively many events potentially dealt with by point 3 would be placed here. The next two points describe events where contact with another important person is broken off, point 8 after a row and point 9 without a row. A friend's decision to move to a distant part of the country would be placed here rather than point 2 if it had been associated with a row with the subject. Point 10 is for events stemming from the subject's romantic susceptibilities which cannot really fit any of points 6–9, (falling in love is hardly really either intentional or negligent). Point 11 we inserted at the last minute – it describes events which derive from the romantic susceptibilities of the subject's partner. Although many such events seem to be 'independent', our threshold has always been so conservative that anything remotely related to the marital *relationship* (as opposed to, say, the majority of the husband's health or work events) was rated only 'possibly independent'. Point 12 for 'illness-related' events can be further extended to a point 13 in projects where the dependent variable may be one type of illness (say, physical) with the intervening variable as another (say, psychiatric).

To spell out in detail the rationales for each of these new points would become tedious; but it must be apparent to anyone familiar with psychiatric orthodoxy about affective disorder that they have a common characteristic. They could be said to tap some quality in the woman *before* the occurrence of the event (say, her carelessness, her tendency to cause rows, a constitutional weakness which produces both physical and psychiatric illness and so on). In that sense it might be maintained that significant findings relating to any one of the new scale points except point 1 would detract from the importance of the severe events in bringing about depression and throw the aetiological ball firmly back into the court of previous personality; that is, it might shift the focus of attention away from the social environment back to the individual's constitution. (But, of course, it should not be forgotten that an event much influenced by someone's 'personality' could still play a direct role in producing depression.) Perhaps the most important feature of the results we obtained using this expanded scale was that the differences between the various depressed groups and the non-depressed comparison group were not affected when degrees of independence were taken into account. As with our previous analyses we use 'experience of at least one severe event of a certain type' rather than looking at overall rates of such events by each group. The latter measure can be an illuminating adjunct to the former but can be misleading on its own in that when overall numbers are small, one woman with 10 possibly independent severe events can swamp another 9 women who each have one independent severe event.

Table 5.2 shows very similar proportions in the three groups of depressed women in Camberwell experiencing the various types of severe event, with of course very much lower proportions among the normal women and borderline cases. In all four groups, even among the non-depressed, the completely independent events (on point 1) are much the most commonly occurring category, most often involving deaths of close relatives and arbitrary decisions by housing authorities or employers. The importance of the social environment is therefore vindicated. Consideration of the figures on point 2 reinforces this conclusion when it is remembered that it is extraordinarily conservative and that most of the events included here almost certainly deserve a rating of '1': for example, a brother's decision to move out of the area probably has nothing to do with the subject's behaviour, but it cannot be completely ruled out that if she had been different in some way he would have been unwilling to contemplate such a move.

Even in those categories of event where there does seem to be some

Table 5.2. *Experience of at least one (or more) severe event of specified types of independence before onset or interview*[a]

Independence	'Endogenous' (N = 63) (%)	Neurotic (N = 49) (%)	Onset cases (N = 37) (%)	Normal and borderline cases (N = 382) (%)
A Independent				
1. Completely independent	35	24	32	9
2. Nearly completely independent	8	8	11	3
3. Lack of care by subject impossible to rule out, but not obvious	3	10	8	1
4. Physical illness to subject	8	18	8	3
B Possibly independent				
5. Subject consents to external event	0	8	3	1
6. Intentional act by subject	8	6	0	2
7. Probably due to carelessness/ negligence	6	6	0	2
8. Rows and breaking off contact	2	6	11	1
9. Breaking off contact without a row	6	6	5	0
10. Subject's own love events	2	0	0	1
11. Subject's partner's love events	5	2	5	0
No severe event[b]	41	35	35	81

The percentages do not sum to 100 because women with several severe events falling into different independence categories have been counted more than once.

[a] The average period before onset for the patient group was 38 weeks so for normal and borderline case women the period taken is 38 weeks before interview.

[b] Some of these of course had major difficulties.

difference between the various groups of women, it is rarely likely to be a difference of aetiological significance given that a number of women have more than one severe event and at least one event falls in a different independence category. For example, patients with neurotic depression seem to have more severe events involving their own physical illness than other patients and onset cases, but more than half of them have other types of severe events as well before onset.

In conclusion then it can be seen that careful use of the independence dimension can increase confidence in some of the general theoretical propositions already outlined about the social and external origins of both endogenous and neurotic depression.

The inclusion of difficulties in a life events schedule

One of the innovative features of the LEDS is the inclusion of measures of ongoing difficulties such as unremitting damp, overcrowded housing or continuous interpersonal neglect, which may or may not have discrete events occurring in association with them. Like events, they are measured on a number of dimensions including one of 'contextual severity' which embodies all the same principles as 'long-term contextual threat' for events.

Some appear to embrace this feature of the LEDS without having thought through its implications. We will deal with some of the resulting issues in the hope of clearing up a certain amount of current confusion which inhibits some from taking full advantage of this innovation.

(*a*) *Time and the causal model*

Many seem to identify the notion of 'vulnerability' with a continuing temporal process and the notion of 'provocation' with occurrence at a particular point in time; they thus find it awkward to include long-term difficulties with provoking agents. The conviction that provocation should be a process that is datable makes a good deal of sense and we have elsewhere discussed evidence that where there is an onset of depression in the setting of a major difficulty without a severe event, it can often be linked to the occurrence of a less threatening event in the few weeks before onset. We have argued that these minor events act to force a person to *reassess* the meaning of an ongoing stressful situation, as when a woman's short stay in hospital for a minor operation like a D and C may bring home with added force the distressing nature of her housing or her marriage (Brown & Harris, 1978*a*: 145). It is, however, her housing or her marriage which leads to the depression, not the D and C as such. Among the 419 women in Camberwell who were not chronic cases, the rate of onset of depression was not significantly different between those with both a severe event *and* a major difficulty (28% or 9/32), those with a severe event but no major difficulty (23% or 15/65), and those with a major difficulty but no severe event (18% or 9/51) in a 38-week period. It would thus appear that severe events and major difficulties operate in a very similar way to produce depression but that the occurrence of both does little to increase the risk following just one of them. A summary measure reflecting the presence of either a severe event *or* major difficulty would thus have a definite predictive advantage over either employed singly. The intuitive hunch on which the LEDS had incorporated difficulties along with events seems therefore to have paid off. Later studies have in general confirmed the appropriateness of this decision.

(b) Aggregation and prediction: the problem of the overlap between severe events and major difficulties

Even when it is accepted that difficulties can be 'provoking', our experience has shown that there is sometimes still a residual feeling that there is something risky in using the combined variable. We argue elsewhere that such wariness about aggregation is often exaggerated beyond all needs of logic (Harris & Brown, 1985); but it is necessary here to point out that analyses which in the interests of some kind of research hygiene avoid combining the two kinds of provoking agent are likely to obtain theoretically misleading results. From the data just cited it will be clear that while they are significantly interrelated the overlap between severe events and major difficulties is only modest. Thus when testing for the impact of life stress in the presence of some other factor (be it one of our cited vulnerability factors or a previous episode of the dependent variable, or some other 'vulnerability' factor), it can be very misleading to deal separately with events and difficulties as it will then appear that many reacting with depression to whichever factor is omitted do so in the absence of stress. To take an example: in an analysis examining the possible buffering role of social support, failure to include those with only a major difficulty among those with a provoking agent will mean that many will appear to develop depression with low social support in the absence of life stress; the effect of lack of social support alone in producing depression will thereby be exaggerated. (One example of a study which only performed separate analyses of severe events and difficulties is Costello's otherwise very careful research in Calgary, 1982.)

(c) Prediction of disorder and dimensions of difficulties

The 'major difficulty' of the Camberwell study identified as increasing risk of depression required a contextual severity on the top three points of a six-point scale, a duration of two or more years before onset or interview, but excluded difficulties relating to the health either of the subject or of other close ties. It was very much a provisional grouping and, although its predictive power for depression was confirmed in the Outer Hebrides data, later users of the LEDS have been encouraged to investigate other possible groupings. Unfortunately results have not always been systematically reported so that different groupings could be compared side by side as Costello did (1982: 333–4). Occasionally, workers have pruned the number of dimensions of difficulties collected and changed the basic ratings so radically that they cannot really be said to have undertaken a replication; the lack of confirmation of a previous result under such circumstances is in no way tantamount to a disconfirmation, though readers may be tempted to see it as such. The apparent failure of health difficulties to increase risk of depression – in Camberwell, the Hebrides and Calgary – is of particular theoretical interest in that it may well relate to the possibility that nursing, either oneself or one's sick relatives, may confer meaning and self-esteem in a way which reduces risk so long as it does not involve any loss of role for the subject. It is thus a pity that Tennant and Bebbington failed to record this dimension in their study in Camberwell (Bebbington *et al.* 1984).

Linking of events and difficulties

Events and difficulties are quite highly interrelated – events often lead to difficulties and difficulties to events. One criticism of the present LEDS is that although we had conceived the measurement of difficulties as an important way of dealing with the 'outcome' of events, we have not pursued this possibility in our analyses. This has probably arisen because of the success of the long-term contextual threat rating in predicting depression. However, the need for a way of systematically linking material on events and difficulties has become clearer. Surtees, in his work on decay periods, has highlighted the importance of considering the longer-term consequences of events outside that of the immediate sequelae dealt with by the long-term threat scale (Surtees, 1980; Surtees & Ingham, 1980). It is after all possible that the long-term threat of an event might clear up only a week or so after the tenth day taken to judge such threat. We had in fact produced indirect evidence that working-class women were less able than middle-class women to resolve difficulties and had a greater proportion continuing for two years or more (Brown & Harris, 1978*a*: 166). And there is every possibility that the greater tendency of difficulties to remain unresolved among working-class women explains a good deal of their greater chance of experiencing chronic depressive disorders at a caseness level.

We have examined the possible links of all 121 severe events occurring to the 220 women in the first Camberwell survey. The link between such events and marked difficulties (1 to 3 on threat and any duration) was for the most part clear – for instance, a husband's acute illness leading to a long bout of unemployment, or a marital separation occurring in the context of a husband's long-term infidelity. However, in some instances the link was more complex. An event was on occasions rated severe because of the presence of a difficulty of a quite different nature – say, the birth of a baby rated severe in the context of financial problems following a husband's imprisonment. Here the *severity* of the event could be said to be due to the difficulty, although the event itself could not in any strict sense be said to have been produced by it. In a few instances the events and difficulties occurred together to bring about a 'high' threat rating in each. One woman, for instance, gave birth to a second child when she was living in too small a flat to cope with two children. If all such complex relationships are classified as severe events stemming from a marked difficulty a clearer picture emerges. Four in ten of the severe events resulted from a marked ongoing difficulty which they then could be said to have helped to perpetuate. (Eighty per cent of the difficulties had lasted at least one year and the majority for considerably longer.) The remaining severe events did not arise from such a difficulty but a quarter of the total led

Figure 5.2. Relationship of severe events and marked difficulties (First Camberwell sample, $N = 220$).

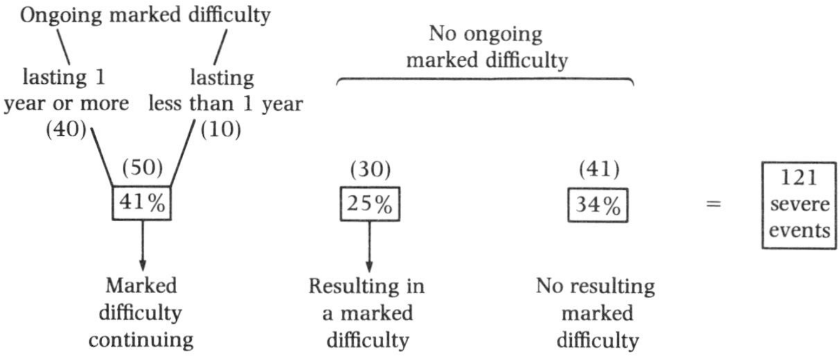

to a marked difficulty, leaving a third which neither arose from or gave rise to such a difficulty (Figure 5.2). The general order of the results is not changed if difficulties of severity '4' (low moderate) are included.

We have now developed a more complex classification scheme to deal with such links, but we believe these results give a reasonable indication of the order of the phenomenon. Its potential importance is underlined by the fact that when all women with children at home in the Camberwell survey are considered, the greater rate of severe events among working-class as compared with middle-class women is cut by approximately four-fifths when the number of ongoing marked difficulties is controlled. (An excess of 54% was reduced to 11%.) One of our interests in the current prospective enquiry is to relate measures of 'support' and 'coping' both to the resolution of ongoing difficulties and to the possibility of such factors reducing the chance of a severe event leading to a marked ongoing difficulty. In other words it is likely that it is class differences in these two factors which explain the original class difference in the links described above.

The new link schedules are designed to simplify the task of counting and specifying types of link between event and event, difficulty and difficulty, and event and difficulty by entering them directly onto the computer. This not only facilitates the study's primary aetiological purpose by helping us to avoid the possibility of double counting in analyses of additive effects (see the next section); it also enables us to compare much more easily the degree of linkage of stressful factors between different demographic groups such as class, age and lifestage groups. The distinctions between different types of link will increase the subtlety of any analyses of additivity, since we are now able to distinguish links due to direct causation from those less direct associations such as 'facilitation' (where a child starting school allows a mother to start a job) or where a difficulty although not causing the occurrence of an event determines its severity (say, a pregnancy which is only severe because of an ongoing financial difficulty).

Problems of design and analysis

Prospective enquiries

Several large-scale prospective enquiries have recently been published dealing with the role of life events and various disorders. Given the effort involved, what they have produced has been disappointing and it is now clear that such studies cannot be fully effective if they rely only on respondent-based measures. It is also clear that costly longitudinal research is not necessarily an effective way to establish temporal order. It is often overlooked that such research is extremely unlikely to obviate the need to reconstruct time order by questioning. Let us assume a design in which social support and psychiatric state are measured at time 1 and life events established for the 6-month period before that, and psychiatric state again at time 2 in an interview 6 months later.

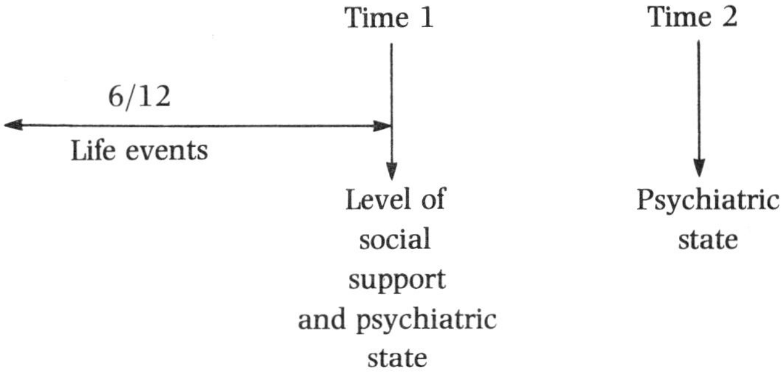

It is still necessary in such a design to establish by skilled questioning the *time order* of events occurring in the 6-month period between time 1 and time 2 and relate these to any onset during that period. (The events in the 6 months before time 1 also have, of course, to be established retrospectively.) It will almost certainly be quite impractical to utilize the prospective design to establish relevant events in an interview taking place *before* the onset has occurred since for many physical and psychiatric conditions the time interval between event and onset is probably only a matter of weeks or even days. But even if the gap were a matter of months rather than weeks, effective prospective research in the sense of picking up events before the disorder occurred would be likely to be ruled out because of the number of interviews that would be necessary in order to be sure of doing this.

Recent prospective studies have re-interviewed subjects after periods ranging from as low as 2 months (Grant *et al.*, 1982), 4 months (Henderson, Byrne & Duncan-Jones, 1981) to one year (Theorell, Lind & Floderus, 1975). All such studies have used checklists to obtain life events and psychiatric state. None has attempted to date onset in the follow-up period and none has therefore followed the design just outlined. Instead, because they ignore events in the intervening time period (since the use of questionnaires seems to rule out accurate dating), such events are never included in their analyses. This almost certainly will lead to a gross underestimate of the aetiological role of events. It appears to have been overlooked that the studies could not hope to be effective in the sense of Meyer & Haggerty's (1962) classic study of streptococcal infections of the throat where children were seen every 2 weeks. (Frequent interviewing was here a practical possibility because such infections are common and the study of a relatively small number of children was all that was necessary to obtain a sufficient number developing the disorder.) The study coming nearest was that of Grant and his colleagues employing a 2-month period (Grant *et al.*, 1982).

We do not wish to suggest that at some stage of a research programme a prospective design may not be both feasible and desirable, albeit combined with retrospective questioning about events and about support actually forthcoming at the time of these events. Such studies become particularly critical when dealing with the role of 'soft' material such as self-evaluation, but it is still necessary to establish how far social support at one point in time is 'mobilised' in a subsequent crisis (Eckenrode & Gore, 1981; Brown *et al.*, 1985*a*).

The aetiological importance of events and difficulties

There has been a good deal of confusion about the importance of the link between life events and difficulties and the onset of specific disorders. Results for the most part have been presented in terms of the apparently straightforward notion of 'variance explained' (r^2), based on squaring the correlation coefficient. The amount 'explained' in these terms by life events is invariably low, usually no more than about 10%, and in studies using checklists it is often a great deal lower. Some reviewers have concluded from this that 'life events are unlikely to have clinical or preventative importance' (e.g. Andrews & Tennant, 1978). The likely pitfall involved in this kind of conclusion can be most easily illustrated by taking an aetiological agent of undisputed importance – cigarette smoking. Although most instances of lung cancer are associated with heavy smoking, much less than 1% of the variance is explained by this link. This surprising failure of the index to reflect the obvious importance of smoking is simple to explain: variance explained takes account of the fact that not only most people with lung cancer are heavy smokers, but also that *most heavy smokers do not have lung cancer*. Since those without greatly outnumber those with lung cancer, the fact that most with lung cancer are heavy smokers gets swamped in any 'two-way' measure of association. This has close parallels with the findings for depression. Although the majority of women developing depression experience a provoking agent before onset, usually involving a major loss or disappointment, most women experiencing such events and difficulties in the population at large do not develop depression. If the practical importance of the aetiological findings for lung cancer and depression are to be assessed, this clearly cannot rest alone on the 'variance explained'. An index is required that reflects the fact that most developing a disorder only do so after the experience of a particular aetiological agent. But given the fact that heavy smoking and severe events are quite common in the general population such an index would need to take account of the fact that agent and disorder will at times be juxtaposed by chance (Cooke & Hole, 1983).

Such alternatives exist (Paykel, 1978). A frequently used index in epidemiological research, Levin's attributable risk per cent (as distinct from the conventional attributable risk) (see Markush, 1977) is a particularly satisfactory index of the importance of an aetiological effect, as it gives the proportion of cases associated with the putative causal risk factor, allowing for the fact that they will in some instances be associated by chance. It is most accurately estimated when there is knowledge of the rate of the putative causal agent in the general population from which the cases are drawn. This cannot be obtained from a matched-comparison type of design: but it can often be estimated from published epidemiological data, or even from the sample under investigation when certain conditions are met (Cole & MacMahon, 1971). In fact the measurement of association '*x*' we have utilised in the Camberwell research is very similar to 'attributable risk per cent'*, being defined as the proportion of those with disorder whose onset was provoked by the specified risk factor (Brown & Harris, 1978*a*: 117–21). A recent review makes clear that the index has been 'discovered' independently on several occasions – in our case by Julian Peto (Markush, 1977). The '*x*' coefficient has been fully discussed and illustrated and we will not go over the same ground. To take an example in terms of the relationship of severe events and major difficulties and onset of depression in the community in Lewis in the Outer Hebrides, 'attributable risk per cent' is 73.4%, '*x*' is 72.9% and 'variance explained' 12%. Another statistic giving the same numerical result from yet another perspective is the prediction logic discussed by Hildebrand and his colleagues as a means of dealing with measures of association in contingency tables. They have argued for the usefulness of making *specific* predictions rather than covering all possible pairs of comparison in a contingency table

* Where the two measures differ is that '*x*' follows the slightly conservative practice of including the proportion of the *total population* with the risk factor (including chronic cases) in the comparison.

(Hildebrand, Laing & Rosenthal, 1977). This involves calculating the expected number in one cell, 'b', of the four-cell contingency table. In the present instance it is necessary to calculate the expected error in predicting onset from knowledge of the presence of a severe event and then to compare this with the actual error.

Onset case in Lewis	Provoking agent Yes	Provoking agent No	
Yes	*a* 13	*b* 3	16
No (excluding chronic cases)	*c* 42	*d* 129	171
	55	132	187

Using the marginal totals giving the actual overall rate of onset to calculate the 'expected' rate of onset in the unexposed group (i.e. $132 \times 16/187 = 11.29$ for 'b') and using the usual proportional reduction in error formula (PRE) we obtain:

$$\frac{\text{expected error} - \text{observed error}}{\text{expected error}} = \frac{11.29\text{–}3.00}{11.29} = 0.734,$$

the same result as 'attributable risk per cent'. That is, taking account of the presence of a provoking agent allows us to improve our prediction of the occurrence of an onset of depression by 73%. Or put in aetiological terms 73% of the onsets of depression are associated with a severe event or major difficulty allowing for the fact that some will have been associated with a severe event by chance.

There has been very little discussion of the shortcomings of 'variance explained' as an index of the impact of 'agents' although warnings can occasionally be found (e.g. Rosenthal & Rubin, 1979). Its common use seems to reflect the much wider ritualistic, almost magical, use of statistics in the social sciences. None-the-less, no one index is likely to be satisfactory and variance explained does reflect a significant issue in life event research. In a strict sense one cannot predict very well from the presence of a provoking agent to the development of depression (or from heavy smoking to lung cancer) and 'predictive' power can often be enhanced by taking into account further factors which potentiate it – say, the amount of social support experienced at the time of an event. A low amount of variance explained can therefore be a useful reminder that even when there is a high attributable risk per cent, or 'x', a great deal more may still be needed to specify the conditions under which the putative causal agent will have an effect. However, the same point can be made by noting the proportion of persons with an appropriate causal agent who do not develop the disorder, and this is perhaps to be preferred as it does not have the same arcane aura as variance explained. Therefore it is in general desirable to take account of a number of indices to understand the aetiological implications of a particular set of results. We merely argue that when considered alone, attributable risk per cent (and relative risk, which we have not dealt with) are less misleading than variance explained.

Additivity in the impact of events and difficulties

Most research on the additivity of events has assumed its importance and, as with the SRE of Holmes & Rahe (1967), incorporated the assumption of additivity into the measurement procedure itself. We have taken the reverse approach: to see first what can be done without the assumption. There is in fact surprisingly little evidence for additivity as far as the onset of depression at a caseness level is concerned. It is the impact of just one event or difficulty of a sufficient severity that appears to be critical. Nothing that has emerged since the original Camberwell survey has led us to change this view. However, there is evidence that additivity plays some role in increasing the severity of depression once onset has occurred and since Surtees has recently approached the question in a quite new way, a general review of present knowledge will perhaps be useful.

Contextual ratings of threat complicate the study of additivity because by taking into account relevant background circumstances, a particular rating may encompass prior events. For example, a birth may be rated severely threatening because a woman's husband has not long before been sent to prison, which has resulted in serious financial problems for her. It might be argued that by taking into account the consequences of the husband's arrest when rating the birth, we will tend to rule out the kind of additivity reflected by the checklist approach which deals with the two events quite independently. If this should be so we are unrepentant as we believe our procedure is a good deal closer to what actually occurs in real life. The impacts of events and difficulties are unlikely to coalesce in a mechanical fashion. They are far more likely to come together in terms of meaning and intimately involve the memory system (Brown, 1983). In this sense additivity certainly does play a role in the onset of depression and it is just this that is taken into account in the contextual ratings. If the woman with a husband in prison develops depression following the birth of her child, it is almost certainly because the 'imprisonment' and 'birth' have been in some degree 'added' in her mind and the birth given a new significance. Therefore questions concerning additivity are probably best formulated in terms of apparently 'unrelated' events and difficulties, in the sense that the severity of threat of the birth of the baby and the husband's imprisonment are 'related' but neither are linked to the woman's mother developing multiple sclerosis about the same time. Fortunately this possibility can be tackled as the contextual ratings ignore events and difficulties that cannot be linked in obvious and commonsense terms. An analysis of 'unrelated' severe events and major difficulties was conducted on the Camberwell material and it was in the light of this that we concluded that there was at best a modest additive effect. Women developing depression had more often experienced *two* or more 'unrelated' events in the 38 weeks before onset than a normal comparison series in the same period – 28% compared with 9%. But it was only 'unrelated' severe events that acted in this way: somewhat surprisingly the consideration of major long-term difficulties did not add anything. Thus although there appears to be some increased risk, the impact of multiple 'unrelated' provoking agents appears to be surprisingly small. In retrospect we believe that our conclusion that the aetiological effect of provoking agents appears to be largely dependent on the meaning derived from a single severe event or major difficulty is basically correct, bearing in mind, as already argued, that 'related' events and difficulties do have an additional additive effect of an unknown (and perhaps unknowable) amount.* A more powerful additive effect would not have been surprising in the sense that the occurrence of yet-another-event-or-difficulty may well lead to a generalisation of hopelessness. The fact that the impact is not greater probably indicates the way in which emotions and memories tend to cluster around a limited number of role identities and activities. We have found helpful here Tomkins' ideas about scripts and nuclear scripts (Tomkins, 1979). We believe that events and difficulties increase risk of depression insofar as they link to core identities and activities (or nuclear scripts in Tomkins' terms) and their additivity in the last analysis is probably determined by such links. Such emphasis, of course, is another way of conceiving of the notion of plans and purposes – but does so by recognising more clearly the emotional and likely long-term development and biographical basis of many key 'plans'.

We do not wish to rule out that additivity may act independently of such

* The original report includes a discussion of the problem of defining 'related' and 'unrelated' events and difficulties and the various kinds of additive mechanism that may be at work (Brown & Harris, 1978*a*: 106–11 and 139–40).

identities, activities and scripts, say, by producing a general feeling of the last straw – 'everything is against me'. But we believe it is more parsimonious theoretically to assume for the present that more specific meaningful links are present and to look for them.

It is important to realise that the analyses of additivity we have reviewed only included severe events and major difficulties. There was no evidence that the general run of events and difficulties added in any way to produce depression, although in a discussion of 'reassessment-forcing' events we did suggest that minor events could bring about depression in someone with an ongoing long-term difficulty (Brown & Harris, 1978*a*: 145). By contrast, Ingham & Miller (1979) have reported evidence for an additive effect, using the LEDS, for both provoking agents in our terms as well as more minor events. However, it is important to note that they dealt with the development of depression as an isolated symptom and thus include people with mere mood changes as well as those with full-blown depression. Furthermore, the additive effect was quite small and needed a large sample to demonstrate it. However, Surtees has since published a series of significant papers using an index of adversity that combines an estimate of the effects of different life events occurring at different times. He calls it a dissipation model as it takes account of the fact that the impact of events will tend to grow less with distance in time from their occurrence. The approach is based on summing the threat ratings of events according to their distance from time of occurrence. It has therefore reopened the additive issue in a quite new way. The approach so far has used events collected by the LEDS and rated in terms of long-term threat (Surtees & Ingham, 1980). The model postulates that the adverse effect produced in an individual subjected to a threatening life event dissipates with time and summates with effects of subsequent events according to their severity. Difficulties are seen to exert a constant effect during the period in which they are present and summate with each other and with life events. The main problem with the approach at present is that it assumes a constant rate of decay for events of the same level of severity (the higher the threat the larger the dissipation period). This is almost certainly inadequate and it is essential ultimately to settle the actual dissipation rates more empirically for each event – perhaps linking outcome of events more clearly to the course of any subsequent difficulty that has stemmed from them (see previous section). There have been some interesting suggestions as to how some events can neutralise the severe threat of previous events (Giel *et al.*, 1978; Tennant *et al.*, 1981*b*). None-the-less the model is a valuable stimulus for further research and has produced interesting results. Broadly, the predictive power of the approach appears to be essentially comparable to that achieved by the earlier Camberwell analysis which uses discrete events and ignored the possibility of 'weighting' threat in terms of distance of onset from occurrence of event. Surtees & Rennie (1983) have utilised in the most recent paper the original Camberwell material and from this it is possible to calculate an 'attributable risk per cent' for severe events of 53% for the dissipation approach and one of 57% where no decay is assumed.* This result is perhaps hardly surprising given the great predictive power of such events. It does not rule out the potential value of a dissipation model but indicates that using the present generation of measures and the arbitrary values concerning dissipation imposed on the material, it is unlikely to add to the *predictive* power of the original results.

Vulnerability factors and provoking agents

There has been increasing interest in variables that mediate between life events and difficulties and the development of depression or other disorders and there has been a number of influential reviews. In terms of our own research the importance of such mediation is illustrated by the fact that only one in five women with a provoking agent in Camberwell went on to develop a depressive disorder at a caseness level; and this ratio may well prove to be even less for those developing an anxiety state following an incident involving serious 'danger'. While genetic and constitutional factors almost certainly play some role, there is now enough evidence to suggest that psychosocial factors are likely to prove critical for the majority of depressive disorders. While a range of indicators have been explored most studies have concentrated on the role of social support (e.g. Lowenthal & Haven, 1968; Brown *et al.*, 1975; Cobb, 1976; Miller, Ingham & Davidson, 1976; Lin *et al.*, 1979; La Rocco, House & French, 1980; Gore, 1981). In the Camberwell research most emphasis was placed on the role of a confiding relationship with a husband or boyfriend and we will concentrate on this because all subsequent studies have dealt with it and most of the research has in any case concentrated on married women with children. Many other factors have been implicated, including those of personality (Hendrie, Lacher & Lennox, 1975; Paykel, 1978). We will not attempt to cover the whole range of factors of possible significance as we are more concerned with the troublesome methodological and theoretical issues that surround this kind of analysis. With this in mind we will largely restrict the review of substantive findings to the role of social support, particularly a confiding relationship with a husband or boyfriend.

* The latter is based on a somewhat longer period than the 38 weeks which we used elsewhere to calculate attributable risk per cent and '*x*' for onset cases and patients.

The recent prospective study by Henderson and his colleagues in Canberra deserves special mention as it undertook important innovations in the measure of social support (1981). As already noted it was a prospective enquiry. While we are convinced that such expensive enquiries are unnecessary for sound research on the aetiological role of life events, they are probably essential if we are to make progress in the study of vulnerability factors. Most of the latter so far identified appear to involve social support in some way and it is difficult to measure this with any subtlety *after* onset of disorder without allowing the possibility of bias. And it is in any case clear that we cannot remain content with the kind of crude indicators utilised in the Camberwell study. The Canberra enquiry is significant because it utilised sophisticated notions concerning forms of social support, particularly influenced by the writings of Robert Weiss, who has delineated major 'provisions of social relationships' (1969, 1973, 1974, 1979). These are 'Attachment', provided by close affectional relationships, 'Social Integration', provided by membership of a network of persons with shared interests, 'Opportunity for Nurturing Others', 'Reassurance of Personal Worth', a 'Sense of Reliable Alliance' (mainly acquired from kin and from obtaining help and advice from informal advisors (Henderson *et al.*, 1981: 31)). The Canberra group has developed an extensive structured 'Interview Schedule for Social Interaction' (ISSI) to reflect such provisions.

Sadly, we do not believe its potential has so far been realised. This is significant because the results themselves are puzzling. The measures of support based on notions of the type of social contact, its presence or absence, and its frequency (called Availability measures) do not relate to the development of psychiatric disorder in the presence of life events; it is only support based on the person's dissatisfaction with the support he or she is receiving that relates to increased risk of psychiatric disorder (called Adequacy measures) (Henderson *et al.*, 1981: 137–55). Interpreting this result in conjunction with correlations found between this dissatisfaction and certain features of personality at follow-up interviews (measured by the Eysenck Personality Inventory), the authors suggest that social support in itself may be unimportant. They argue that because the Adequacy measure of support is entirely based on the respondent's evaluation of his or her relationships, there is the possibility that 'personality' factors which have nothing to do with support are the reason for the measure's ability to predict the occurrence of psychiatric disorder, since they relate separately both to satisfaction and disorder.

However, while we would not wish to rule out the role of 'personality' factors (Brown, Harris & Bifulco, 1985*c*), a closer look at the indices of support employed make it quite unnecessary to entertain the kind of radical interpretation put forward by the investigators. The main index dealing with availability of support is concerned with attachment and is based on only 8 of the 100 or so questions in the schedule. Six of the eight involve issues of attachment (feel very close, share happiness, know someone very well, etc.). One question deals with satisfaction (whether there are persons who really appreciate the respondent) and only one question deals with confiding. (Do you have someone you can share your most private feelings with (confide in) or not?) Although for each question the respondent was permitted to record more than one person, only one was used in the index. It therefore probably has a number of serious limitations. First, since it has been ability to confide (especially in a husband and boyfriend) that has been shown to play the most critical role in the development of depression, it is odd that only one question deals with it. Second, the phenomenon of attachment is not distinguished from *provisions* of practical help, emotional support and advice, accorded by close relationships. A good case can be made that attachment purely and simply in the sense of persons to whom one feels close will not necessarily protect against depression and in certain circumstances may be associated with increased risk (O'Connor & Brown, 1984). Various aspects of support need to be more clearly distinguished. Third, since only one person is counted for each question the index can only provide an approximate indication of the numbers to whom the respondent feels close. (The authors note 'much of the data obtained in the Attachment Table (where all data on such persons was recorded) have not yet been fully utilised by us as a source of predictor variables' – O'Connor & Brown, 1984: 37).

The second index concerned with availability of social integration is equally curious since its 16 items conflate four dimensions of relationships conceived to be theoretically distinct. Although multivariate analysis enabled the authors to conclude that a general dimension of 'Social Integration' could be formed by the combination of acquaintance, friendship, reassurance of warmth and reliable alliance, the only fully convincing demonstration that information was not lost would be to relate each dimension separately to the risk of developing psychiatric disorder. It should be added that, as already noted, there is some suggestion from cross-sectional studies that the kind of general relationships reflected in this index (e.g. whether there are six or more people with whom the subject can exchange a word or two in shops and such like on most days) do not protect from the development of a definite depressive disorder (e.g. Brown & Harris, 1978*a*: 173–9; Surtees, 1980: 76).

Finally, and perhaps more critically, actual support received in a crisis is not recorded. Expected support is by no means always mobilised (Eckenrode & Gore 1981); and failure to receive 'expected' support may well lead to an even higher rate of disorder than when there were no grounds to expect it (Brown *et al.*, 1985*a*). We therefore conclude that it is likely that the two indices of availability of support confound too many distinct dimensions and fail to distinguish clearly enough the different types of relationship (spouse, same sex friend, parent, etc.) to provide a definitive test of the vulnerability hypothesis. It follows that the fact that the two 'subjective' measures related to the development of depression may simply be due to the fact that paradoxically they were more effective indicators of the actual objective factors crucial for protection against disorder. (However, since the measures of life events and psychiatric disorder were also respondent-based and 'subjective' there is the possibility that the obtained links were a function of 'response sets'.)

In our own current prospective study in Islington we are using certain new measures of social support developed in this unit by Pat O'Connor and others (O'Connor & Brown, 1984). We have been particularly concerned to stay at the level of detailed specific dimensions of support, rating each dimension for as many different individuals as appear relevant in the life of the interviewee: thus one subject may have a series of ratings for each of three 'very close others', and each of four 'resource others' (felt by the subject to be less close than 'very close others'), a husband and a lover, while another subject may have only one 'resource other' rated. The dimensions cover similar sorts of areas to the ISSI but more attention is paid to confiding, emotional support and dependency than to the more amorphous notion of attachment. There is a whole section on the subject's self-evaluation, which brings us much closer to measuring the crucial intervening variable in our model, 'self-esteem'. In order to substantiate our claim that social support has an impact on self-esteem we need to consider certain dimensions which bridge the gap between the measures of support and those of self-evaluation: these are 'felt competence', 'helplessness', 'identity enhancement' and 'identity destruction' which are rated for each of the crucial relationships mentioned above, as well as for certain critical role areas such as motherhood, work and external arenas (the latter referring to the wider network of contacts and activities such as pub-going, sports clubs, bingo friends and so on).

Causal modelling and vulnerability

We have already noted the particular kind of mediating role involved in a vulnerability model: that lack of support (or other relevant factors) only increases risk of depression in the presence of provoking agents, but that the latter have an effect even when lack of support is not present.

The vulnerability model is most easily illustrated by a diagram plotting the percentage developing depression in a given period of time in terms of the four possible combinations of provoking agent and vulnerability factor. The figures in brackets represent proportions of women developing depression in a recent Canadian study (Costello, 1982).

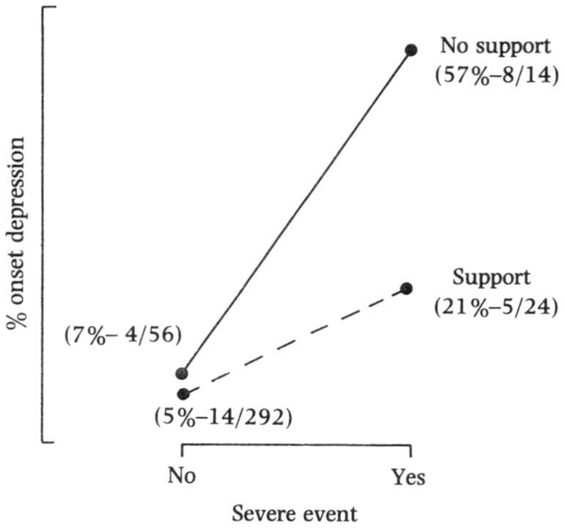

D. Cooke (personal communication) has noted three other possible models; we will discuss them in terms of severe event and support although, of course, they are all of general relevance.

Mutual potentiation model. For mutual potentiation both lack of support and severe event increase risk in each other's presence and risk is low if either factor is absent.

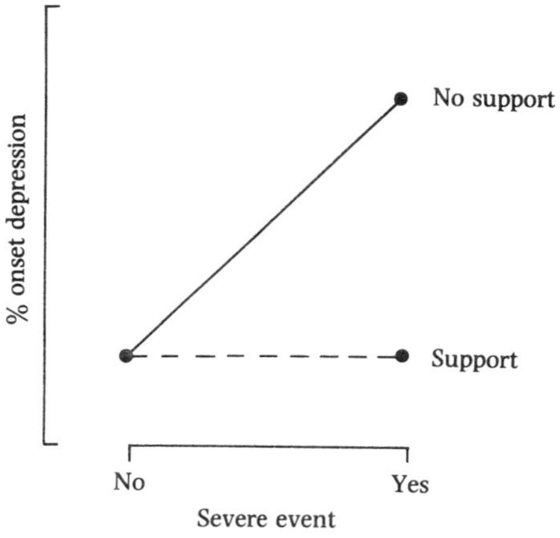

Complex synergistic model. For the complex model lack of support and severe event both increase risk but in addition their joint occurrence produces a disproportionately increased risk. (Cooke calls this a synergistic model, but we would argue that synergism is a more general concept which includes all the models just outlined.)

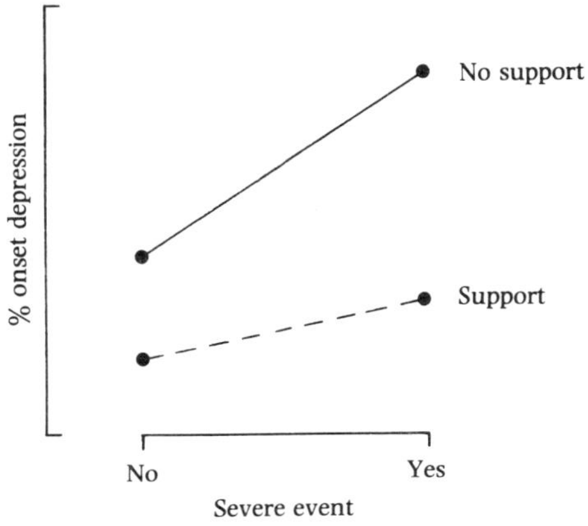

Independent causes model. For the independent causes model lack of support increases risk irrespective of severe event which contributes an independent effect. The effect on risk of their joint occurrence is no more than would be expected from a combination of each independent effect.

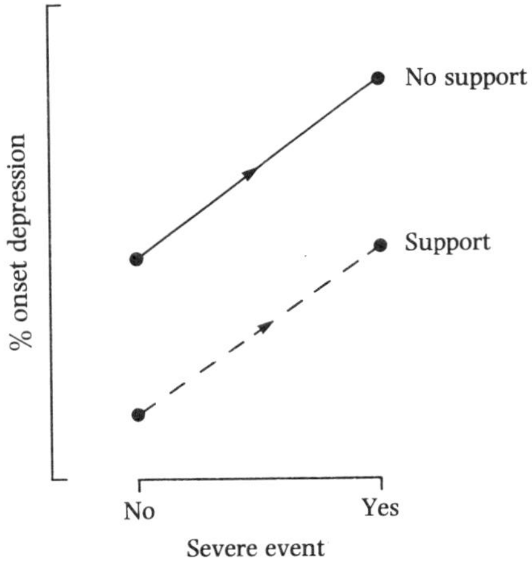

Any of the first three models would be of considerable theoretical and practical interest: the fourth independent causes model would merely suggest that a further 'provoking agent' has been discovered. (It should be noted that at this point of our presentation we have dealt in all four models with the relationship between variables only in additive terms. Multiplicative models will be introduced later.) Somewhat surprisingly there is good evidence that the vulnerability model may be the one of importance for depression. We say surprisingly because a number of shortcomings in measurement and design will tend to militate against finding support for the model and to result in support for one of the other three. Although we believe we have met a series of potential shortcomings in measurement and design which would militate against confirming the vulnerability model, there is one still built into our approach. The vulnerability model depends on there being no or little difference in depression between women high and low on vulnerability without a provoking agent. But because the contextual ratings are conservative there can be no doubt that at times some with a genuine 'provoking' factor which has led to depression are classified as *not* having a provoking agent. For example, in our original report one of these exceptions had had a marked marital difficulty lasting *only 18 months* (thus not major) involving a total change in the husband's personality after an accident. It would therefore not be surprising if there was a slight difference between the women high and low on vulnerability in the 'no provoking agent' group. Of course, in terms of our earlier discussion this also underlines the importance of definition and measurement of provoking agents for an adequate test of the vulnerability model and for depression. Katschnig (1980) has demonstrated that for a group of young people who have attempted suicide, high scores on Holmes & Rahe's SRE are uncorrelated with the presence or not of a provoking agent, using the LEDS, and therefore quite different results may occur using such an instrument.

There are a series of further shortcomings in design and measurement, which we believe we have met in our approach, but which if uncorrected would militate against the confirmation of the vulnerability model. The first of these concerns the dating of onset. Perhaps the most surprising weakness of many of the studies testing for the role of support is the neglect of the time dimension since the need for the provoking agent to occur *prior* to onset of depression is central to *any* aetiological model. If the time period under study for possible provoking agents is a year, a measure of prevalence of disorder, say, in the month before interview, is quite inadequate for two reasons. First, certain people may have experienced a provoking agent much earlier in the year covered by the enquiry, have developed a depressive disorder and then have improved by the time of interview – at least from major manifestations. But by dealing with only the month before interview such persons will be classified along with those who have remained symptom-free throughout the year. This would clearly lead to an underestimate of any impact of provoking agents. Second, and more important, certain respondents, although manifesting clear symptomatology, will be unsuitable for inclusion because the duration of their symptoms has been so long-standing that investigation of any potential aetiological factors would need to start way before the period of the year chosen for the study. Unfortunately about half of all depressive disorders found in the general population are chronic conditions, which, albeit often fluctuating, date from outside the year before interview – and often many years earlier. One of the first essential steps then must be to separate those with such chronic conditions from those who had an onset in the time period of interest.

The importance of this distinction can be illustrated by the example of lack of confiding or intimacy. If this is truly a vulnerability factor, rather than a provoking variable in its own right, then it should show little or no association with risk of depressive disorder without the presence of a defined provoking agent. This does in fact hold for women in Camberwell and in the Outer Hebrides when only onset cases are compared with women without depression. However, when chronic cases are examined the vulnerability factor appears to be playing a more independent and separate role. Since the numbers of onset and chronic cases in the year are almost identical their combination will largely obscure the onset result and the investigator would probably decide that there was evidence for only a complex synergistic not a vulnerability model (see figure 7.2 in Brown, 1981).

There are probably two reasons why the inclusion of chronic cases will tend to suggest that lack of intimacy does not just play an intervening role between provoking agents and depression and both are consistent with our causal model. It is highly likely that since the original onset of the chronic conditions the rate of severe events and major difficulties has tended to return from the high level reached just before onset, while the level for vulnerability remains just as high, thus diminishing the overall proportion with both provoking agent and vulnerability factor and increasing the proportion with vulnerability factors alone. Second, lack of intimacy or other forms of shortcoming in social support can themselves be produced by the chronic depressive condition – obvious examples being a woman's withdrawal from a job and social contacts outside the home consequent upon the self-depreciative and anergic features of the episode itself. This would tend to reduce the numbers in the group with provoking agent and without vulnerability factor, thus underestimating the aetiological role of the former as compared with the latter.

As critical as time order in aetiological research, and something almost as commonly neglected, is the need to take account of severity and diagnosis. The idea that aetiological factors will be discovered which apply uniformly to all types of psychiatric disorder is almost certainly illusory. And almost equally illusory is the idea that it might be possible to develop a general uniform criterion for caseness regardless of type of disorder. Several studies have now shown important differences in the way in which case and borderline case conditions of depression are brought about by social factors. While both often follow a major loss or disappointment, the presence of a vulnerability factor only increases the risk of a disorder at the *case* level of severity. The presence of vulnerability factors does not increase the risk of a borderline case condition occurring. Indeed, in research in the Outer Hebrides, women developing borderline case conditions have *fewer* vulnerability factors than ordinary women. The reason for this seemingly odd result appears clear enough: the presence of a major loss or disappointment without the presence of a vulnerability factor tends to lead to a borderline case rather than a true case condition.

Given the sensitivity of the vulnerability model to measurement and design issues it is notable that six of the eight studies that appear to have kept closely to the requirements we have outlined have produced comparable results to our original enquiry and therefore impressive support for the vulnerability model in the terms in which it was originally formulated. In addition, a closely related study by Paykel *et al.* (1980) has produced comparable findings and one by Murphy (1982) with the elderly fits the model if the criteria for intimacy are extended to cover all sources of confiding (see Table 5.3). The only real exception is the Camberwell study carried out by Bebbington and his colleagues. We have no explanation for this discrepancy, although this particular study has produced a whole series of discrepant results and in that sense this particular result is less surprising (Bebbington *et al.*, 1984).

However, even before the completion of any of these 10 studies a good deal of controversy had arisen from two papers emerging from the MRC Social Psychiatry Research Unit about our original findings and the points they raise there are thus applicable to each of the replications in the table (Tennant & Bebbington, 1978; Bebbington, 1980). (See also our replies, Brown & Harris, 1978*b*, 1980.) The effect of the papers has undoubtedly been to increase awareness of the complexities involved in the statistical

Table 5.3. *Onset caseness depression, intimacy with husband and presence of a severe event or major difficulty*

	Provoking agent			No provoking agent		
	No intimacy (%)	Intimacy (%)		No intimacy (%)	Intimacy (%)	
Strict replication						
(a) Severe events or major difficulty						
Brown & Harris (1978*a*) (Camberwell)	32 (24/76)	10 (9/88)	$P < 0.001$	3 (2/62)	1 (2/193)	ns
Campbell (1982) (Oxford)	50 (8/16)	13 (2/15)	$P < 0.05$	9 (1/11)	0 (0/29)	ns
Cope (1983) (Oxford)	40 (4/10)	13 (1/8)	ns	17 (1/6)	7 (1/15)	ns
Brown & Prudo (1981) (Lewis)	36 (8/22)	15 (5/33)	ns	5 (2/40)	1 (1/92)	ns
Bebbington *et al.* (1984) (Camberwell)	22 (8/37)	24 (5/21)	ns	11 (5/45)	6 (3/49)	ns
G. Parry (personal communication) (Sheffield)	31 (8/26)	10 (5/49)	$P < 0.05$	10 (2/19)	5 (5/98)	ns
R. A. Finlay-Jones (personal communication) (Regents Park, London)	45 (24/53)	17 (4/23)	$P < 0.05$	8 (3/36)	3 (1/39)	ns
(b) Severe events only						
Costello (1982) (Calgary)	57 (8/14)	21 (5/24)	$P < 0.05$	7 (4/56)	5 (14/292)	ns
Martin (1982)[a] (Manchester)	73 (8/11)	14 (2/14)	$P < 0.01$	40 (2/5)	4 (2/5)	$P < 0{\cdot}01$
Total (a and b)	38 (102/268)	14 (39/285)	—	7 (20/277)	3 (28/845)	ns
Closely related studies						
Paykel *et al.* (1980)[b] (South London)	82 (9/11)	24 (8/34)	$P < 0.001$	14 (1/7)	12 (6/52)	ns
Murphy[c] (1982) (North London)	35 (6/17)	11 (10/90)	$P < 0.02$	0 (0/19)	3 (2/74)	ns

[a] A study of a series of women covering a pregnancy and a birth in every instance.
[b] Study of post-partum women. One or more undesirable events and poor communication with husband.
[c] Elderly sample of both sexes. Severe event or major difficulty. Low intimacy = no confiding with anyone, i.e. not only husband

analysis of contingency tables, but in the short term they have led to a good deal of confusion.

The key issue is whether lack of support (or any other factor) has an independent effect in increasing risk of depression or only increases risk in the presence of a provoking agent. Tennant & Bebbington concluded on the basis of our material that 'the social variables involved do not segregate into "vulnerability factors" and "provoking agents". Both categories of variables affect the risk of disorder independently of the other' (Tennant & Bebbington, 1978: 574); and that 'vulnerability factors have an effect somewhat similar to the separate provoking effect of life events' (p. 573). In other words they assert that vulnerability factors act statistically as provoking agents.

It is important to recognise that it is usually possible to *see* from such diagrams or tables what kind of mediating role is being played by a third factor such as social support. Statistical analysis is most critical in providing initial tests of the differences involved and the importance of such tests is likely to lessen as results are replicated and numbers increase. Indeed, such tests of *significance* can easily in these circumstances distract the investigator from his main task of evaluating the likely *size* of the effects involved and the most likely mode of influence; as with increasing numbers quite small differences in size of effect are likely to be significant, but possibly substantively trivial. Therefore in discussing the controversy that has resulted from Tennant & Bebbington's claims it is wise to bear constantly in mind the results summarised in Table 5.3. They obviously do provide a powerful prima-facie case for the vulnerability model.

We believe there are two responses to Tennant & Bebbington's claim. The first is *pragmatic*: it does not say that they are wrong but that their description is far less informative than one emphasising the importance of the joint effect of vulnerability factor and provoking agent. The second *theoretical* approach is stronger and asserts that Tennant & Bebbington's is not a reasonable test of a vulnerability model.

(*1*) *Pragmatic reply*. One problem with Tennant & Bebbington's criticism is their failure to appreciate that certain assumptions about the world are typically already built into statistical techniques; whether or not it is reasonable to go along with these assumptions cannot then be settled by statistical arguments depending on these very assumptions. Statistical procedures often handle interactive effects differently and such effects are central to the models we have outlined.

It has been traditional in the social sciences to see interaction in terms of an *additive* model as already assumed in the figure presented earlier describing the vulnerability model (p. 145). Let A and B represent two independent factors and a, b, c and d represent proportions of a third dependent factor C in the four cells formed by the combination of A and B:

		A: Yes	A: No
B	Yes	a	b
	No	c	d

The independent effect of A is $(c-d)$ and B is $(b-d)$; d is subtracted in each instance as it represents the state of affairs when neither A nor B occur. Thus a simple additive effect will be $(c-d)+(b-d)$. Interaction represents the excess in terms of a proportion when these terms plus what would be expected in any case without them (i.e. d) is subtracted from the effect when A and B occur together (Galtung, 1967: 415):

$$\text{Excess ('interaction')} = a - [(b-d)+(c-d)+d].$$

For the Camberwell material the independent effects are 9% for provoking agent and 2% for lack of intimacy and the effect when neither provoking agent nor lack of intimacy is present is 1%. When both A and B are present 32% became cases of depression (top line of Table 5.3). Therefore the excess or interactive effect of provoking agent and vulnerability factor when occurring together is 20% – i.e. $32-[(10-1)+(3-1)+1)]$. This is quite sufficient to establish a general case for the vulnerability model – although not, of course, to deal with the issue of statistical significance.

However, there is an alternative way of considering interaction in which effects are *multiplied* rather than added. The independent effects of A and B are obtained by dividing b and c respectively by d (i.e. b/d and c/d), since any effect of A or B is seen as multiplying the effect of d alone. In order to establish what would happen given a straightforward multiplicative model the independent effects are multiplied with each other and then with $d: c/d \times b/d \times d = 3/1 \times 10/1 \times 1$ which gives 30%. Therefore multiplicative interaction is represented by any excess over 30% in the cell representing the joint effect of A and B (i.e. cell a). In the present instance since 32% is very little different from 30%, there is no interaction (multiplicative) and the two approaches therefore give quite different answers concerning the presence of interactive effects.

In passing it should be noted again that the four diagrams set out earlier, which are the conventional way of representing the relationship of two variables to a third, are additive in nature. In order to represent a multiplicative perspective a logarithmic scale would have to be used on the Y-axis if the convention of representing independent effects by parallel lines is to be preserved.

The original paper by Tennant & Bebbington failed to recognise that the ordinary log-linear approach they employed reflects only multiplicative effects. Everitt & Smith (1979) have confirmed that if the alternative linear modelling methods based on an additive approach (such as GSK) are used, interaction is present in this Camberwell data. They state that the choice between models using the two different types of interaction cannot be settled in statistical terms but none-the-less show a preference for a multiplicative approach – as does Bebbington, (this volume). However, recent opinion in epidemiology has emphasised how much information can be lost by ignoring additive interaction (Rothman, 1974, 1976, 1978; Blot & Day, 1978).

In pragmatic terms it is, we believe, more informative to use an additive approach for three reasons.

(i) It would be quite misleading to conclude (with Tennant & Bebbington) that provoking agents and vulnerability factors act in comparable ways statistically. We saw earlier that there was little or no evidence that *two* provoking agents increase risk more than just one and yet the impact of one provoking agent and one vulnerability factor far exceeds the effect of one provoking agent. We believe it is most parsimonious to see this reflected in an additive model in which provoking agent and vulnerability factor are seen as having an interactive effect.

(ii) The assessment of multiplicative interaction places critical importance on the ratio b/d – that is, on women developing depression when they have no provoking agent but lack social support compared with those developing depression with no provoking agent but with social support. But because the former women are so very rare (see third column, Table 5.4), effects emphasised by a multiplicative model are bound to rely on a very small number of cases. For example, in the results shown earlier in the vulnerability model diagram the difference between columns three and four, 7% (no provoking agent and lack of support) and 5% (no provoking agent and no lack of support), entirely disappears if the first category loses *one* of its four cases – i.e. 4/56 (7%) becomes 3/55 (5%). In practice, as we have argued earlier, any errors are likely to be biased in favour of a model attributing a direct effect to a vulnerability factor: in other words, some cases in column three actually might have experienced an event which had 'provoked' a reaction of hopelessness but because of the conservative nature of the contextual threat ratings discussed earlier, this event was not rated severe and they were thus counted as having no provoking agent (see Brown & Harris, 1978*a*: 147–9). This would make reliance on such small numbers even more equivocal. It should also be noted that the consequences of such minor fluctuations in cell frequencies are trivial for an additive approach.

(iii) An additive model has the merit of emphasising that in practice (*a*) onset cases are rare when there is lack of support but no provoking agent, (*b*) the great majority of onset cases occur when provoking agent and lack of support occur together, and (*c*) that a substantial number occur when provoking agent occurs alone.

(2) *Theoretical reply*. There is a second, stronger reply that emphasises the irrelevance of many traditional statistical tests for a strict test of the vulnerability model. Surtees (1980) has made clear that any approach which assumes in advance that the support factor has an effect both with and without a provoking agent is bound to militate somewhat against the confirmation of a vulnerability model which specifies that in the absence of a provoking agent a vulnerability factor has little effect. Rutter with this in mind goes so far as to see the controversy as pointless: 'The controversy lacks point because the crux of the issue does not lie in the particular sort of statistical interaction found, but rather in the simpler notion that there are vulnerability variables which have a negligible effect in the absence of stressors, but a significant effect in the presence of stressors; an effect, that is, which exceeds both the effect of the stressor on its own and also the sum of the separate effects of the vulnerability factor and the stressors when they occur in isolation. The chief limitation of the multi-variate statistics usually employed to test for this interactive effect is that they use as their starting-point the assessment of whether the vulnerability factor shows a significant main effect. Unfortunately, this is not the same as determining whether the variable has an effect in the absence of the stressor – the one datum crucial to the hypothesis (see Brown and Harris, 1978*b*; Rutter, 1979). As a result, the usual multivariate statistics are inappropriate for testing for this particular sort of vulnerability or protective effect' (Rutter, 1981). One can add that if a vulnerability model holds, the issue of type of interaction is irrelevant: if there is no main effect for the vulnerability factor, strictly speaking there is no 'interaction' because there is no effect to interact with that of the provoking agent and thus debate about whether it is additive or multiplicative becomes irrelevant. What, of

course, is relevant is the assessment of the 'potentiation' of the effect of the provoking agent by the vulnerability factor.

There are, we believe, two ways forward given this strict view. The first is simply to deal with the $2 \times 2 \times 2$ table as we did in the original report in terms of two 2×2 tables (we repeated this in Table 5.3). This has much to commend it as it stays close to the data and the reader is led to focus on the substantive questions at issue. Indeed, the salient relationships between the variables are most readily apparent in this form. As we have seen in Table 5.3, showing the original Camberwell results, lack of support has virtually no effect in the absence of a severe event while in the presence of a provoking agent the effect is pronounced.

However, a second, more systematic approach is in fact contained within Bishop, Fienberg & Holland's (1975) account of log-linear analysis where they discuss an approach developed by Worcester (1971). This represents one way of avoiding the narrow restriction to hierarchical models in conventional log-linear analysis where one is prohibited from suggesting models in which a three-factor interaction term is posited in the absence of one or both of the main effect terms. To illustrate: if the mutual potentiation model is true, that is, where neither variable *on its own* has an effect on depression, the use of a hierarchical approach might well none-the-less mistakenly demonstrate powerful main effects and no significant interaction.

If by simple inspection of the data, it is clear that either the vulnerability or mutual potentiation models appear plausible, then one is well advised not to restrict oneself solely to hierarchical models. Using Worcester's non-hierarchical approach the vulnerability model fits the original Camberwell data very well. Furthermore, it can be shown that in the case of a vulnerability model the goodness of fit test for the whole model reduces to the X^2 for the two right-hand columns in Table 5.3 (i.e.risk of depression by presence and absence of support when no provoking agent is present), and the X^2 in the two left-hand columns (i.e. risk of depression by presence and absence of support in presence of provoking agent) is a test of significance of the interaction term itself (Eales, 1983). Of course, where there are replications, tests of significance can be given somewhat less importance and this simplification enables one to see at a glance that all the studies reviewed in the table (other than that by Bebbington and his colleagues) support the vulnerability model.

For the purist this procedure may not always solve the problem 'which is the right model?' since one may still be left with quite a difficult task in choosing between two models, if the X^2 values are low relative to the degrees of freedom for each model. On the other hand it certainly must solve the related problem 'is a vulnerability or mutual potentiation model out of the question?'. Using Worcester's model we analysed the Camberwell data on which Tennant & Bebbington based their 1978 conclusion that a vulnerability model was out of the question. Table 5.4 compares the goodness of fit of their original model and the Worcester model and allows us to conclude that they were no less 'premature' in their decision that a vulnerability model was out of the question than we were supposed to be in deciding that it was relevant (Everitt & Smith, 1979).

In conclusion it should perhaps be stated that we have never been particularly wedded to a *pure* vulnerability model and do not think it would be of any practical or theoretical importance if a vulnerability factor such as lack of intimacy did have a small independent effect. However, we have so far been intrigued that the evidence supporting a pure vulnerability model has been so impressive – not least because, as already argued, errors in rating would tend to militate against such support. Support is so impressive that, as we have seen, a strict non-hierarchical statistical test of the model which Bishop and colleagues have shown can be formulated in a log-linear framework (1975: 111–14) does show a close fit. We therefore have no doubt that it is at present the most accurate and useful way of describing the kind of results summarised in Table 5.3 concerning lack of support. We also believe that the kind of simple X^2 statistical tests presented in that table are unlikely to mislead the reader who studies the tabular results in detail. Moreover, we have seen that a non-hierarchical

Table 5.4. *Analyses of the association between unemployment (A), provoking agent (B) and caseness (C). Models 1–5 by hierarchical analysis (see Tennant & Bebbington, 1978); models 6–8 by Worcester's less restricted method (1971)*

Model	Parameters included				LRX^2	Degrees of freedom
1	AB	AC	BC	ABC	0	0
2	AB	AC	BC	—	1.67	1
3	AB	AC	—	—	20.52	2
4	AB	—	BC	—	5.77	2
5	—	AC	BC	—	1.69	2
6	—	—	BC	ABC	1.01	2
7	AB	—	—	ABC	7.27	2
8	AB	—	BC	ABC	0.98	1

approach does provide a fully appropriate means of formally testing the model.

Failure to replicate. Given acceptance of additive and non-hierarchical models and given the impressive replications of the results for lack of intimacy with husband or boyfriend, it is still necessary to consider several recent studies that have been cited as providing negative evidence for the vulnerability model. A distinction must be made between failure to replicate and disagreement about the statistical and theoretical *interpretation* of the results. For example, we have seen (Table 5.3) that Costello's (1982) Calgary study provides exactly the same support for a vulnerability model as the original Camberwell results and yet the study itself concluded that it provided no support and this conclusion was repeated by Wing & Bebbington in a recent review (1982). In fact this is entirely the result of employing a log-linear analysis which, as already seen, cannot be used in a straightforward way to test a vulnerability model. It also underlines the importance of looking at results independently of statistical tests: surely it should at least have been noted that the actual results were an almost perfect *replication* of the original study.

If the issue of statistical treatment is henceforth set aside, there remain four criteria concerning measurement and design that must be met for a satisfactory replication of the Camberwell vulnerability model. To our knowledge seven studies other than those already cited considered the role of 'stressors' and 'support' in the development of depression and in doing so produced evidence of some relevance for testing the vulnerability model. (Most refer explicitly to their work's relevance for testing the model in terms of intimacy with husband). All conclude that there is no support for the vulnerability model or wish to amend it in important ways. (One exception is a study by Roy (1978) which, since it did not examine for the presence of a 'stressor', has been excluded as it does not reach even minimal criteria for an adequate test.) Table 5.5 reviews the studies in terms of the four criteria. It is notable that all but one fail to exclude chronic conditions and all have at least two major shortcomings. For example, the study by Solomon & Bromet (1982), cited by Wing & Bebbington (1982) as failing to support the vulnerability model, merely established the presence of depression during the year before interview, ignoring any date of onset in the year or whether it was present at the start of the year (i.e. was 'chronic'); the measure of support from husband was adequate but the measurement of provoking agents was not.

Table 5.5. *Minimal criteria for a test of the vulnerability model and some recent studies*

	Solomon & Bromet (1982) (Pennsylvania)	Miller *et al.* (1976) (Edinburgh)	Aneshensel & Stone (1982) (Los Angeles)	Frydman (1981) (Australia)	Andrews *et al.* (1978) (Sydney)	Lin *et al.* (1979) (Washington)	Henderson *et al.* (1981) (Canberra)
Exclusion of chronic conditions	No	No	No	No	No	No	
Distinction between 'case' and 'borderline case'		No		No	No	No	No
Appropriate measurement of provoking agents	No			No	No	No	No
Appropriate measurement of vulnerability factors			No	No	No	No	?

Some further considerations on the interaction between provoking agents and vulnerability factors

(*a*) *Bias and contamination through the rating procedure*

Tennant, Bebbington & Hurry (1981*a*) in a general discussion of life events raise a potentially serious criticism of the contextual approach. They argue that the overlap between two types of causal factor in this model is too great for a true test of the vulnerability model: 'The contextual rating of an event is based on social data which also serve as "independent" antecedent variables. . . This procedure would tend to produce an association between life events [they mean severe long-term contextual threat events] and other antecedent variables which would not be empirical, and would thus overestimate the causal role of "life events" in illness.' This is a fair point and deserves serious consideration. They are suggesting that raters will produce an association between vulnerability factor and provoking agent which is 'illicit' because the rules for rating contextual threat specify that certain otherwise minor threat events will be rated severe because of the presence of a vulnerability factor and this would tend to confound any conclusions about the relative roles of provoking agent and vulnerability factor.

This possibility merits two comments. First, the rules very rarely make such a specification; second, when they do it is not 'illicit' in the way implied. Starting with the first, it is necessary to emphasise that the sorts of things relevant for rating contextual threat rarely coincide exactly with definitions of the vulnerability factors. For example, the presence of *any* young children at home will increase the threatfulness of a financial difficulty but the presence of *three* children under 14 (the vulnerability factor) would not be crucial for deciding the severity of the difficulty, say, compared with two or four children. Similarly the subject's own employment is only of crucial relevance to threat ratings if there is no other wage earner in the family, a rare phenomenon in female samples. In our Camberwell sample there were only 15 single parents, and more than half of these were working. And even when the subject *is* the 'chief wage earner' mere lack of employment is not the feature which raises the threat rating of events: it is any financial or interpersonal tension difficulty associated with the lack of employment which has this impact on the long-term contextual threat. It will not be difficult for readers to agree that loss of mother before 11 is so much out of the current context that it almost never affects a threat rating in contemporary life in this crucial way.

The fourth vulnerability factor, lack of a confiding relationship in husband or boyfriend has the strongest potential link with contextual threat, but even that role is not strong. Very often the existence of a *major* marital difficulty forms the background context which puts an event (such as a pregnancy of subject or a loss of job by husband) up into severe threat when it would otherwise be minor threat. However, greater 'objective' evidence of marital disturbance than mere lack of confiding (say, of violence or of neglect) is required for a marital difficulty to be rated major. Only 12% of the Camberwell women with a 'non-a' relationship (i.e. no close confiding relationship with husband) had a *major* marital difficulty, that is a provoking agent. So what of lack of confiding on its own? When does it influence threat ratings? There is the quite clear rule, and one which operates regularly, that when a subject has only one confidant the loss of that confidant is more severe on threat than when she already has an alternative confidant. Thus a woman whose female confidant friend moves to Birmingham with the result that she can only visit her once every few months whereas she previously saw her twice a week will be rated differently on the severity of this 'interaction change' event according to whether she has another confidant nearby or not. If she has another female confidant *and* she confides in her husband it will not be a severely threatening interaction change. If she has no other confidant (neither husband nor female friend) it will be registered as severe, thus as a provoking agent. It is thus clear that in rating the threat of loss of confidant events, one may be required by the rules to consider the vulnerability factor of not confiding in husband/boyfriend. But how often does this in fact occur?

To answer this we considered our original ratings. We asked ourselves whether or not, in rating each severe event *or* major difficulty, knowledge of either lack of intimacy with husband, three or more children under 14 at home, or lack of employment would be likely to have determined the fact that they were given these particular threat ratings. Or, put another way, was the event or difficulty and its immediate context enough to have classified it severely threatening without either direct knowledge of the presence of one of the vulnerability factors, or a reasonable hunch that it was present – for example, from being told that the two did not get on well and had not had sexual intercourse for several years.

The results of the exercise were surprisingly clearcut. We considered that only a few of the severe events and difficulties *could* have been influenced in this way. For instance, one severe event consisted of a husband returning to live at home unexpectedly because of chronic arthritis, after working at sea for many years. The couple had got on very badly in the past and his staying at home would be likely to cause financial problems. Here we felt we would have implicitly taken into account lack of confiding, although the difficulty in the relationship had far broader ramifications. Much the same can be concluded about a severe threat to another woman whose mother-in-law living next door was her only confidant and who moved out of London with the result that they could only see each other once every 6 weeks. We felt that we would again implicitly have taken into account the lack of a confiding relationship with her husband. But by the same kind of argument we could exclude many from risk of contamination. For example, the confidant of one woman, a man, had been seen almost daily for 20 years (he was married and felt he could not separate from his handicapped wife); when he died the woman had no other close confidant. This was excluded from the risk of contamination as we argued that it would have been rated as a severe event even if she had had a confiding relationship with a husband. We used a similar logic with a housing problem when we could argue that the difficulty would certainly be a major one even if the subject had only one or two, not three, children under 14 (the vulnerability factor). In the first Camberwell sample we considered that at most only 5 of the 97 women with a provoking agent had this potential contamination and even this is probably an overestimate as our judgments were conservative in the sense of including women where there was any doubt at all as to the possibility of contamination. We therefore conclude that the kind of bias Tennant and his colleagues appear to have had in mind could not have played an important part in our results, particularly if it is recalled that it would have occurred for normal women as well as those developing depression.

It is necessary to make a final point before leaving this topic. Tennant & Bebbington confuse two things when they comment on the possible illicit conclusions. The first, which is quite fair, and has already been covered, is that such contamination will radically threaten a proper choice between models assessing the relative contribution of each type of variable. The second is implicit in their comment: 'As it stands, Brown's measures might be more accurately described as a measure of general 'social stress' rather than as a "life events" measure per se' and this point must be rejected. It suggests that somehow 'pure' life event measures are superior to measures of general social stress. Few epidemiologists have the proof or disproof of the vulnerability model as their main purpose; most are in business to predict illness and thus if a measure of 'general social stress' should turn out to have superior predictive power to a sterilised measure of 'life events *per se*' it is to be preferred for that particular task rather than facing all-round rejection on grounds of some 'impurity'. In fact it is just such 'impurity' which we would maintain is the merit of the contextual approach. As Tomkins notes concerning a somewhat similar problem in the measurement of emotion: 'the pursuit of purity and decontamination of ambiguity is not without a serious price when it pulls apart what nature has joined together' (Tomkins, 1981: 314).

At this point it may be fruitful to repeat some points touched on earlier in connection with long-term difficulties which have direct bearing on this issue of the complexity of the experience of stress. First, one of the advantages of the LEDS over other instruments is, we believe, its measurement of difficulties. Second, we acknowledge the frequent links between difficulties and events but rather than trying to get rid of them by changing the instrument, we see their successful reflection in the measures as likely to enhance understanding. Third, we acknowledge the frequency with which the existence of certain long-term difficulties is actually built into the rules for raising the threat of certain events (e.g. a pregnancy to the subject is usually not in itself judged a severe event but if there is a major marital or housing difficulty it will usually become so by definition). This is the feature which so alarmed Tennant & Bebbington but, of course, since we put major difficulties into the same 'box' as severe events in our model (the provoking agent box), there is no good reason for alarm about the overlap between events and difficulties as there might be between provoking agents and vulnerability factors.

One further 'contamination' which is occasionally mentioned is that between lack of intimacy and marital status (Waring *et al.*, 1980). We do not regard this as a contamination but accept it as an inevitable overlap, and attribute the higher prevalence of depression among the widowed, divorced and separated to the lesser frequency of intimate relationships. But for the record it should be said that when only married women were selected the vulnerability model still obtained for intimacy (the percentage of onsets of depression which would fall into the four columns of Table 5.3 were 34% (16/47), 10% (8/81), 6% (2/34) and 1% (2/186). It can be seen from this that the degree of overlap is not that great anyway. As many as 59% (81/138) of those who lacked 'a' intimate relationships were actually married.

(*b*) *Bias stemming from the analysis*

Another possibility of bias stemming from the confounding of provoking agent and vulnerability factor arises from the data analysis itself. If vulnerability factors tend to be linked with the occurrence of more than one provoking agent (see section on additivity, p. 138), these, rather than the vulnerability factor itself, may be the reason for the increased risk of depression. A recent direct check on this possibility did not suggest it was of any significance although further checks should be made (Brown & Prudo, 1981: 596).

Before leaving the topic of vulnerability it may be important to repeat the point that there will very often be more than one vulnerability factor in a model. The discussions here have been couched in terms of presence or absence of one particular factor mainly for the sake of simplicity since examples of tables with more than three dimensions are less easy to follow. However, it is essential to consider more complex situations. One straightforward approach is merely to consider whether the person has *at least one* of the listed vulnerability factors. One of the results which originally confirmed our confidence in the distinction between provoking agents and these other factors was obtained when we applied just such a generalised dimension. When women in Camberwell with a provoking agent but no vulnerability factor are compared with those with at least one vulnerability factor but no provoking agent, the former had a higher rate of depression – 11% (4/35) versus 1% (2/151). Admittedly numbers are small, but there is nothing to shake our conviction that the two types of factor are not interchangeable in terms of producing depression.

Another implication of the existence of more than one vulnerability factor is that analyses of their additivity can contribute to model building. For example, when women with a provoking agent and *one* vulnerability factor were compared with those who had two or more vulnerability factors but no provoking agent, there was, again, nothing to suggest that the two types of factor had comparable effects – 12% (10/83) of the former developed depression compared with only 3% (1/39) of the latter. In this context it may be worth reminding the reader of the very different results we obtained from the similar exercise comparing effects of severe events and major difficulties which confirmed our decision to include both with provoking agents despite the difficulties having no discrete occurrence in time (see p. 140).

Cross-cultural research

'Cross-cultural' research is not ruled out by a contextual approach. In fact over 30 research centres have had at least one person trained in the LEDS and many have been from outside the United Kingdom – for example, from Australia, Austria, Canada, Eire, Germany, Italy and the United States. It or a closely similar version has been employed in a range of cultures – for example, in the Outer Hebrides, Vienna, Nairobi, Prague, Aarhus, Chandigarh in India, several places in Germany and Italy, and Calgary in Canada. First, it can be stated that we have received no report other than from India that there have been significant difficulties in applying the life events section of the LEDS (Day *et al.*, 1982). We do not suggest that in the 'translation' of the ratings cultural factors can be ignored; nor that certain events do not differ in significance – for example, in our own experience in the Outer Hebrides loss of job and resulting unemployment of anyone in the immediate family appeared to trouble women less than in London (Brown & Prudo, 1981; Prudo *et al.*, 1981). What is clear is that the contextual approach is surprisingly flexible in coping with such variations. In the Hebrides the fact that there was often some work on the croft and that many of the men had multiple jobs was almost certainly reflected in our ratings. A more dramatic example concerns the small study in Kenya for which events were rated blind by our own unit (Vadher & Ndetei, 1981). It was still culturally acceptable for husbands to obtain second wives and several of the women had experienced this. However, it was clear that the circumstances surrounding some of the marriages had departed significantly from traditional practice and that the event had some of the feel of the western practice of taking a mistress with its implication of rejection of the wife. In our blind ratings we rated such events severe and they all turned out in fact to antedate a serious depressive disorder.

However, we do not wish to underplay potential difficulties. For example, what is the significance in a peasant culture if all the children in a family decide to work away from the family land and how should account be taken of the great emphasis in certain rural areas of Europe of the virginity of a woman if she is to make an acceptable marriage (e.g. Cutileiro, 1971)? Moreover, in the setting of developing countries in particular, it is likely to prove far easier to transfer the part of the LEDS concerned with discrete crises than that dealing with ongoing difficulties such as poor or overcrowded housing. For example, a recent study in a rural community in south Portugal showed that somewhat over half of the dwellings were without glass windows, running water, a butane cooker, lavatory, plaster ceilings, bath and tiled floor (Jenkins *et al.*, 1979: 39). Standards developed in London would suggest these villagers had major housing problems, a judgment almost certainly out of keeping with local feelings.

While it would be ill-judged to underplay the apparent success of these early cross-cultural studies there is a need for a general strategy to deal with apparent anomalies. We suggest that in the first place the standards developed in London should be applied, although for 'new' events such as instances of polygamous marriage in Nairobi rating examples must be extended and some consideration taken of local practice. This step is essential to provide some kind of touchstone for cultural differences. However, in addition, whenever it appears appropriate, parallel ratings should be developed that are more sensitive to local values and experience. For these it may be necessary to take more account of self-reports of response than is strictly allowed by the contextual approach. Almost certainly something like this will be required to deal with difficulties: it is unclear how far it will be necessary for events. Some such procedure appears to have been necessary in the Indian enquiry although not to the extent that some might have envisaged (Day *et al.*, 1982).

Some substantive issues

So far we have concentrated on issues of method and design and dealt with substantive findings as a backdrop to these. We will end by discussing some such issues in their own right. Two, concerning early loss of a parent and social class, have been involved in recent controversy in the sense of how far results have been replicated. The third, concerning the nature of the depressive disorders studied, has proved controversial less because of conflicting findings than because of the inherent complexity of the issues and perhaps the understandable tendency for psychiatrists to be sceptical about any aetiological theory that places critical importance on the role of psychosocial factors in the severest depressive conditions.

In the course of discussing certain methodological issues we have referred on several occasions to substantive results confirming the role of confiding as a vulnerability factor. Before turning to the role of loss of mother in childhood, it may be fruitful to remind the reader of the general stance we take on the role of vulnerability factors and to say a few words about the other two (employment and three or more children at home under 14). In general we see these factors as relatively crude indicators of some underlying process, such as low self-esteem or mastery, which is where the source of depression lies, rather than as straightforward causes of depression in their own right. Although the intimacy rating is less crude in this sense we have consistently argued that it may not necessarily be confiding as such which is critical. At the moment we would argue no more than that it is likely to be a reasonably good indicator of the feelings of self-worth and security which a woman receives from the relationship. The prospective study in Islington is designed to explore exactly what is involved: for example, is it support at the time of the crisis, is it the tension-relieving quality of a good, long-term sexual relationship, or is it the long-term identity enhancement of an approving confidant which provides the protection? Employment and three or more children under 14 at home are even more atheoretical indicators, and so one would expect them to be highly sensitive to any changes in population where cultural or subcultural variations may powerfully influence their relationship to the underlying process. There is thus likely to be more difficulty in obtaining replications for these two factors. The elucidation of the role of lack of employment was particularly complicated in the Camberwell research: it only emerged when considered in the light of the other three factors. Warr & Parry (1982) have a useful review of the whole topic and we will not attempt to go over the same ground. They note the complexities and call for improved research along the lines of a conceptual framework which they develop. The relationship of lack of employment to depression has been a particularly unstable finding and we fully concur with their conclusions. However, despite the difficulties of empirical research we continue to be impressed by the tremendous difference a job can apparently make to a woman both in helping to avoid the consequences of a major loss or disappointment and in helping to reduce the severity and length of a particular depressive illness. This leaves the role of having three or more children under 14 living at home. It is obvious that the impact of such a factor is particularly likely to be dependent on the more general context of a woman's life, on social provisions of nursery schools and free reliable contraception. It is enough to bear in mind its likely interaction with social class; not only will the resources of a middle-class woman be superior but she will more probably deliberately have chosen to have three or more children. Results are also likely to be influenced by the fact that women living as single parents are particularly likely to suffer from depression and yet tend to have fewer children than other women (e.g. Brown & Harris, 1978*a*; Surtees *et al.*, 1983). There have been some reports of replication of this particular result (e.g. Brown & Prudo, 1981; Campbell, Cope & Teasdale, 1983), but the need to move beyond the highly atheoretical indicator of number of children is obvious.

Vulnerability and replication: early loss of mother

The aetiological model isolated in the original Camberwell enquiry included early loss of mother before 11; the aggregate term 'loss' combined deaths with any separation for a minimum of one year except for war-time evacuation. The omission of the latter was for pragmatic reasons, and in current research we are aiming to look at this category more thoroughly. Along with this impact upon incidence went a greater prevalence of depression among such women in the general population, but a higher rate among the patient series just failed to reach statistical significance. Since then, two recent reviews dealing with loss of parent in childhood have been sceptical about the presence of any aetiological effect (Crook & Eliot, 1980; Tennant, Bebbington & Hurry, 1980*a*); although the group at the Institute of Psychiatry have recently somewhat modified their entirely negative conclusion (Tennant *et al.*, 1982*a*). Only one recent review finds evidence to be more convincing (Lloyd, 1980: 534).

None-the-less, two further population studies carried out in Islington and Walthamstow have produced unequivocal evidence for the importance of early loss of mother. The Walthamstow enquiry was designed especially to tackle the question of early loss and over 3000 women were screened to provide instances of such loss. Those with early loss of mother by death, or separation for at least one year, had a significantly higher rate of current depression at a caseness level and this held for losses up to the age of 17 and for working-class and middle-class women. Those with a loss before 11 had a higher rate than those with a loss between 11 and 17, although this did not reach statistical significance. Differences for loss of father did not reach statistical significance, although there was some hint that loss of a father by separation may somewhat increase risk of later depression (Brown *et al.*, 1985).

The Islington prospective survey has involved the study of some 400, largely working-class, women with at least one child living at home. Those with an early loss of mother experienced double the prevalence of depression at a caseness level. Again the high rate of depression among those losing a mother between 11 and 17 suggests that our original Camberwell cut-off at age 11 may have been rather too hastily adopted.

Given these three results from large-scale London-based enquiries it is necessary to ask why other published studies have been so inconsistent and how seriously the scepticism of the recent reviews should be taken? It is necessary at once to recognise the frequent shortcomings of design which may well have produced both negative and positive findings (Granville-Grossman, 1968). It is also worth emphasising the crudity of many efforts to measure early loss. A research report by one of the recent set of reviewers, for example, merely states that separations from a parent of two weeks or more were unrelated to current psychiatric disorder among a random sample of men and women in Camberwell in south London (Tennant *et al.*, 1980*b*). There is nothing, that we are aware of, suggesting that a separation of such a short length would be correlated with any long-term consequences. However, undoubtedly the greatest shortcoming has been failure to take account of the highly complex chain of experience that must link loss of a parent and later depression, and of the fact that if populations are studied where factors which provide crucial intervening links tend to be lacking, then the association between loss of a parent and depression in adult life is bound to be low. There has, for example, been a general failure to recognise the importance of the key final link – that most episodes of depression appear to result from *current* adversity whatever the contribution of early experience to vulnerability.

Given that early loss of a parent acts as a vulnerability factor, it is likely to show a relatively low association with prevalence of depression in any population with a low rate of provoking agents. This is because a vulnerability factor cannot act without the presence of a provoking agent. Furthermore, since risk of depression increases with the number of vulnerability factors, early loss of a mother will be more highly associated with depression in any population in which such loss is correlated with other vulnerability factors such as having three or more children under 14 living at home. In Camberwell, at least, both points hold for working-class women – they more often experienced provoking agents and vulnerability factors, and among them early loss of mother was more highly correlated with the other vulnerability factors, and it is therefore perhaps not surprising that the link between early loss of mother and depression clearly held only among working-class women.* Very few other *population* surveys have considered the long-term effect of losing a parent. The midtown survey in New York reported by Langner & Michael (1963) is the only one to our knowledge which gives results in terms of social class. Only loss of mother, not of father, related to current psychiatric state and the association for loss of mother by death held only for 'lower-class' women. This social-class effect seen in London and New York is probably enough to explain the negative results obtained in a recent small, but well-conducted survey by John Birtchnell of women whose mothers had died in childhood and who were currently living in the Chichester area of West Sussex, a notably prosperous English county town (Birtchnell, 1980).

Findings concerning early loss will, therefore, almost certainly vary with the social composition of the population studied – in general, the lower the rate of provoking agents and the vulnerability factors other than early loss, the lower will be the association between early loss and current depression. However, it is still necessary to consider another study with seemingly negative results as it was carried out in the same location as our first

* 58% (15/26) of working-class women with a loss of mother before 11 were cases compared with 20% (43/214) without such a loss ($P < 0.001$). Figures for middle-class women were 14% (2/14) and 8% (16/204) respectively (ns).

enquiry, Camberwell, and thus cannot be accounted for by varying rates of severe life events and different class compositions between populations (Bebbington *et al.*, 1981*a*). One complication in coming to terms with this study is that the results have been presented in five papers often in rather differing ways, both in terms of the measures of loss and in terms of statistical methods. In some of their more recent publications (Tennant *et al.*, 1982*a, b*) the authors seem to be moving towards the conclusion that there do exist some effects of childhood loss of parent upon depression in adult life. At any rate, it is likely that their earlier failure to detect effects of separations could be due, as already noted, to their having taken too short a duration of separation at that time (Tennant *et al.*, 1980*b*). Moreover, their claim that early death of mother is unrelated to adult morbidity is contradicted by their own data. This shows a higher rate for those who are cases for those with maternal death both at 0–10 and 11–18 but neither on its own reaches statistical significance (Tennant *et al.*, 1981*c*: table 2, p. 311). However, if the two loss groups are combined the difference between maternal-loss and maternal-no-loss groups is statistically significant (7% of non-cases having a loss of mother and 14% of cases, $P < 0.05$; this has been confirmed by personal communication with Tennant).

The mode of the impact of early loss is undoubtedly complex and on the basis of the research in Walthamstow we have emphasised the role of untoward experiences such as lack of adequate care by surrogate parents *after* the loss in influencing long-term cognitive sets such as helplessness, and the woman's social class position. Experiences such as premarital pregnancy which are related to early loss of mother, and the way of coping with them, must provide an important part of any final explanation (Brown *et al.*, 1985*c*). It is too soon to be sure how far early loss of mother acts as a vulnerability factor in the sense formulated in the original Camberwell enquiry; this has not yet been directly re-examined. None-the-less, that it has some long-term impact is becoming increasingly less controversial – but this must not be seen in absolute terms. Just what is found concerning early loss will almost certainly depend on the nature of the population studied. Studies of women in inner city areas have produced the most clearcut findings and this might well be linked with certain selective processes: perhaps women whose experiences following loss of a mother were the most unpleasant and least well coped with tend to be the women who are to be found in inner city areas – further, the higher rate of provoking agents in such areas is likely to highlight any underlying greater vulnerability.

Social class position

Given the great complexity of experiences of inequality and other correlates of class position, what justification is there for the general use of the crude and arbitrary methods of measurement of class based on indicators like occupation? For example, should occupation be the sole measure of class, or should it be combined with or displaced by income, educational attainment, possession of car and telephone, subscription to certain attitudes, or even by a subjective definition of class by the interviewee himself? In fact for studies of psychiatric disorder and distress, at least, the same associations emerge whatever index is used (Kessler, 1982). For the Camberwell material it mattered remarkably little what indicator was taken – eight measures ranging from occupation of household head to a woman's educational level gave similar results with the 'lower' groups having the highest rate of disorder (Brown & Harris, 1982*c*: table 1).

There are several excellent reviews of the relationship of social class and mental disorder. Particularly notable are those produced by the Dohrenwends who conclude that most studies show the greater prevalence of psychiatric disorder in the lower social classes and this also holds for affective disorder (Dohrenwend & Dohrenwend, 1969, 1974; Dohrenwend, 1975). A more recent review reached the same conclusion about depression (Bebbington, 1978). Studies in North America have largely used questionnaire-type instruments. These give results that agree in broad terms with those of standardised clinical-type interview instruments, such as the Present State Examination (PSE) and the Schedule for Affective Disorders and Schizophrenia–Research Diagnostic Criteria (SADS–RDC) (Spitzer, Endicott & Robins, 1978; Wing, Cooper & Sartorius, 1974). However, such self-report questionnaires almost certainly overestimate the overall prevalence of disorder, because a number of individuals who report high scores do not suffer from psychiatric disorder (Finlay-Jones & Murphy, 1979). Furthermore they probably cannot be used to distinguish conditions, such as depression, anxiety and phobia, and obsessional disorder. However, because depressive phenomena seem to be the most common of psychiatric disorders, at least in urban settings, they probably provide a rough index of the distribution of depression. Two studies in the United States using such questionnaires have shown sizable class differences (Warheit, Holzer & Schwab, 1973; Comstock & Helsing, 1976). The first population survey in North America using a clinical-type interview (SADS–RDC) has also shown social class differences in 'minor depression' but the trend does not reach significance for 'major depression' (Weissman & Myers, 1979).

Unfortunately, because it was part of a long-term prospective study with some fallout over the years, and because the SADS–RDC was only employed on the last wave of interviews, the percentage of the original sample actually interviewed was low (511 of 938, or 54%). It is possible that this high rate of drop-out would introduce some bias into the conclusions based upon the remainder.

Clinical-type interviews have been more commonly employed in Great Britain, and they also show much higher working-class rates of disorder (Richman, 1974, 1976; Rutter *et al.*, 1975; Rutter & Quinton, 1977). Our own survey, using the PSE on a random sample of 458 women living in Camberwell in southeast London, showed that affective disorder (depression in particular) was much more common among working-class women: 23% were considered to be cases in the 3 months before the interview, compared to only 6% of middle-class women.

An important survey has just been published concerning the prevalence of psychiatric disorder in a random sample of 576 women living in an Edinburgh community, using the PSE and the SADS to which RDC can be applied. Large and statistically significant class differences emerged using all instruments and the authors see the work as a confirmation of the class differences revealed in the Camberwell survey (Surtees *et al.*, 1983).

To our knowledge there is only one large-scale population survey of an urban population, using clinical-type measures, that has failed to find a social class difference. Bebbington and his colleagues (1981*a*) did not find a significant difference in rates of morbidity between social classes, using the PSE–Index of Definition (ID) system to measure psychiatric disorder in Camberwell – in fact a significant difference *was* obtained for men and the trend for women was in the anticipated direction (for one measure of disorder 11% and 18% (Bebbington *et al.*, 1981*a*: table 10) and for an alternative measure 13% and 21%). None-the-less it is an unexpected result. Surtees and his colleagues suggest that it may be related to certain differences in procedure – they used staff revisits and a case-weighting procedure but their sample was relatively small ($N = 161$) and, of course, the same differences would reach significance with larger samples – for example, the last result reaches significance if the sample is doubled to 322. Perhaps, therefore, too much should not be made of their findings given the general agreement of a very wide range of studies. However, the fact that they also failed to find any difference between case rates for married and for separated/divorced/widowed women suggests that they were dealing with a very unusual sample since this difference has been universally found (Briscoe & Smith, 1973; Gove, 1973; Bachrach, 1975;

Bloom, Asher & White, 1978, etc.). While we see the study as providing no justification for controversy at present, we believe that it would be highly misleading to expect such class differences as a matter of course. Studies in rural populations, for example, have tended not to show class differences (e.g. Leighton, Hagnell & Leighton, 1971). We confirmed this in a study in two rural samples of women in the Outer Hebrides and argued that, while there were important differences *within* the population, these only emerged when demographic-like variables reflecting *integration* into the traditional culture and way of life rather than social class were employed (Brown & Prudo, 1981; Prudo *et al.*, 1981).

It should be emphasised again that in claiming that social class is not of importance in explaining rates of psychiatric disorder in the Outer Hebrides, we refer to measures based on occupation. We do not claim that social class viewed in more fundamental terms is unimportant. Indeed, the high rate of psychiatric disorder among women living in council housing suggests that there is an important social class component. Such women tend not only to be the least integrated into the traditional culture, but also to be the most likely of all women on the island to have undergone the kind of crises and difficulties experienced by working-class women in Camberwell (Brown & Prudo, 1981; Prudo *et al.*, 1984).

Moreover, we would also expect differences to emerge when comparing urban populations. There is some reason to believe that rates of disorder in Walthamstow in North London may be a good deal lower than in Islington to the south, an inner city area with more obvious social problems. It is also possible that in certain central areas of London, middle-class women might experience particularly high rates of affective disorder (e.g. Finlay-Jones & Brown, 1981). While speculative, these points underline our view that class differences should be a spur to the development of causal models and theory, and that it is highly misleading to concentrate too much on the fact of replication as such. A result based on a crude indicator such as social class should only be considered as a failure in terms of replication if differences in rates of disorder in the population do not coincide with differences in the distribution of underlying factors of known aetiological significance such as the experience of provoking agents.

Interpretations of the dependent variable in life event studies

Although this essay is primarily concerned with life events, the way in which particular conceptions of a dependent variable can radically affect the evaluation of results deserves some comment, particularly in view of

Paul Bebbington's chapter in this volume. He seems to suggest that research based on community studies has little relevance for furthering the understanding of depression in psychiatric patients. This opinion seems to derive from two kinds of argument: first, that studies of depressed *patients* have not shown an aetiological role for life events, and second, that cases of depression in the community are not 'real' but only instances of distress. We will deal with each point in turn.

(a) Are depressed patients somehow different?

The study of psychiatric patients is, of course, subject to all the problems faced by community studies. Has a suitable threshold of severity been established for life events (such as severe long-term contextual threat)? Are difficulties included? Have 'possibly independent' events been ignored? Has the additivity of events been assumed rather than demonstrated? Has due attention been paid to the date of onset and to diagnosis? We have so far considered all but the last two questions. Paradoxically, the rigorous description of symptoms enforced upon those doing community research is not always employed in research among clinic attenders, while this probably does not result in the inclusion of anything more than a handful of subthreshold cases (borderline cases in our terms or minor depressions in RDC terms), it means that research with patients often omits to give detailed symptom pictures. In our experience the distinction between the diagnosis of primary depressive disorder and anxiety states with secondary depression is often unclear, and the boundaries between the two can vary strikingly between clinicians. The same seems to apply to three other categories, the schizo-affective and personality disorders, and post-partum depression. In view of the conclusion that events of lesser severity are required to produce schizophrenic onset (see p. 121) and of the possibility that hormonal factors may place many post-partum depressions immediately following birth in a distinct diagnostic category, some detailed discussion of the symptoms would clearly be helpful before conclusions about the role of life events in causing primary depression can be drawn with any validity from samples of psychiatric patients. It is our impression that many patients with affective disorders have been suffering for months with clearcut symptoms before they are referred to psychiatric hospitals and concern with dating of onset is even more essential. Unless this is done in a precise and standardised way, there is always the danger that a point in time quite close to the start of treatment will be arbitrarily chosen as the date of onset. This tendency will be enhanced if the clinician has been trained to be suspicious of any data about symptoms based on a recall

Table 5.6. *Summary of recent studies of life events and onset of depression among psychiatric patients*

Source	Number of		Proportion with at least one event			
	Patients	Comparison group	Patients (%)	Comparison group (%)	Period covered	Type of event
Paykel *et al.* (1969) (New Haven)	185	185	44	17	6 months	'Undesirable'
Brown & Harris (1978*a*) (London)	114	382	61	19	8 months	'Severe threat'[d]
Barrett (1979) (Boston)	130	—	58	—	6 months	'Undesirable'
Glassner *et al.* (1979) (New York)	25[a]	25	56	16	12 months	'Major role loss'
Fava *et al.* (1981) (Padua)	40	40	73	30	6 months	'Uncontrollable'
Benjaminsen (1981) (Odense, Denmark)	89	—	63	—	6 months	'Severe loss'
Vahder & Ndetei (1981) (Nairobi)	30	40	67	8	12 months	'Severe threat'[d]
Murphy (1982) (London)	100[b]	168	48	23	12 months	'Severe threat'[d]
Katschnig *et al.* (1981) (Vienna)	176[e]	—	42[e]	—	12 months	'Severe threat'[d]
Bebbington *et al.* (1981*b*) (London)	45[c]	257	18	10	3 months	'Marked and moderate threat – independent events'

[a] Manic-depressive, bipolar sample.
[b] Elderly sample aged 65–87 years.
[c] Includes some anxiety states.
[d] Either independent or possibly independent events.
[e] Special analysis for this chapter.

period of more than one month. (It is ironic how often this refusal to trust retrospective data prevents the exclusion of events and vulnerability factors which have developed *after* onset of symptoms and are thus irrelevant for their aetiology.)

Table 5.6 summarises the results of recent studies which meet the criteria specified for both the measures of life events and attention to the dependent variable. As can be seen the proportion with at least one of the specified types of events among patients in all but one of these studies is similar to that found in community 'cases' and provides no justification for the belief that there is something which sets patients apart and requires a quite different aetiological model. The only exception is the recent report by Bebbington *et al.* (1981*b*); however, they failed to include 'possibly independent' events, took a period of only 3 months and their specification of onset date and symptom picture is unclear. There is every likelihood that those differences are enough to explain their quite discrepant results. A similar study at roughly the same time by Katschnig *et al.* (1981) found that only 86 of the 176 psychiatric patients had as long as 6 months symptom-free before the index episode of the project, suggesting that unless great care is taken patient samples may contain substantial numbers of chronic cases and thus distort a clear picture of aetiology (see p. 234).

(*b*) *Are community cases somehow different?*

Bebbington and his colleagues also suggested in the same report (1981*b*) that cases in the community are only examples of distress. It is not so much the use of the term 'distress' in contrast to, say, 'disease', on which attention should be focused, but upon the word 'only'. David Goldberg (1982) in discussing general practice attenders contrasts distress requiring intervention from distress not requiring intervention; the former clearly does not have the same implication as the phrase 'only distress'. It would probably be wise to shift our focus for the moment away from the word 'distress', and from debate about the boundaries of the disease concept and consider the problem in its straightforward form: in what way could cases in the community differ so radically from patients that factors bringing about their depressions are irrelevant for depressed patients? It can hardly be a straightforward issue of severity since, whatever the instrument (be it SADS–RDC or Index of Definition for the PSE), thresholds for distinguishing cases from non-cases have been set with the notion of a comparable severity with psychiatric patients explicitly in mind. The Bedford College caseness threshold falls, if anything, at a higher severity level than the SADS–RDC or ID (Dean, Surtees & Sashidharan 1983; Brown, Craig &

Harris, 1985*b*). Of course, given everyone reaches a certain minimal threshold of severity, there can be differences in severity above it between community cases and patients. Our own five-point measure of severity certainly suggested that in-patients were on the whole more severely disturbed than out-patients, but severity among out-patients was barely higher than among the community cases. Far from seeing such a gradation in severity (above a certain threshold) as a reason to set apart a separate aetiological model – at least for in-patients – we found that such variation in severity could be incorporated into our aetiological model. We developed a notion of change-point in severity of symptoms in order to take account of marked changes in severity after original onset, usually taking place over a matter of days. We found that out-patients and in-patients did not differ in severity at point of first onset but that in-patients become more severely ill because of subsequent worsenings of their condition in most instances involving only one change-point. It was further shown that these subsequent changes tended to be brought about by the same kind of severe events so often involved in bringing about the original onset (Brown & Harris, 1978*a*: chapter 13).

If severity does not explain the fundamental difference suggested between patients and community cases, perhaps it might be a matter of duration. In an earlier report Tennant & Bebbington (1978) refer to 'transient situational disturbances', a term which appears to have been the forerunner of their usage of 'only distress'. Unfortunately it would be necessary to follow patients and community cases prospectively in order to distinguish genuine recoveries from fluctuations in an ongoing episode, and such data is not available; but the retrospective data already collected has important implications which should not be ignored. In all of our eight studies (Camberwell I and II, North Uist, Lewis, Walthamstow a and b, Regents Park, Islington) there were as many women with episodes which they claimed had lasted more than 12 months as those with new onsets during the previous year. Data from other research units in Britain suggests much the same result (e.g. Campbell, 1982; Bebbington *et al.*, 1984). There is some suggestion that in more prosperous populations studied in the Commonwealth the ratio of chronic to onset cases is somewhat lower but still substantial (Henderson *et al.*, 1981: 121; Costello, 1982). Therefore it is clear that a considerable proportion of cases are anything but transient, and it is in any case worth pointing out that the definition of 'transient situational disturbance' in the ninth edition of the Internal Classification of Disease (ICD) (category 307) extends only to hours or days rather than months.

A third possibility is that *type* of symptom is the crucial discriminating feature between community cases and patients; there is certainly evidence that the proportion of 'psychotic' symptom pictures is low in a random community sample. However, it does not follow that the number of community cases with vegetative symptoms such as sleep disturbance, early waking, loss of appetite, weight or libido, is also low. In any case if the different rates of 'psychotic' symptom pictures are to be taken as the grounds for proposing two aetiological models, then neurotic patients should obviously be considered along with the community case model and this does not seem to be part of the particular strategy proposed by Bebbington and his colleagues.

Symptom formation, or the determination of the types of symptoms in a particular syndrome, has been one of the foci of our overall model (Brown & Harris, 1978*a*, particularly chapter 14). In our samples, however, it was not rates of provoking agents or vulnerability factors which distinguished *patients* diagnosed as 'endogenous' from those diagnosed 'neurotic'. This has been confirmed by a number of studies of patient samples (Leff, Roatch & Bunney, 1970; Paykel, Prusoff & Klerman, 1971; Thomson & Hendrie, 1972; Hirschfeld, 1981; Katschnig *et al.*, p. 234 this volume). Nor could we find any relationship among our *community* cases between these independent variables and the patterning of symptoms, unlike Cooke (1980, 1981). It is perhaps worth noting, however, that although employing Paykel's life event interview Cooke only used a Total Life Stress score of the kind discussed earlier rather than the experience of at least one exit or undesirable event as Paykel also did. In our samples other psychosocial 'symptom formation factors', did appear to relate not only to the well-known psychotic–neurotic distinction but also to the degree to which anxiety accompanied depression (Prudo *et al.*, 1981, 1984). This led us to suggest that *style* of attachment to others is a trait which shapes the symptom picture of affective disorder in both community and hospital samples. But hypotheses of this sort can only be properly investigated when comparable ratings of patient and community samples are made in one overall study: to do otherwise at this stage of knowledge would not allow the hypothesis that they differ to be systematically confirmed or refuted.

It is important to emphasise that we are not arguing against the notion that some 'depressions' might differ from others in the factors required to explain them: there is, for example, mounting evidence for a strong genetic contribution to bipolar but not unipolar conditions (Bertelsen, Harvald & Haugue, 1977). We do argue that it would be highly misleading to suggest that the boundaries between these different 'depressions' coincide with the division between community cases and psychiatric patients. When the idiosyncratic nature of many referrals by general practitioners to psychiatrists is considered (Goldberg & Huxley, 1980), it would in any case seem unlikely that patient status could prove a more useful variable than, say, symptom type, previous episode, prior personality, past experience of major loss, attachment style and current events, difficulties and vulnerability factors.

The conviction that the status of the patient is of such rare and central importance is understandable in terms of the historical development of medical thinking but in the 1980s deserves to be supplemented by the conviction that the causal models of epidemiology and sociology are adjuncts not threats to traditional psychiatry. For it is hard to resist the conclusion that despite the internationally accepted progress in the development of diagnostic interviews such as the PSE, the SADS–RDC, DSM-III and Diagnostic Interview Schedule there is still a certain reluctance to relinquish the old approach – one relying not on symptoms alone but on weighting them according to the nature of the circumstances in which they arise. Category 309 of the ninth edition of the ICD, exhibits just such a reluctance: a quite new 'adjustment reaction' is introduced without it being made clear anywhere how it relates to distinctions such as 'minor' versus 'major depression', 'borderline case' versus 'case' and so on; there is merely the implication that there is something to which adjustment is required. It suggests that certain symptomatic reactions to events and difficulties are less serious than 'depression' (ICD, 300.4) but more serious than 'transient situational disturbances' (ICD, 307), but how this might be decided is left quite open. Such vagueness can only be irritating to research workers struggling against the confusions and circularity which result when causal assumptions are built into diagnostic definitions instead of being examined independently (Blumenthal, 1971; Ní Brolcháin, 1979). But a broader, sociological, perspective would suggest that more than mere conservatism is involved. There is probably some failure to meet an important need on the part of recent research, however admirable the clarity of the new diagnostic criteria. One possibility is that since the primary focus of physicians is upon practical intervention, they will have difficulty in adjusting their perspective and practice until recent advances in aetiological theory are supplemented by parallel developments concerning treatment, recovery and relapse. Another possible explanation is that although physicians are quite capable of translating theories about onset into theories about the rate of recovery, this will only be satisfactory if the original theories (about onset) include all the variables which they are accustomed to use, albeit in an intuitive and unsystematic way, in their daily clinical practice. We might speculate, for example, that the crucial features upon which general practitioners base decisions to refer patients to a psychiatric department involve personality and coping strategies, neither of which has received as much detailed exploration as adversity and social support. (Although the Eysenck Personality Inventory may garnish a large number of research projects, use of that type of instrument as such rarely contributes any fundamental additional insight. At present it tends to serve as a residual explanation when doubts arise about other variables – Henderson *et al.*, 1981.) Normative judgments about how patients are coping with adversity and whether they exaggerate or downplay events are probably what is at the heart of the recent distinction between 'depression' and 'adjustment reaction'. Those who react 'abnormally' (that is unusually) would probably be less likely to obtain an 'adjustment reaction' diagnosis in the average general practice surgery than those who despite an equal number of symptoms appear to be trying to cope sensibly without denial or hyperbole, and who, it might well be thought, may therefore be expected to recover spontaneously before too long.

The solution to this kind of muddle is, of course, to encompass the whole range of depressive phenomena in research. For it is only when the totality of these disorders (including what we have called borderline cases) is examined using a full range of variables from demographic, through life events, social support, other vulnerability factors (including childhood experience), personality, coping strategies and physiological susceptibility that the question 'Aren't psychiatric patients different from depressives found in population surveys?' can be answered in an informed way. We have no doubt that when the matter is settled there will be found to be a very substantial overlap between patients and community 'cases'.

Conclusions

It has become a ritual to end reviews such as this with a call for integrated research projects which will span the full range of variables relevant for conditions with a multifactorial aetiology. It was not ritual which led us to make such a call at the end of the last section in the context of topics such as coping, personality and physiological susceptibility. Though it is beyond the scope of this review to describe them, we have been developing measures of the first two for use in our more recent studies. We have also trained a number of workers to use the LEDS in their research into the physiology of depressive disorders. But extension of width will have no value if the depth of the information is curtailed to compensate for the additional expenditure of resources, be it time or money. It has been the intention of this chapter to emphasise above all else the importance of depth of understanding. We see this as the contribution of contextual measurement and of semi-structured interviewing, that without any loss of statistical comparability between classes or groups, one can describe with reliability something of the most private experiences of the soul.

References

Andrews, G. & Tennant, C. (1978). Being upset and becoming ill: an appraisal of the relation between life events and physical illness. *Medical Journal of Australia*, **1**, 324–7.

Andrews, G., Tennant, C., Hawson, D. & Vaillant, G. (1978). Life event stress, social support, coping style, and risk of psychological impairment. *Journal of Nervous and Mental Disease*, **166**, 307–16.

Aneshensel, C. S. & Stone, J. D. (1982). Stress and depression. A test of the buffering model of social support. *Archives of General Psychiatry*, **39**, 1392–6.

Bachrach, L. L. (1975). *Marital status and mental disorder: an analytical review. National Institute of Mental Health*, Series D, No. 3, 1–23. US Department of Health, Education and Welfare.

Barrett, J. E. (1979). The relationship of life events to the onset of neurotic disorders. In *Stress and mental disorders*, ed. J. E. Barrett, pp. 87–109. New York: Raven Press.

Bebbington, P. E. (1978). The epidemiology of depressive disorder. *Culture, Medicine and Psychiatry*, **2**, 297–341.

Bebbington, P. E. (1980). Causal models and logical interference in epidemiological psychiatry. Letter to editor in *British Journal of Psychiatry*, **136**, 317–25.

Bebbington, P., Hurry, J., Tennant, C., Sturt, E. & Wing, J. K. (1981*a*). Epidemiology of mental disorders in Camberwell. *Psychological Medicine*, **11**, 561–79.

Bebbington, P., Sturt, E., Tennant, C. & Hurry, J. (1984). Misfortune and resilience: a replication of the work of Brown & Harris. *Psychological Medicine*, **14**, 347–63.

Bebbington, P., Tennant, C. & Hurry, J. (1981*b*). Adversity and the nature of psychiatric disorder in the community. *Journal of Affective Disorders*, **3**, 345–66.

Benjaminsen, S. (1981). Stressful life events preceding the onset of neurotic depression. *Psychological Medicine*, **11**, 369–78.

Bertelsen, A., Harvald, B. & Haugue, M. (1977). A Danish twin study of manic depressive disorders. *British Journal of Psychiatry*, **130**, 330–51.

Birtchnell, J. (1980). Women whose mothers died in childhood: an outcome study. *Psychological Medicine*, **10**, 699–713.

Bishop, Y. M. M., Fienberg, S. E. & Holland, P. W. (1975). *Discrete multivariate analysis: theory and practice*. Cambridge, Massachussets & London: MIT Press.

Bloom, B. L., Asher, S. J. & White, S. W. (1978). Marital disruption as a stressor: a review and analysis. *Psychological Bulletin*, **85**, 867–94.

Blot, W. J. & Day, N. E. (1978). Synergism and interaction: are they equivalent? *American Journal of Epidemiology*, **110**, 99–100.

Blumenthal, M. (1971). Heterogeneity and research on depressive disorders. *Archives of General Psychiatry*, **24**, 971–8.

Brim, O. G. & Ryff, C. D. (1980). On the properties of life events. In *Life-span development and behaviour, vol. 3*, ed. P. B. Baltes & O. G. Brim, pp. 367–88. London: Academic Press.

Briscoe, C. W. & Smith, M. (1973). Depression and marital turmoil. *Archives of General Psychiatry*, **29**, 812–17.

Brown, G. W. (1981). Life events, psychiatric disorder and physical illness. *Journal of Psychosomatic Research*, **25**, 461–73.

Brown, G. W. (1983). Accounts, meaning and causality. In *Accounts and action*, ed. N. Gilbert & P. Abell, pp. 35–68. Aldershot: Gower Publications.

Brown, G. W., Andrews, B., Bifulco, A., Adler, Z. & Bridge, L. (1985*a*). Social support, self-esteem and depression. MS.

Brown, G. W. & Birley, J. L. T. (1968). Crises and life changes and the onset of schizophrenia. *Journal of Health and Social Behaviour*, **9**, 203–14.

Brown, G. W., Birley, J. L. T. & Wing, J. K. (1972). Influence of family life on the course of schizophrenic disorders: a replication. *British Journal of Psychiatry*, **121**, 241–58.

Brown, G. W., Craig, T. K. J. & Harris, T. O. (1985*b*). Depression: Distress or Disease? Some epidemiological considerations. *British Journal of Psychiatry*, **147**, 612–22.

Brown, G. W. & Davidson, S. (1978). Social class, psychiatric disorder of mothers and accidents to children. *The Lancet*, 18 February, 378–80.

Brown, G. W. & Harris, T. O. (1978*a*). *Social origins of depression: a study of psychiatric disorder in women*. London: Tavistock; New York: Free Press.

Brown, G. W. & Harris, T. (1978*b*). Social origins of depression: a reply. *Psychological Medicine*, **8**, 577–88.

Brown, G. W. & Harris, T. (1980). Further comments on the vulnerability model. *British Journal of Psychiatry*, **137**, 584–5.

Brown, G. W. & Harris, T. (1982*a*). Fall-off in the reporting of life events. *Social Psychiatry*, **17**, 23–8.

Brown, G. W. & Harris, T. (1982*b*). Disease, distress and depression: a comment. *Journal of Affective Disorders*, **4**, 1–8.

Brown, G. W. & Harris, T. (1982*c*). Social class and psychiatric disorder. In *Culture and psychopathology*, ed. Ihsan Al-Issa, pp. 125–56. Baltimore: University Park Press.

Brown, G. W., Harris, T. O. & Bifulco, A. (1985*c*). Long-term effect of early loss of parent. In *Depression in childhood: developmental perspectives*, ed. M. Rutter, C. Izard & P. Read, pp. 251–96. New York: Guildford Press.

Brown, G. W., Harris, T. O. & Peto, J. (1973). Life events and psychiatric disorders. Part 2. Nature of causal link. *Psychological Medicine*, **3**, 159–76.

Brown, G. W., Ní Bhrolcháin, M. & Harris, T. O. (1975). Social class and psychiatric disturbance among women in an urban population. *Sociology*, **9**, 225–54.

Brown, G. W. & Prudo, R. (1981). Psychiatric disorder in a rural and an urban population. 1. Aetiology of depression. *Psychological Medicine*, **11**, 581–99.

Campbell, E. (1982). Vulnerability to depression and cognitive predisposition: psychosocial correlates of Brown and Harris's vulnerability factors. Paper presented *British Psychological Society Annual Conference, April, 1982*.

Campbell, E., Cope, S. & Teasdale, J. (1983). Social factors and affective disorder: an investigation of Brown and Harris's model. *British Journal of Psychiatry*, **143**, 548–53.

Cobb, S. (1976). Social support as a moderator of life stress. *Psychosomatic Medicine*, **38**, 300–14.

Cole, P. & MacMahon, B. (1971). Attributable risk percent in case-control studies. *British Journal of Preventive and Social Medicine*, **25**, 242–4.

Comstock, G. W. & Helsing, K. J. (1976). Symptoms of depression in two communities. *Psychological Medicine*, **6**, 551–63.

Connolly, J. (1976). Life events before myocardial infarction. *Journal of Human Stress*, **2**, 3–17.

Cook, T. D. & Campbell, D. T. (1979). *Quasi-experimentation: design and analysis issues for field studies*. Chicago: Rand McNally.

Cooke, D. (1980). The structure of depression found in the general population. *Psychological Medicine*, **10**, 455–63.

Cooke, D. (1981). Life events and syndromes of depression in the general population. *Social Psychiatry*, **16**, 181–6.

Cooke, D. J. & Hole, D. J. (1983). Aetiological importance of stressful life events. *British Journal of Psychiatry*, **143**, 397–400.

Cope, S. (1983). Social and psychiatric disturbance in working-class women with young children in Oxford city. MS.

Costello, C. G. (1982). Social factors associated with depression: a retrospective community study. *Psychological Medicine*, **12**, 329–39.

Craig, T. K. J. & Brown, G. W. (1984*a*). Life events, meaning and physical illness: a review. In *Health care and human behaviour*, ed. A. Steptoe & A. Matthews, pp. 7–39. London: Academic Press.

Craig, T. K. J. & Brown, G. W. (1984*b*). Goal-frustration and life events in the aetiology of painful gastrointestinal disorder. *Journal of Psychosomatic Research*, **28**(5), 411–21.

Creed, F. (1981). Life events and appendicectomy. *The Lancet*, 27 June, 1381–5.

Crook, T. & Eliot, J. (1980). Parental death during childhood and adult depression: a critical review of the literature. *Psychological Bulletin*, **87**, 252–9.

Cutileiro, J. (1971). *A Portuguese rural society*. Oxford: Oxford University Press.

Day, R., Nielsen, J. A. & Korten, A. (1982). Life events and the onset of acute schizophrenic episodes: a cross-national study of Czechoslovakian, Danish, and Indian patients. MS.

Dean, C., Surtees, P. G. & Sashidharan, S. P. (1983). Comparison of research diagnostic systems in an Edinburgh community sample. *British Journal of Psychiatry*, **142**, 247–56.

Dohrenwend, B. P. (1975). Sociocultural and social–psychological factors in the genesis of mental disorders. *Journal of Health and Social Behaviour*, **16**, 365–92.

Dohrenwend, B. P. & Dohrenwend, B. S. (1969). *Social status and psychological disorder: a causal inquiry*. New York: John Wiley.

Dohrenwend, B. P. & Dohrenwend, B. S. (1974). Psychiatric disorders in urban settings. In *American handbook of psychiatry, vol.* II, *Child and adolescent psychiatry, sociocultural and community psychiatry*, ed. G. Caplin, pp. 000–000. New York: Basic Books.

Eales, M. (1983). Limitations of hierarchical model fitting in the analysis of causal systems. MS.

Eckenrode, J. & Gore, S. (1981). Stressful events and social supports: the significance of context. In *Social networks and social support in community mental health*, ed. B. H. Gottlieb, pp. 43–68. Beverly Hills, California: Sage.

Everitt, B. S. & Smith, A. M. R. (1979). Interactions in contingency tables: a brief discussion of alternative definitions. *Psychological Medicine*, **9**, 581–3.

Fava, G. A., Munari, F., Pavan, L. & Kellner, R. (1981). Life events and depression. *Journal of Affective Disorders*, **3**, 159–65.

Finlay-Jones, R. (1981). Showing that life events are a cause of depression – a review. *Australian and New Zealand Journal of Psychiatry*, **15**, 229–38.

Finlay-Jones, R. & Brown, G. W. (1981). Types of stressful life event and the onset of anxiety and depressive disorders. *Psychological Medicine*, **11**, 803–15.

Finlay-Jones, R. A. & Murphy, E. (1979). Severity of psychiatric disorder and the 30-item general health questionnaire. *British Journal of Psychiatry*, **134**, 609–16.

Frydman, M. I. (1981). Social support, life events and psychiatric symptoms: a study of direct, conditional and interaction effects. *Social Psychiatry*, **16**, 69–78.

Galtung, J. (1967). *Theory and methods of social research*. London: Allen & Unwin.

Giel, R., Ten Horn, G. H. M. M., Ormel, J., Schudel, W. J. & Wiersma, D. (1978). Mental illness, neuroticism and life events in a Dutch village sample: a follow-up. *Psychological Medicine*, **8**, 235–43.

Glassner, B., Haldipur, C. V. & Dessauersmith, J. (1979). Role loss and working-class manic depression. *Journal of Nervous and Mental Disorders*, **167**, 530–41.

Goldberg, D. (1982). The concept of a psychiatric 'case' in general practice. *Social Psychiatry*, **17**, 61–5.

Goldberg, D. & Huxley, P. (1980). *Mental illness in the community: the pathway to psychiatric care*. London: Tavistock.

Gore, S. (1981). Stress-buffering functions of social supports: an appraisal and classification of research models. In *Stressful life events and their contexts*, ed. B. S. Dohrenwend & B. P. Dohrenwend, pp. 202–220. New York: Prodist.

Gove, W. R. (1973). Sex, marital status and morality. *American Journal of Sociology*, **79**, 45–67.

Grant, I., Yager, J., Sweetwood, H. L. & Olsen, M. S. (1982). Life events and symptoms: Fourier analysis of time series from a three-year prospective inquiry. *Archives of General Psychiatry*, **39**, 598–605.

Granville-Grossman, K. L. (1968). The early environment of affective disorder. In *Recent developments in affective disorders*, ed. A. Coppen & A. Walk, pp. 65–80. London: Headley Brothers.

Harris, T. O. & Brown, G. W. (1985). Interpreting data in aetiological studies: pitfalls and ambiguities. *British Journal of Psychiatry*, **147**, 5–15.

Henderson, S., Byrne, D. G. & Duncan-Jones, P. (1981). *Neurosis and the social environment*. London: Academic Press.

Hendrie, H. D., Lacher, D. & Lennox, K. (1975). Personality trait and symptom correlates of life change in a psychiatric population. *Journal of Psychosomatic Research*, **19**, 203–8.

Hildebrand, D. K., Laing, J. D. & Rosenthal, H. (1977). *Analysis of ordinal data*. Beverly Hills: Sage Publications.

Hirschfeld, R. M. A. (1981). Situational depression: validity of the concept. *British Journal of Psychiatry*, **139**, 297–305.

Holmes, Th. H. & Rahe, R. H. (1967). The Social Readjustment Rating Scale. *Journal of Psychosomatic Research*, **11**: 213–18.

Hudgens, R. W., Morrison, H. R. & Barchaa, R. G. (1967). Life events and onset of primary affective disorders. *Archives of General Psychiatry*, **16**, 134–45.

Hudgens, R. W., Robins, E. & Delong, W. B. (1970). The reporting of recent stress in the lives of psychiatric patients. *British Journal of Psychiatry*, **117**, 635–43.

Hultsch, D. F. & Plemons, J. K. (1979). Life events and life-span development. In *Life-span Development and Behaviour* (vol. 2), ed. P. B. Baltes & O. G. Brim, Jr, pp. 1–31. New York: Academic Press.

Ingham, J. G. & Miller, P. McC. (1979). Symptom prevalence and severity in a general practice population. *Journal of Epidemiology and Community Health*, **33**, 191–8.

Jenkins, C. D., Hurst, M. W. & Rose, R. M. (1979). Life changes – do people really remember? *Archives of General Psychiatry*, **36**, 379–84.

Kasl, S. V., Evans, A. S. & Neiderman, J. C. (1979). Psychosocial risk factors in the development of infectious mononucleosis. *Psychosomatic Medicine*, **41**, 445–66.

Katschnig, H. (1980). Measuring life stress: a comparison of two methods. In *The suicide syndrome*, ed. R. Farmer & S. Hirsch, pp. 116–23. London: Croom Helm.

Katschnig, H., Brandl-Nebehay, A., Fuchs-Robetin, G., Seelig, P., Eichberger, G., Strobl, R. & Sint, P. P. (1981). *Lebensverändernde Erignisse, psychosoziale Dispositionen und depressive Verstimmungszustände.* Wien: Psychiatrische Universitätsklinik.

Kessler, R. C. (1982). Socioeconomic status and psychological distress. *American Sociological Review*, **47**, 752–63.

Langner, T. S. & Michael, S. T. (1963). *Life stress and mental health.* London: Collier Macmillan.

La Rocco, J. M., House, J. S. & French, J. R. P. (1980). Social support, occupational stress and health. *Journal of Health and Social Behaviour*, **21**, 202–18.

Leff, J. & Vaughn, C. (1980). The interaction of life events and relatives' expressed emotion in schizophrenia and depressive neurosis. *British Journal of Psychiatry*, **136**, 146–53.

Leff, J. & Vaughn, C. (1983). *Expressed emotion in families – its significance for mental illness.* MS.

Leff, J., Roatch, J. F. & Bunney, W. E. (1970). Environmental factors preceding the onset of severe depressions. *Psychiatry*, **33**, 293–311.

Leighton, D. C., Hagnell, O. & Leighton, A. H. (1971). Psychiatric disorder in a Swedish and a Canadian community: an exploratory study. *Social Science and Medicine*, **5**, 189–209.

Lin, N., Ensel, W. M., Simeone, R. S. & Kuo, W. (1979). Social support, stressful life events, and illness. *Journal of Health and Social Behaviour*, **20**, 108–19.

Lloyd, C. (1980). Life events and depressive disorder reviewed. 1. Events as predisposing factors. *Archives of General Psychiatry*, **37**, 529–35.

Lowenthal, M. E. & Haven, C. (1968). Interaction and adaptation: intimacy as a critical variable. *American Sociological Review*, **33**, 20–30.

Markush, R. E. (1977). Levin's attributable risk statistic for analytic studies and vital statistics. *American Journal of Epidemiology*, **105**, 401–7.

Martin, C. J. (1982). Psychosocial stress and puerperal psychiatric disorder. Presented to the Maré Society.

Meyer, R. J. & Haggerty, R. J. (1962). Streptococcal infections in families. *Pediatrics*, **29**, 539–49.

Miller, P. McC. & Ingham, J. G. (1983). Dimensions of experience. *Psychological Medicine*, **13**, 417–29.

Miller, P. McC. & Ingham, J. G. (1986). Dimensions of experience and symptomatology. *Journal of Psychosomatic Research* (in press).

Miller, P. McC., Ingham, J. G. & Davidson, S. (1976). Life events, symptoms and social support. *Journal of Psychosomatic Research*, **20**, 512–22.
Murphy, E. (1982). Social origins of depression in old age. *British Journal of Psychiatry*, **141**, 135–42.
Murphy, E. & Brown, G. W. (1980). Life events, psychiatric disturbance and physical illness. *British Journal of Psychiatry*, **136**, 326–38.
Neilson, E. M. & Brown, G. W. (1984). Psychological factors in physical disorders: a preliminary report to the ESRC.
Ní Bhrolcháin, M. (1979). Psychotic and neurotic depression. 1. Some points of method. *British Journal of Psychiatry*, **134**, 87–93.
O'Connor, P. & Brown, G. W. (1984). Supportive relationships: fact or fancy? *Journal of Social and Personal Relationships*, **1**, 159–75.
Parry, G., Shapiro, D. & Davies, L. (1981). Reliability of life-event ratings: an independent replication. *British Journal of Clinical Psychology*, **20**, 133–4.
Paykel, E. S. (1974). Recent life events and clinical depression. In *Life stress and illness*, ed. E. K. E. Gunderson & R. D. Rahe, pp. 134–63. Illinois: Charles C. Thomas.
Paykel, E. S. (1978). Contribution of life events to causation of psychiatric illness. *Psychological Medicine*, **8**, 245–53.
Paykel, E. S. (1983). Methodological aspects of life events research. *Journal of Psychosomatic Research*, **27**, 341–52.
Paykel, E. S., Emms, E. M., Fletcher, J. & Rassaby, E. S. (1980). Life events and social support in puerperal depression. *British Journal of Psychiatry*, **136**, 339–46.
Paykel, E. S., Myers, J. K., Dienelt, M. N., Klerman, G. L., Lindenthal, J. J. & Pepper, M. P. (1969). Life events and depression: a controlled study. *Archives of General Psychiatry*, **21**, 753–60.
Paykel, E. S., Prusoff, B. A. & Klerman, G. L. (1971). The endogenous–neurotic continuum in depression, rater independence and factor distribution. *Journal of Psychiatric Research*, **8**, 73–90.
Prudo, R., Brown, G. W., Harris, T. & Dowland, J. (1981). Psychiatric disorder in a rural and an urban population. 2. Sensitivity to loss. *Psychological Medicine*, **11**, 601–16.
Prudo, R., Harris, T. & Brown, G. W. (1984). Psychiatric disorder in a rural and an urban population. 3. Life events, social integration and the morphology of affective disorders. *Psychological Medicine*, **14**, 327–45.
Richman, N. (1974). The effects of housing on pre-school children and their mothers. *Developmental Medicine and Child Neurology*, **16**, 53–8.
Richman, N. (1976). Depression in mothers of pre-school children. *Journal of Child Psychology and Psychiatry*, **17**, 75–8.
Rosenthal, R. & Rubin, D. B. (1979). A note on percent variance explained as a measure of the importance of effects. *Journal of Applied Social Psychology*, **5**, 395–6.
Rothman, K. J. (1974). Synergy and antagonism in cause–effect relationships. *American Journal of Epidemiology*, **99**, 385–8.
Rothman, K. J. (1976). The estimation of synergy or antagonism. *American Journal of Epidemiology*, **103**, 506–11.
Rothman, K. J. (1978). Occam's razor pares the choice among statistical models. *American Journal of Epidemiology*, **108**, 347–9.
Roy, A. (1978). Vulnerability factors and depression in women. *British Journal of Psychiatry*, **133**, 106–10.
Rutter, M. (1979). Protective factors in children's response to stress and disadvantage. In

Primary prevention of psychopathology, vol. 3, *social competence in children*, ed. M. W. Kent & J. E. Rolf, pp. 49–74. Hanover, New Hampshire: University Press of New England.

Rutter, M. (1981). Stress, coping and development: some issues and questions. *Journal of Child Psychology and Psychiatry*, **22**, 323–54.

Rutter, M. & Quinton, D. (1977). Psychiatric disorder – ecological factors and concepts of causation. In *Ecological factors in human development*, ed. H. McGurk, pp. 173–87. Amsterdam: North Holland.

Rutter, M., Yule, B., Quinton, D., Rowlands, O., Yule, W. & Berger, M. (1975). Attainment and adjustment in two geographical areas. III. Some factors accounting for area differences. *British Journal of Psychiatry*, **126**, 520–33.

Sarason, I. G., de Monchaux, C. & Hunt, J. (1975). Methodological issues of the assessment of lifestress. In *Parameters of emotion*, ed. L. Levi. New York: Raven Press.

Schmid, I., Scharfetter, C. & Binder, J. (1981). Lebensereignisse in Abhängigkeit von soziodemographishen Variables. *Social Psychiatry*, **16**, 63–8.

Solomon, Z. & Bromet, E. (1982). The role of social factors in affective disorder: an assessment of the vulnerability model of Brown and his colleagues. *Psychological Medicine*, **12**, 123–30.

Spitzer, R. L., Endicott, J. & Robins, E. (1978). Research diagnostic criteria: rationale and reliability. *Archives of General Psychiatry*, **35**, 773–82.

Surtees, P. G. (1980). Social support, residual adversity and depressive outcome. *Social Psychiatry*, **15**, 71–80.

Surtees, P. G., Dean, C., Ingham, J. G., Kreitman, N. B., Miller, P. McC. & Sashidharan, S. P. (1983). Psychiatric disorder in women in an Edinburgh community: associations with demographic factors. *British Journal of Psychiatry*, **142**, 238–46.

Surtees, P. G. & Ingham, J. G. (1980). Life stress and depressive outcome: application of a dissipation model to life events. *Social Psychiatry*, **15**, 21–31.

Surtees, P. G. & Rennie, D. (1983). Adversity and the onset of psychiatric disorder in women. *Social Psychiatry*, **18**, 37–44.

Tennant, C. & Bebbington, P. (1978). The social causation of depression: a critique of the work of Brown and his colleagues. *Psychological Medicine*, **8**, 565–75.

Tennant, C., Bebbington, P. & Hurry, J. (1980*a*). Parental death in childhood and risk of adult depressive disorders: a review. *Psychological Medicine*, **10**, 289–99.

Tennant, C., Bebbington, P. & Hurry, J. (1981*a*). The role of life events in depressive illness: is there a substantial causal relation? *Psychological Medicine*, **11**, 379–89.

Tennant, C., Bebbington, P. & Hurry, J. (1981*b*). The short-term outcome of neurotic disorders in the community: the relation of remission to clinical factors and to neutralizing life events. *British Journal of Psychiatry*, **139**, 213–20.

Tennant, C., Bebbington, P. & Hurry, J. (1982*a*). Social experiences in childhood and adult psychiatric morbidity: a multiple regression analysis. *Psychological Medicine*, **12**, 321–7.

Tennant, C., Hurry, J. & Bebbington, P. (1980*b*). Parent–child separations during childhood: their relation to adult psychiatric morbidity and to referral: preliminary findings. *Acta Psychiatrica Scandinavica*, **285**, 324–31.

Tennant, C., Hurry, J. & Bebbington, P. (1982*b*). The relation of childhood separation experiences to adult depressive and anxiety states. *British Journal of Psychiatry*, **141**, 475–82.

Tennant, C., Smith, A., Bebbington, P. & Hurry, J. (1979). The contextual threat of life events: the concept and its reliability. *Psychological Medicine*, **9**, 525–8.

Tennant, C., Smith, A., Bebbington, P. & Hurry, J. (1981*c*). Parental loss in childhood. *Archives of General Psychiatry*, **38**, 309–14.

Theorell, T., Lind, E. & Floderus, B. (1975). The relationship of disturbing life-changes and emotions to the early development of myocardial infarction and other serious illnesses. *International Journal of Epidemiology*, **4**, 281–93.

Thomson, K. C. & Hendrie, H. C. (1972). Environmental stress in primary depressive illness. *Archives of General Psychiatry*, **26**, 130–32.

Tomkins, S. S. (1979). Script theory: differential magnification of affects. In *Nebraska Symposium on Motivation*, vol. 26, ed. H. E. Howe, Jr & R. A. Dienstbier, pp. 201–36. Lincoln: University of Nebraska Press.

Tomkins, S. S. (1981). The quest for primary motives: biography and autobiography of an idea. *Journal of Personality and Social Psychology*, **41**, 306–29.

Vadher, A. & Ndetei, D. M. (1981). Life events and depression in a Kenyan setting. *British Journal of Psychiatry*, **139**, 134–7.

Vaughn, C. & Leff, J. P. (1976). The influence of family and social factors on the course of psychiatric illness. A comparison of schizophrenic and depressed neurotic patients. *British Journal of Psychiatry*, **129**, 125–37.

Warheit, G., Holzer, C., III, & Schwab, J. (1973). An analysis of social class and racial differences in depressive symptom-aetiology: a community study. *Journal of Health and Social Behaviour*, **4**, 921–99.

Waring, E. M., Tillman, M. P., Frelick, L., Russell, L. & Weisz, G. (1980). Concepts of intimacy in the general population. *Journal of Nervous and Mental Disorders*, **168**, 471–4.

Warr, P. & Parry, G. (1982). Paid employment and women's psychological well-being. *Psychological Bulletin*, **91**, 498–516.

Weiss, R. S. (1969). The fund of sociability. *Transaction*, July/August, 36–43.

Weiss, R. S. (1973). *Loneliness: the experience of emotional and social isolation*. Cambridge, Massachussets: MIT Press.

Weiss, R. S. (1974). The provision of social relationships. In *Doing unto others*, ed. Z. Rubin, pp. 17–26. Englewood Cliffs, New Jersey: Prentice Hall.

Weiss, R. S. (1979). *Going it alone*. New York: Basic Books.

Weissman, M. M. & Myers, J. K. (1979). Affective disorders in a U.S. urban community. *Archives of General Psychiatry*, **35**, 1304–11.

Wershow, H. J. & Reinhart, G. (1974). Life change and hospitalization – a heretical view. *Journal of Psychosomatic Research*, **18**, 393–401.

Wing, J. K. & Bebbington, P. (1982). Epidemiology of depressive disorders in the community. *Journal of Affective Disorders*, **4**, 331–45.

Wing, J. K., Cooper, J. E. & Satorius, N. (1974). *The measurement and classification of psychiatric symptoms: an instruction manual for the Present State Examination and CATEGO programme*. London: Cambridge University Press.

Wing, J. K. & Sturt, E. (1978). *The PSE-ID-CATEGO system – a supplementary manual*. London: Institute of Psychiatry (mimeo).

Worcester, J. (1971). The relative odds in the 2^3 contingency table. *American Journal of Epidemiology*, **93**, 145–9.

World Health Organisation (1978). *Mental disorders: glossary and guide to their classification in accordance with the ninth revision of the International Classification of Diseases*. Geneva: WHO.

Yager, J., Grant, I., Sweetwood, H. L. & Gerst, M. (1981). Life-event reports by psychiatric patients, non-patients, and their partners. *Archives of General Psychiatry*, **38**, 343–7.

6

Establishing causal links – recent controversies

P. BEBBINGTON

Life event research in psychiatry is no longer new. However, major conceptual and methodological difficulties remain and must be overcome before more than tentative conclusions can be drawn. In the author's view, the resulting proliferation of reviews requires no apology, as conceptual discussion is a prerequisite for advances in this field of investigation. In this chapter, an attempt to relate the difficulties of this type of research to the methods used in pursuing it will be made, with emphasis on those for establishing the occurrence of life events. There are basically two techniques which have been employed. The first is based upon a finite and predetermined inventory which seeks to cover at least the majority of potential events (e.g. Holmes & Rahe, 1967; Paykel, Prusoff & Uhlenhuth, 1971; Tennant & Andrews, 1976; Dohrenwend *et al.*, 1978; Sarason, Johnson & Siegel, 1978). The second is based on decisions following a wide-ranging and semi-structured interview and was developed by Brown and his colleagues as a result of his criticisms of the inventory approach (Brown, 1974). Inventories have a considerable cost advantage when presented in questionnaire form. However, we shall see that the requirements of life event research in psychiatry are such that the procedure cannot produce useful results unless it is considerably supplemented.

The study of potentially causal associations must follow decisions about the creation of dependent variables from the subject matter of psychiatry. There are, of course, no absolute *a priori* criteria for these decisions. However, the information obtained from a given study can have value only in the light of what has gone before. This implies that existing categories should not be abandoned before their usefulness has been fully explored and their inadequacies clearly exposed.

Traditionally, psychiatry has been a branch of medicine and shares the particular scientific approach of that discipline. This lies essentially in the use of disease theories. Syndromes, once demarcated, can be used to test theories of causation and treatment. If these theories are not corroborated, the syndromes on which they are based can be abandoned and the clinical phenomena regrouped, hopefully in more useful forms. This procedure is a powerful technique for the extension of knowledge (Wing, 1977).

This approach is also that of psychiatry. By analogy with the symptoms and signs of physical disease, psychological symptoms and signs are defined and used to construct syndromes which form the basis of the various disease theories in psychiatry. The diagnosis of psychiatric disorders follows a hierarchical procedure. When organic psychopathology has been discounted, schizophrenia lies at the top of the diagnostic hierarchy as there are symptoms of schizophrenia which are regarded as pathognomonic, clinching the diagnosis even when symptoms of disorders lower down in the hierarchy are present. The disease concept of schizophrenia has, of course, been widely criticised, often through a misunderstanding of the nature of the medical approach which underlies it. This merely claims that it is useful to group the phenomena in this way, an empirical rather than a conceptual issue. If this position is accepted, the disease concept, at least of acute schizophrenia, is one of the least controversial for life events research in psychiatry.

The use of disease categories leads naturally to a consideration of the concept of onset, insofar as at the very least there must be a point in time at which the category is entered. For any association to be regarded as causal the cause must precede the effect, and hence the only life events which might qualify are those which happened before onset. It is safest to assume that onset precedes, perhaps considerably, the time when the disease becomes diagnosable, and conditions which begin insidiously may pose major problems of assessment. Some of the difficulties surrounding the definition of onset, using schizophrenia as an example, have been reviewed by von Cranach, Eberlein & Holl (1981). Considerable effort must therefore be made to date both life events and onset as accurately as possible. This requirement does not very much increase the onerousness of life event histories obtained at interview. It does mean that the mere presentation of an inventory of events must be supplemented by close questioning about timing, and this helps to dissipate the apparent cost advantage of this method. If this is not done, there is a real danger that events may be accepted as causes which are in fact purely the *result* of affective disturbance, arising from the subject's response to changed mood and functioning. This danger in fact applies whether qualitative or quantitative methods are used to describe symptoms, so a close assessment of their development over time is necessary whichever method is chosen.

Some authors have gone further in attempting to circumvent this problem. Paykel (1974) provides a separate analysis for events which appear to be outside the subject's control, accidents in the true sense of the word, although this apparently simple judgment is often ambiguous, particularly with events which have been obtained by checklist rather than interview. The more detailed and less limited material obtained through their interviews enabled Brown & Harris (1978*a*) to develop and apply their concept of 'independence'. In the original version of this judgment, three categories were recognised: those events which were 'logically' independent of the influence of the subject's disorder, although they might nevertheless (unlike Paykel's 'uncontrolled' category) represent actions of the subject, such as taking an exam at the end of a recognised course of instruction; 'dependent' events, which were likely to have arisen from the subject's responses to his disorder; and an intermediate category of 'possibly independent' events which could have been illness-dependent, although there was no evidence that this was true. This is a very conservative approach to life event data when comparisons are made between ill and normal subjects, as few of the latter are likely to have events rated as dependent. Nevertheless, Brown and his colleagues have felt the need for considerable elaboration of this original format.

Life event research has also been directed at psychiatric phenomena which are not conceptualised as disease, for instance attempted suicide. Particular difficulties arise from this in the case of affective disturbances, which have been defined and measured both in terms of an undifferentiated departure from normal mood and in terms of a disease category. The first approach usually relies on the total number of symptoms as a measure of severity, information which is often obtained by questionnaire. No attempt is made to establish inclusion and exclusion criteria which could support a differential diagnosis. There is nevertheless nothing intrinsically invalid in taking this approach. What is invalid is the legerdemain of those researchers and reviewers who interpret the results of such studies in terms of the categories that psychiatrists traditionally use to group depressive phenomena. Many community studies have used such methods. The wide spread of affective symptoms in the community and the potential differences between factors determining disorder and those leading to referral mean that such studies are of considerable significance in the investigation of the causes of depression. It is only recently that researchers have come to use the relatively expensive procedures necessary to establish symptom-based categories for the purpose of testing disease theories of affective disorders (Wing, 1976; Brown & Harris, 1978*a*; Weissman & Myers, 1978; Bebbington *et al.*, 1981*a*; Henderson, Byrne & Duncan-Jones, 1981). There are, of course, several of these, corresponding to various symptomatic subdivisions. Like any disease theories they are tentative, and have been in a particular state of flux over recent years.

Disease theories of affective disorder can be contrasted with the concept of distress, an important idea which people in general use to give meaning to their emotional experience but one which is also used by psychiatrists. This idea is primarily a quantitative one: by and large, people are upset in proportion to the degree of misfortune they suffer. It therefore appears to demand methods of assessment which give undifferentiated measures of affective disturbance. It would, of course, be possible to use a categorical approach, defining 'cases' of distress but this would be a secondary elaboration of the concept.

To an extent, the distinction between the concept of emotional distress and the concept of depressive illness is a distinction of matter: disturbances so minor that no one would consider placing them in a disease category are readily understood as emotional reactions to untoward circumstances. However, the two concepts are considerably more intertwined than this would suggest, and although they are recognised and distinguished by psychiatrists, the implications of the distinction for research have not been fully appreciated. In particular, it has not been made clear what information would enable us to decide that the distinction is genuinely useful.

Disease theories of depression in their current form go back at least to the nineteenth century. In this form, depression is actually defined in terms of life events but in a negative way. The main points can be obtained from the writing of Griesinger (1861). Depressive illness is to be distinguished from normal emotional experience. It *may* be distinguished by having no apparent psychosocial precipitant. Where a psychosocial precipitant does exist, depressive illness may be distinguished by the severity of the symptoms, by its protraction, by an apparent autonomy, and by symptoms which are qualitatively different from those which appear in 'normal' distress. Bucknill & Tuke (1879: 216) add to this formulation the concept of 'incubation', in which the relationship between the concepts of stress and of depressive illness is apparent: a normal emotional response to an event gradually transforms into an autonomous and protracted depressive illness.

All of these assertions emphasise the distinction between depressive illness and normal emotional responses to events. Whilst this distinction may represent the application of considerable clinical intuition, it cannot be said to have been validated. Nevertheless. the separation remains a central idea in the psychiatry of affective disturbances. It is, for example, incorporated into the latest revision of the International Classification of

Disease (World Health Organisation, 1978) which specifically separates the 'depressive adjustment reactions' from depressive neurosis on the basis of the nature of the relationship to stress. It is also commonly the basis of overall models of affective illness (e.g. Akiskal & McKinney, 1975; Depue, Monroe & Shackman, 1979).

This separation of depressive illness from normal emotional responses to events presupposes that the latter can be defined. What range and combinations of symptoms seem reasonable in the light of a given set of stressful circumstances? Paykel (1982) has argued that the need for such a judgment makes the current concept of affective illness an unsatisfactory one. There are two complementary ways in which a reply to this contention can be sought. The first requires a consideration of the way in which life events are quantified. The dimension 'stressfulness' or 'threat' seems to have a higher predictive validity than measures of the social change inherent in the event (Mueller, Edwards & Yarvis, 1977). This concept of stressfulness is rarely defined but seems to refer to the capacity of a given event to elicit an unpleasant emotional response. If this is assumed, some evidence of the reliability and validity of measures of threat can be derived from Brown's (1974) use of the panel technique. This is based upon information obtained at the interview described above. The interviewer presents vignettes of events to a panel of raters, together with information about social circumstances. The event is then rated by consensus, and with training these ratings can be made with considerable reliability (Tennant *et al.*, 1979). In view of the concept of threat which is used as the basis of this rating, it appears therefore that people *can* make reliable guesses at the range of normal emotional response to events, at least within their own culture. Moreover, because these ratings agree quite closely with the estimations that normal subjects make of their actual responses to these events, the ratings also appear to be valid (Brown & Harris, 1978*a*: 113). This implies that it might well be possible to distinguish the normal emotional response from depressive illness, although it may often be difficult in marginal cases.

The second line of investigation is to seek concomitant variation in the pattern of affective symptoms and the pattern of the relationship with adversity. In fact the requirement that there should be symptomatic differences between depressive illness and emotional distress can at best only be approximately true. Relapses in someone who has previously suffered an episode with the clinical features suggestive of a severe depressive illness may, if mild or seen early, show none of these severe symptoms. Secondly, it must be demonstrated that illness and distress have different relationships with adverse circumstances.

Ideally, research diagnostic instruments should rely solely upon symptoms to provide a classification without reference to aetiology (Wing, Cooper & Sartorius, 1974; Spitzer & Endicott, 1978). They can then be used to validate the distinction between depressive illness and emotional distress, providing that their subclassifications of affective disturbance are likely to be roughly equivalent to the expected symptomatic differences between them, and also that their threshold for classifying affective disturbance is sufficiently low to permit the inclusion of an adequate number of potential cases of distress. These requirements are probably met by the Present State Examination–Index of Identification–CATEGO (PSE–ID–CATEGO) system if cases are designated as those of ID level 5 and above. (Wing, 1976, 1980).

The empirical evidence for their distinction along these lines is so far equivocal and in any case poses considerable problems of statistical analysis. Bebbington, Tennant & Hurry (1981*b*) did find in their sample that syndromes typified by pathological guilt, retardation or agitation, in comparison with syndromes without these symptoms, occurred in people who were relatively unlikely to have experienced adversity in the preceding 3 months. On the other hand, the careful study of Katschnig and his colleagues (1981) failed to reveal significantly different relationships with adversity among groups of depressives distinguished as 'endogenous' or 'neurotic' in a variety of ways. (See also the chapter by Katschnig, Pakesch & Egger-Zeidner, this volume, p. 234.) Other studies have major defects of method or reporting which preclude definite conclusions and the issue remains open.

If the distinction between distress and depressive illness cannot be made on grounds *both* of the symptom picture and of the relation to adversity, it can, of course, always be made on *either* of these grounds. However, unless conditions distinguished on only one of these bases do not differ in other ways (such as family history or response to treatment) the separation is not of use. In particular, if the only distinction between distress and depressive illness was in terms of symptoms, it becomes merely an arbitrary prejudice against the reactivity of the severer forms, or in favour of that of the milder forms of disturbance. Finally, if at the end of the day all we can conclude is that events produce distress, this tells us something about our measure of life events (that it is valid) but very little about the nature of distress: it is not very surprising that life events which people think are likely to be distressing are often found to distress people. It would be much more interesting if the presuppositions of the nineteenth-century psychiatrists concerning the relation between depressive illness and upsetting events were substantiated. Nevertheless, as suggested above, this relationship between symptoms and adversity is *not* crucial to the validation of disease theories of depression.

A further problem which applies to many disorders of uncertain aetiology, both physical and psychiatric, but which is most acute in considering the effects of life events upon affective disturbance, is that the researcher shares his research hypothesis with his subjects. People suffering from lowered mood are only too ready to explain it in terms of their circumstances. Their search after meaning may lead them to an unwarrantable magnification of the significance of the events they have experienced. Moreover, depressed mood of itself tends to reduce the tolerance of people to their circumstances and is likely therefore to enhance their estimation of events. These two effects of depressed mood are likely to lead to subjects with depression remembering more events, especially if negative, and, probably more significantly, assessing them as more stressful. It is clear that, in general, people forget events: this can be shown by the amount of information added by using another informant close to the subject and by the demonstration of a fall-off in recall as the time of events becomes more distant. For most investigations using predetermined lists of events, whether presented visually or verbally, the information added by a further informant is around 30% (Schless & Mendels, 1978; Yager *et al.*, 1981). Likewise, the decrement in recall using such means appears to be around 5% of remembered material per month. (Uhlenhuth *et al.*, 1977; Jenkins, Hurst & Rose, 1979). On both of these grounds, the semi-structured interview performs rather better. Brown and his colleagues (1973) report that additional informants added only 10% to the material already recorded from the subject through this procedure. With the exception of Schmid, Scharfetter & Binder (1981), the reduction in recall over time also seems less, at any rate for severe events (Bebbington *et al.*, 1981*b*; Brown & Harris, 1982). Few workers have reported on the important possibility that depressives remember more events. One line of evidence is provided by observing differences between depressives and normals in recording mild events which are unlikely to have been important in the onset of affective disturbance. Brown and his colleagues (1973) did not show a difference, whilst in the results of Bebbington and his colleagues (1981*b*) the difference is marked. If depressives do recall more events, this would, of course, confound the relationship between events and affective disturbance. As severe events are likely to be remembered by most people, the contextual rating of threat employed by Brown has a further role in restraining this potential confusion. This is because the contextual rating is used not merely to assess severity, but also to determine which events (the most threatening) are used in the analysis.

The subject's own judgment of the *severity* of an event may also contaminate the finding of an association between adversity and disorder. The two different ways of obtaining event histories solve this problem in different ways. When predetermined inventories are used, the stress rating of an event is obtained by averaging the ratings ascribed by a sample of the general population. Such samples have usually been chosen for convenience rather than for representativeness. The rating involves subjects making a judgment of the distress the event would occasion either to themselves or to the traditional 'man on the Clapham omnibus'. Such judgments are in essence culture bound (Hough, Fairbank & Garcia, 1976). They also have the disadvantage that there is no possibility of allowing for the individual circumstances surrounding individual events.

In the 'panel' technique developed by Brown (1974), the raters have no knowledge of the subject's actual response to the event or psychiatric state, thus eliminating as far as possible the effects of the 'search after meaning' and the 'black spectacles' described above. The raters may, however, ask questions which clarify the objective implications of the event: e.g. did the son who has left home make a major contribution to the household income? Although this method probably avoids most of the contamination from interpretations of events by the subject, it does not eliminate all of it, as the reporting of the *context* of the event is obtained from what the subject says and may have been presented to the interviewer in a way to maximise the significance of the event. This degree of objectivity attained by the panel technique has a cost. Only a crude assessment of the meaning the event has for the subject can be ascribed by a consideration of his current circumstances. Some authors have argued that the meanings of events are so individual that only the subject's assessment can have validity. The author's view is that there must be a trade-off between contamination by subjective overvaluation of events and the loss of the fine detail of individual circumstances, and that the contextual rating of threat developed by Brown and his colleagues eliminates most of the former at least cost to the latter. Although the differences which arise through using subjective and objective ratings may not be great, they may be crucial.

A major problem for accounts of affective symptoms in terms of the experience of adversity is the finding that, on average, measures of adversity do not account for more than 10% of the variance of these symptoms (Andrews & Tennant, 1978). This is not surprising as it is quite apparent that not all individuals respond equally badly to events which appear to be equally distressing. However, it immediately raises the issue of what modifies the impact of events.

Kessler (1979) has clearly set out the possibilities. On one hand, events may be modified by the social circumstances of the individual at the time of the event. Such social circumstances affect the practical implications and hence the meaning of the event for the subject. On the other hand, there may be particular attributes of the individual which affect his vulnerability to the effects of psychosocial stress. One possible group of these attributes consists of those which are readily observable in the way the individual copes with the practical and emotional effects of an event. This in turn may be ascribed to the effects of current or earlier circumstances or to constitutional factors. In cases where no abnormality of handling an event is evidence, covert factors affecting its impact may be postulated. There is no *a priori* reason why these factors should not relate to former experiences of the person, but implicit in the disease theory of depression described above has been a predilection in favour of constitutional explanations. One reason for this is the appearance of symptoms which are not usually seen in ordinary sorrow or apprehension, those that Griesinger calls the 'other accessory affections'. It is felt by many that the emergence of such symptoms must reflect an underlying diathesis. However, once more there is no reason why this is necessarily so and attempts have been made to offer an environmental explanation for these qualitatively different symptoms. An example is the suggestion of Brown, Harris & Copeland (1977) that the nature of early loss may affect the symptomatic form of later disorders.

As has already been suggested above, the distinction between depressive illness and distress symptoms does not depend exclusively on the different part that misfortune might play in their onset. If no difference were found, the concept of depressive illness, syndromally defined, could still have validity if it were shown that the unexplained variance was accounted for by factors different from those important in emotional distress. These factors either act independently or would themselves determine the susceptibility of the subject to life events or difficulties. A biological basis for depressive illness is best sought through genetic studies, as biological markers such as the Dexamethasone Suppression Test may merely be correlates of symptoms rather than correlates of the causes of symptoms. The ideal study would be one which investigated social, psychological and genetic factors simultaneously as determinants of risk and of vulnerability to life events. Because research workers tend to be specialised creatures, such a study would be difficult to organise. It is nevertheless the only way to explore the important interactions between these variables which many have postulated.

Brown's measure of contextual threat is probably the best method of investigating the interaction between life events and psychological attributes or genetic influences. It does, however, have a disadvantage in the study of the modifying influence of social factors on the effects of life events, as the measure takes account of social factors in the rating of the severity of the event. The method consists of the rater using his experience to construct hypotheses about the impact of single events. Although certain broad principles apply to this procedure, the rating is based on the individual circumstances of the event and, as such, the precise use of other social factors cannot be specified. This means that in some cases tests of interaction between particular social factors and life events will be contaminated, and to an unknowable degree. The effect of contamination depends on the *actual* effects of life events and a given factor, rated independently; the frequency of life events and of given levels of the social factor; the frequency of cases; and the degree of contamination. Where the social factor in question, life events and cases are all relatively infrequent, the tendency would be for contamination to minimise the actual degree of interaction. In principle, this difficulty could, however, be obviated if the rater remained blind to the particular social factors being studied.

Studies of distinctions of three or more variables lead to particular problems of statistical analysis, especially if it is postulated that one factor modifies the relationship between the other two. There are two ways of approaching this analysis. Frydman (1981) has clarified the terminology by emphasising the distinction between 'conditional effects' and 'interactions'. A conditional effect exists when the presence of a modifying variable reveals a relationship which does not occur in its absence. This is essentially an additive model of modification. An interaction is said to occur when the presence of the modifying variable acts to increase the relative risk of disorder from the presence of the primary independent variable. Such an interaction can be tested for using the technique of log-linear analysis (see Everitt, 1977) and is multiplicative. There has been argument about which of these analyses is superior (Brown & Harris 1978*b*; Tennant & Bebbington, 1978; Everitt & Smith, 1979; Bebbington, 1980). The author's own opinion is that the additive model carries some dangers. It basically involves the partition of a $2 \times 2 \times 2$ contingency table into two 2×2 tables distinguished by the level of a given variable of the original three. This permits the postulation of complementary predictions, depending on which variable is used to make the partition. The author has set out the various possibilities elsewhere (Bebbington, 1980) where he has also shown it is possible on the same data set to refute some predictions whilst confirming others. The author now thinks this anomaly arises because of the nature of the statistical test involved (X^2) rather than because of a logical paradox. There are other statistical reasons for preferring to study interactions rather than conditional effects (Everitt & Smith, 1979). On balance, the author is inclined to agree with Frydman (1981) that both types of analysis should be reported when the distributions of three variables is being presented.

It is apparent even from this discussion, limited as it is to relatively few issues, that the knowledge obtained from studies of life events, particularly in depression, remains hedged about with qualifications. Some of the difficulties are insuperable for all practical purposes. Others, however, are not and the next generation of studies, especially if they adopt an integrated approach towards biological and social factors, will see considerable advances in our knowledge.

References

Akiskal, H. S. & McKinney, W. T., Jr (1975). Overview of recent research in depression: integration of ten conceptual models into a comprehensive clinical frame. *Archives of General Psychiatry*, **32**, 285–305.

Andrews, G. & Tennant, C. (1978). Life event stress and psychiatric illness. *Psychological Medicine*, **8**, 545–9.

Bebbington, P. E. (1980). Causal models and logical inference in epidemiological psychiatry. *British Journal of Psychiatry*, **136**, 317–25.

Bebbington, P., Hurry, J., Tennant, C., Sturt, E. & Wing, J. K. (1981*a*). The epidemiology of mental disorders in Camberwell. *Psychological Medicine*, **11**, 561–80.

Bebbington, P. E., Tennant, C. & Hurry, J. (1981*b*). Life events and the nature of psychiatric disorder in the community. *Journal of Affective Disorders*, **3**, 345–66.

Brown, G. W. (1974). Meaning, measurement and stress of life events. In *Stressful life events: their nature and effects*, ed. B. S. Dohrenwend & B. P. Dohrenwend), pp. 217–43. New York: John Wiley.

Brown, G. W. & Harris, T. (1978*a*). *The social origins of depression*. London: Tavistock.

Brown, G. W. & Harris, T. (1978*b*). Social origins of depression: a reply. *Psychological Medicine*, **8**, 577–88.

Brown, G. W. & Harris, T. (1982). Fall-off in the reporting of life events. *Social Psychiatry*, **17**, 23–8.

Brown, G. W., Harris, T. O. & Copeland, J. R. (1977). Depression and loss. *British Journal of Psychiatry*, **130**, 1–18.

Brown, G. W., Sklair, F., Harris, T. & Birley, J. L. T. (1973). Life events and psychiatric disorders. Part 2. Nature of the causal link. *Psychological Medicine*, **3**, 159–76.

Bucknill, J. C. & Tuke, D. H. (1879). *A manual of psychological medicine*. London: Churchill.

von Cranach, M., Eberlein, R. & Holl, B. (1981). The concept of onset in psychiatry. In *What is a case? The problem of definition in psychiatric community surveys*, ed. J. K. Wing, P. E. Bebbington & L. N. Robins, pp. 155–60. London: Grant McIntyre.

Depue, R. A., Monroe, S. M. & Shackman, S. L. (1979). The psychobiology of human disease: implications for conceptualising the depressive disorders. In *The psychobiology of the depressive disorders: implications for the effects of stress*, ed. R. A. Depue, pp. 3–22. New York: Academic Press.

Dohrenwend, B. S., Krasnoff, L., Askenasy, A. R. & Dohrenwend, B. P. (1978). Exemplification of a method for scaling life events: the PERI life events scale. *Journal of Health and Social Behaviour*, **19**, 205–29.

Everitt, B. S. (1977). *The analysis of contingency tables*. London: Chapman & Hall.

Everitt, B. S. & Smith, A. M. R. (1979). Interactions in contingency tables: a brief discussion of alternative definitions. *Psychological Medicine*, **9**, 581–3.

Frydman, M. I. (1981). Social support, life events and psychiatric symptoms: a study of direct, conditional and interaction effects. *Social Psychiatry*, **16**, 69–78.

Griesinger, W. (1861). *Die Pathologie und Therapie der Psychischen Krankheiten*, 2nd edition. Braunschweig: Wreden. (Translated as *Mental pathology and therapeutics* by C. L. Robertson & J. Rutherford (1867). London: New Sydenham Society.)

Henderson, A. S., Byrne, D. G. & Duncan-Jones, P. (1981). *Neurosis and the social environment*. Sydney: Academic Press.

Holmes, Th. H. & Rahe, R. H. (1967). The Social Readjustment Rating Scale. *Journal of Psychosomatic Research*, **11**, 213–18.

Hough, R. L., Fairbank, D. T. & Garcia, A. M. (1976). Problems in the ratio measurement of life stress. *Journal of Health and Social Behaviour*, **17**, 70–82.

Jenkins, C. D., Hurst, M. W. & Rose, R. M. (1979). Life changes: do people really remember? *Archives of General Psychiatry*, **36**, 379–84.

Katschnig, H., Brandl-Nebehay, A., Fuchs-Robetin, G., Seelig, P., Eichberger, G., Strobl, R. & Sint, P. P. (1981). *Lebensverändernde Ereignisse, Psychosoziale Dispositionen und Depressive Verstimmungzustände*. Wien: Abteilung für Sozialpsychiatrie und Dokumentation, Psychiatrische Universitätsklinik.

Kessler, R. C. (1979). A strategy for studying differential vulnerability to the psychological consequences of stress. *Journal of Health and Social Behaviour*, **20**, 100–8.

Mueller, D. P., Edwards, D. W. & Yarvis, R. M. (1977). Stressful life events and psychiatric symptomatology: change or undesirability. *Journal of Health and Social Behaviour*, **18**, 307–17.

Paykel, E. S. (1974). Life stress and psychiatric disorder: applications of the clinical approach. In: *Stressful life events: their nature and effects*, ed. B. S. Dohrenwend & B. P. Dohrenwend, pp. 135–49. New York: John Wiley.

Paykel, E. S. (1982). Social and psychological causes of affective psychosis. In *Handbook of psychiatry*, vol. III, ed. J. K. Wing, pp. 141–6. Cambridge University Press.

Paykel, E. S., Prusoff, B. A. & Uhlenhuth, E. H. (1971). Scaling of life events. *Archives of General Psychiatry*, **25**, 340–7.

Sarason, I. G., Johnson, J. H. & Siegel, J. M. (1978). Assessing the impact of life changes: development of the Life Experiences Survey. *Journal of Consulting and Clinical Psychology*, **46**, 932–46.

Schless, A. P. & Mendels, J. (1978). The value of interviewing family and friends in assessing life stressors. *Archives of General Psychiatry*, **35**, 565–7.

Schmid, I., Scharfetter, C. & Binder, J. (1981). Lebensereignisse in Abhängigkeit von sozio-demographischen Variablen. Eine Erhebung an einer Stichprobe aus der Normalpopulation mittels der Brown'schen Inventars. *Social Psychiatry*, **16**, 63–8.

Spitzer, R. L. & Endicott, J. (1978). *Schedule for Affective Disorders and Schizophrenia – life–time version*, third edition. New York State Department of Mental Hygiene, New York State Psychiatric Institute, Biometrics Research.

Tennant, C. & Andrews, G. (1976). A scale to measure the stress of life events. *Australian and New Zealand Journal of Psychiatry*, **10**, 27–33.

Tennant, C. & Bebbington, P. (1978). The social causation of depression: a critique of the work of Brown and his colleagues. *Psychological Medicine*, **8**, 565–75.

Tennant, C., Smith, A., Bebbington, P. & Hurry, J. (1979). The contextual threat of life events: the concept and its reliability. *Psychological Medicine*, **9**, 525–8.

Uhlenhuth, E., Balter, M. D., Lipman, R. S. & Haberman, S. J. (1977). Remembering life events. In *The origins and course of psychopathology*, ed. J. S. Strauss, H. M. Babigian & M. Roff, pp. 117–32. New York: Plenum Press.

Weissman, M. M. & Myers, J. (1978). Affective disorders in a United States urban community: the use of Research Diagnostic Criteria in an epidemiological survey. *Archives of General Psychiatry*, **35**, 1304–14.

Wing, J. K. (1976). A technique for studying psychiatric morbidity in in-patient and out-patient series and in general population samples. *Psychological Medicine*, **6**, 665–71.

Wing, J. K. (1977). The limits of standardisation. In *Psychiatric diagnosis*, ed. V. M. Rakoff, H. Stances & H. B. Kedward, pp. 84–108. New York: Brunner/Mazel.

Wing, J. K. (1980). The use of the Present State Examination in general population surveys. *Acta Psychiatrica Scandinavica*, Suppl. 285, 230–40.

Wing, J. K., Cooper, J. E. Sartorius, N. (1974). *The measurement and classification of psychiatric symptoms*. Cambridge University Press.

World Health Organisation (1978). *Mental disorders: glossary and guide to their classification in accordance with the ninth revision of the International Classification of Diseases*. Geneva: WHO.

Yager, J., Grant, I., Sweetwood, H. L. & Gerst, M. (1981). Life events reported by psychiatric patients, non-patients and their partners. *Archives of General Psychiatry*, **38**, 343–7.

7

Life stress and depressive subtypes: a review of present diagnostic criteria and recent research results

H. KATSCHNIG, G. PAKESCH & E. EGGER-ZEIDNER

The confusion continues

The identification of an 'endogenous' factor in the first factor analytic study on depression by Hamilton & White (1959) marks the beginning of a period of research on the up to then mainly dogmatically discussed thesis of the binary nature of depressive disorders. Is it justified to distinguish a 'real depressive disease', characterised by a morbid process in the brain and variably named 'endogenous', 'melancholic', or 'psychotic', from a more or less 'normal' variant of mood, called 'reactive', 'psychogenic' or 'neurotic', and supposed to be dependent on environmental influences? Or are we simply dealing with different degrees of severity of one and the same depressive disorder?

With the development of new data collection methods and new techniques of data analysis, these and related questions have increasingly been subjected to empirical study in the past 25 years. However, the answers provided by empirical research to date are ambiguous and seem indeed to have obscured the issue even further.

On the one hand, the classification of depression has become more complicated since Hamilton & White's (1959) study. The classical dichotomy of 'endogenous' (i.e. biologically caused) versus 'reactive' (i.e. psychosocially determined) depression has been questioned by new evidence, favouring either a 'unitarian' view (Kendell, 1968) or extending the number of identifiable depressive subtypes to three or four (e.g. Overall *et al.*, 1966; Paykel, 1971). Furthermore, influential classification systems such as the latest revision of the International Classification of Diseases (ICD-9, World Health Organisation 1978) and the 'Diagnostic and Statistical Manual-III' (DSM-III) of the American Psychiatric Association (1980), depart substantially from the traditional dichotomy. Finally, matters have been made more complicated by proposals for alternative classification models, replacing the categorical approach by a dimensional (Eysenck, 1970) or a hierarchical one (Foulds, 1973).

While on the one hand the 'contemporary confusion' in the classification of depression so brilliantly described by Kendell (1976) is thus increasing, a reverse trend towards maintaining or reviving the simple categorical endogenous/reactive dichotomy can also be observed in recent years. Originating from the detection of neuroendocrine abnormalities in some depressive patients (e.g. Carroll, Martin & Davies, 1968), there has developed in the past decade a whole new branch of psychiatric research which tries to identify 'biological markers' in the 'endogenous' subtype of depression as opposed to 'reactive' depressives or normal controls. Since the clinical demarcation of a group of depressive disorders, suspected to be of biological origin, from a 'non-biological' group constitutes the necessary first step in such a search for biological markers, the availability of new biological research techniques has obviously tempted research workers to continue to think in the simple categorical endogenous/reactive dichotomy. In doing so they are harking back to earlier workers such as Kraepelin, who in the seventh edition of his textbook (1904) introduced the separate category of 'psychogenic neurosis' and in the eighth edition (1913, p. 1389) used that of 'psychogenic depression', or Kurt Schneider (1959), who clearly distinguished the functional psychoses, presumed to be the consequence of a morbid process in the nervous system, from 'abnormal reactions to emotional impressions', judged by him to be 'abnormal varieties of sane mental life'.

In one way or another, the concept of reactivity in its broadest sense – implying that social factors produce, trigger, or maintain depression – is of central importance in most attempts at subdividing depressive disorders. Even if a 'reactive' type of depression is not explicitly defined, the demarcation of a 'biological' type in many diagnostic criteria requires a specific judgment about the *absence* of relevant psychosocial influences. In most such diagnostic decisions the life event methodology now available (see Katschnig, p. 74, this volume) is not used; instead, judgments about reactivity and the presence or absence of 'social factors' are typically made on intuitive or commonsense grounds (which contrasts unfavourably with the now-common habit of standardised data collection in the field of psychopathological information).

It is the purpose of this article to describe and evaluate critically the use of the concepts of reactivity and life stress in present diagnostic formulations and in research on depressive subtypes, thus supplementing the historical review presented by Cooper in this volume (p. 1). For illustrative purposes we will refer repeatedly to a study of 176 depressed in-patients carried out in Vienna between 1977 and 1980 (Katschnig, 1984*a*,*b*;

Katschnig *et al.*, 1981; Katschnig & Seelig, 1985)*. In this study standardised assessment and rating techniques were employed both for psychiatric variables (for which an expanded version of the 'Present State Examination' by Wing, Cooper & Sartorius (1974) was used) and for life stress (where the London 'Life Event and Difficulty Schedule' by Brown (1974) was employed; see Katschnig, p. 74, this volume; and Brown & Harris, p. 107, this volume). Since psychopathological and life stress data were elicited by different teams of interviewers, these variables were not (as is frequently the case) already confounded with one another at the data collection stage and could therefore be analysed independently from one another.

Depressive subtypes in present diagnostic criteria

In order to understand better the role of the concept of reactivity in currently employed diagnostic formulations of subtypes of depressive disorders, it will be useful to review first some recent developments in psychiatric classification. Subsequently the most widely used and important contemporary diagnostic formulations for subtypes of depression will be analysed in terms of their use of the concepts of reactivity and life stress.

New developments in psychiatric classification

Five new developments in psychiatric classification, which can be contrasted with five traditional approaches, will be briefly discussed here: (1) the use of 'operational' diagnostic criteria as opposed to the traditional 'paradigmatic' approach; (2) the 'multiaxial' versus the 'uniaxial' approach; (3) the development and use of 'compromise' classification systems as opposed to the use of specific 'school systems'; (4) the 'polydiagnostic' versus the 'monodiagnostic' approach; and finally (5) attempts at empirical validation of psychiatric diagnoses versus the traditional dogmatic approach.

Operational criteria versus paradigmatic diagnosis

It is always tempting and sometimes fascinating to reduce and classify complex phenomena into a handful of categories or even just two classes. Depression has not escaped this fate, and most diagnostic formulations incorporate in one way or the other the 'biological/psychosocial' dichotomy put forward by classical psychiatric writers. Such simplifications are possible because the scientific basis for the classification of the functional psychiatric disorders is still very weak. In fact, this basis is still largely

* Supported by Grant Si 236 of the 'Deutsche Forschungsgemeinschaft'.

pragmatic, that is, it is rooted in the practical purpose of guiding and orientating psychiatric clinicians and researchers in their still largely unstructured fields of action and knowledge, where simple classifications are required. Thus, clinicians make their therapeutic decisions after assigning patients to diagnostic classes, while research workers make use of diagnostic criteria to establish groups of patients to be studied.

In everyday clinical practice the pressure to arrive at therapeutic decisions furthers a paradigmatic form of classifying, allowing the clinician to assign most of his patients to a diagnostic group and leaving as few patients as possible undiagnosed – at the cost of establishing heterogeneous diagnostic groups. Textbook definitions of mental disorders are typical for such paradigmatic descriptions. The paradigmatical way of assigning patients to diagnostic categories is subject to many random influences. It could, e.g., be demonstrated that the diagnosis of 'endogenous' depression showed a threefold increase between 1949 and 1959 for patients admitted to the Psychiatric Clinic of the University of Vienna (Hofmann *et al.*, 1971). This can probably be attributed to the availability of a new biological treatment, the anti-depressant drugs, introduced into clinical practice in the second half of the 1950s and putting clinicians under pressure to assign patients suffering from unclear depressive syndromes to a diagnostic group for which a new and promising therapy was available.

Research workers, on the other hand, in order to identify correlations between syndromes and aetiological or therapeutic variables must aim at arriving at as homogeneous a group of patients as possible without creating too much 'noise' by the inclusion of patients who, in fact, belong to a different diagnostic class. The growing awareness of psychiatrists of this methodological problem has led, in the last 15 years, to the formulation of so-called 'operational criteria' (or 'diagnostic algorithms') for specific psychiatric diagnostic classes. For the sake of homogeneity, these criteria must leave a smaller or larger number of patients undiagnosed. Disease entities defined for research purposes by such operational criteria are, however, just as arbitrary as the clinical entities employed in everyday practice; it is simply hoped that such operationalisation will facilitate their validation or their refutation through external variables. Thus the new operational criteria are only 'hypotheses' about the existence of disease entities, in the same sense that the paradigmatic clinical disease entities are only 'working' assumptions, which allow a preliminary structuring of the field of mental disorders for the purpose of their management.

Life stress and/or reactivity play an important role in most paradigmatic and operational definitions of depressive subtypes, as will be demonstrated below. However, while the symptomatological elements of operational diagnostic criteria for depression are at least in some instances clearly defined, life stress is not, and in both 'paradigmatic' and 'operational' definitions of depressive subtypes, usually simple commonsense judgments about 'reactivity' and 'stress' are employed.

'Multiaxial' and 'uniaxial' approaches to psychiatric diagnosis

The simultaneous diagnostic assessment of a psychiatric patient on several so-called 'axes' – such as clinical syndrome, course and outcome, aetiological factors, associated social disabilities etc. – represents one of the most promising new trends in psychiatric classification (Mezzich, 1979). As opposed to the traditional 'uniaxial' approach, implying the provision of a single axis – the disease axis – for diagnostic description of a psychiatric patient, the 'multiaxial' approach allows different areas which do not necessarily correlate with one another to be assessed independently. This is of special interest for the classification of depression, since, e.g., the 'multiaxial' approach allows one to describe a syndrome as 'melancholic' on the psychopathological axis and at the same time to rate the involvement of stress in its onset on an aetiological/pathogenetic axis separately from the clinical picture. In a later section of this chapter (p. 231) the usefulness of this approach for the classification of depression will be shown.

The 'multiaxial' approach has advantages both for scientific research – where it helps to disentangle different aspects of a diagnostic concept – and for clinical practice, where management decisions can be related to separate assessments of a patient's condition on different axes. This is especially important in community psychiatry, where social disabilities warrant a separate evaluation from the clinical picture. The practical application of multiaxial diagnostic systems becomes problematic if the number of axes becomes too large. Mezzich, Fabrega & Mezzich (1985) have identified 21 axes used in or proposed for multiaxial diagnostic systems developed since Essen-Möller & Wohlfart (1947) first introduced the idea.

The DSM-III of the American Psychiatric Association (1980) is the best known 'multiaxial diagnostic system', providing five axes (clinical syndrome, personality disorders, physical disorders and conditions, severity of psychosocial stressors, highest level of adaptive functioning in the past year). Although the separate 'stress' axis does have its merits, the DSM-III has some serious deficiencies, such as interaxis overlap, which do in fact prevent its correct use as a multiaxial system (Berner, Katschnig & Lenz, 1983*b*; Cooper, p. 24, this volume).

Compromise classification systems

Until recently the ICD of the World Health Organisation has been the only widely and internationally used diagnostic system in psychiatry. Its section V (mental disorders) has been developed as part of a comprehensive classification system for all diseases and has been translated into many languages. Its recent ninth revision (ICD-9; World Health Organisation, 1978) now has a formidable rival in the shape of the American DSM-III, which is being propagated vigorously outside the United States of America. Both systems have a decisive weakness: although they have contributed, and indeed still do contribute, to unifying diagnostic terms around the world and providing at least some basic common notion of the main psychiatric disorders, the structure of each system and the definitions of specific diagnoses are the result of compromises reached in discussions of large committees. Political considerations, chance majorities and even personal predilections of committee members have led to the inclusion or exclusion of specific diagnoses or terms or have at least coloured their definition. There is thus no clear theoretical principle behind these classification systems; instead, they constitute a patchwork of theoretical considerations of many different origins leading to a number of logical weaknesses which theoretically based systems do not have. The most deplorable fact, however, is that the ICD-9 and DSM-III by the very fact of being *two* different compromise classification systems contribute to creating even more confusion. Unfortunately, from present auguries, it seems improbable that the major differences will be resolved in the ICD-10 and DSM-IV.

The 'polydiagnostic' approach

A number of studies has been carried out in recent years in which research populations have been defined not just by one but by several specific diagnostic formulations simultaneously (e.g. Brockington, Kendell & Leff, 1978). This research strategy has been called the 'polydiagnostic' approach (Berner & Katschnig, 1983; Katschnig & Berner, 1985). It has been contrasted with the 'compromise' approach and, in fact, has been suggested as an alternative to it. It allows specific diagnostic formulations of different schools to be used alongside each other in one and the same research project. It could be shown that such an approach is feasible without too much additional effort and that it is worthwhile, since different definitions of one and the same concept not only yield different numbers of cases but also only partially overlap (see p. 226). It was also demonstrated that correlations with external variables do vary from one specific diagnostic formulation to another. Thus, Katschnig *et al.* (1981; see also Katschnig, 1984*a,b*; Katschnig & Seelig, 1985) showed that, while a correlation existed between the ICD-8 'neurotic depression' and preceding life stress, a number of other formulations for neurotic depression did not show such a correlation (see p. 234). The 'polydiagnostic' approach is recommended in order to clarify discrepancies between results of studies employing only one – but from study to study different – specific diagnostic formulation for one and the same concept. In order to promote the idea of using several diagnostic formulations simultaneously, we have recently compiled and commented on 15 diagnostic formulations for schizophrenia and 11 for affective psychoses (Berner *et al.*, 1983*a*).

Empirical validation of psychiatric diagnosis

Only recently can a trend be observed in psychiatric research to 'validate' specific definitions of psychiatric diagnoses by testing correlations with external variables. As opposed to the traditional approach, which relies on 'theory and argument' (Lewis, 1971), this approach employs the measurement of external variables and the search for their association with specific diagnostic formulations. This type of research has particularly developed in the field of depression, where a large number of studies has already been carried out in order to identify biological correlates of 'endogenous' depression, or – in fewer studies – to look for a possible association between life events and the neurotic subtype of depression. Course of the illness, familial aggregation data and other variables have also been employed in validation. In later sections of this article we will deal especially with attempts to validate diagnostic subtypes of depression through biological markers and through measures of life stress.

The International Classification of Diseases

The ICD is still the most widely employed and influential psychiatric classification system. In a recent survey carried out in Austria, Germany and Switzerland, at least 70% of psychiatric in-patient units were found to use it in daily routine (Berner *et al.*, 1983*b*). The ICD was basically developed for statistical reporting of data generated in clinical practice, but is also incorrectly used for defining research populations or reporting research data. It is uniaxial and incorporates definitions which clearly belong to the paradigmatical approach. The description of 'neurotic depression' (category 300.4) is a typical example for this 'paradigmatical' character of ICD definitions:

> . . . a neurotic disorder characterized by disproportionate depression which has usually recognisably ensued on a distressing

> experience; it does not include among its features delusions or hallucinations, and there is often preoccupation with the psychic trauma which preceded the illnesses, e.g. loss of a cherished person or possession. Anxiety is also frequently present and mixed states of anxiety and depression should be included here. The distinction between depressive neurosis and psychosis should be made not only upon the degree of depression but also on the presence or absence of other neurotic and psychotic characteristics and upon the degree of disturbance of the patient's behaviour.

'Depressive reaction' and 'reactive depression' are given as inclusion terms, indicating that emphasis is put on the 'distressing experience'; however, psychopathology and severity of symptoms also play a role as inclusion or exclusion criteria, reflecting the classical disease concept of a specific link between aetiology and symptomatology. The use of words like 'usually', 'often', and 'frequently', is typical for a paradigmatical definition; one can easily imagine that very different patients are grouped under 'neurotic depression', especially since no provision at all is made for a valid and reliable evaluation of what constitutes a psychic trauma.

In the ninth revision of the ICD the problem of separating neurotic depression from a number of other reactive depressive states arises; these include 'brief depressive reaction' (309.0: 'states of depression, not specifiable as manic-depressive, psychotic or neurotic, generally transient, in which the depressive symptoms are usually closely related in time and content to some stressful event'): 'prolonged depressive reaction' (309.1: 'states of depression, not specifiable as manic-depressive, psychotic or neurotic, generally long-lasting, usually developing in association with prolonged exposure to a stressful situation'); and 'acute reaction to stress with predominant disturbance of emotions' (308.0: 'very transient disorders of any severity and nature which occur in individuals without any apparent mental disorder in response to exceptional physical or mental stress, such as natural catastrophe, and which usually subsides within hours or days'). Again, also in these formulations it is completely open to the clinician's personal judgment what to regard as a stressful event or situation.

While it may not be helpful to have so many categories for coding reactive depressive states in the 'neurotic disorders' section of the ICD, the provision of two distinct categories for the psychotic form of depression seems at first glance to be very useful: in addition to the classical 'psychotic' or 'endogenous' type of depression (296.1: manic-depressive psychoses, depressed type, or 296.3: manic-depressive psychoses, circular type but currently depressed) and under the overall category of 'other non-organic psychoses' (298), category 298.0 ('depressive type') is defined as

> . . . a depressive psychosis which can be similar in its symptoms to manic depressive psychosis, depressed type (296.1), but is apparently provoked by saddening stress, such as a bereavement or a severe disappointment or frustration. There may be less diurnal variation of symptoms than in 296.1, and the delusions are more often understandable in the context of the life experiences. There is usually a serious disturbance of behaviour, e.g., major suicidal attempt.

In the general description of the group of 'other non-organic psychoses', it is stated that these psychotic conditions are 'largely or entirely attributable to recent life experience' (in ICD-8 they were, therefore, more correctly called 'reactive depressive psychosis'). Thus, the ICD – largely under Scandinavian influence (see Cooper, p. 22, this volume) – allows a 'psychotic symptomatology' to be classed together with provoking life stress and consequently the terms 'reactive depressive psychosis' and 'psychogenic depressive psychosis' are given as inclusion terms. Again, no clearcut definition is given of what constitutes a stress, and the remark that category ICD 298 'should not be used for the wider range of psychoses in which environmental factors play some (but not the *major*) part in etiology' makes the situation very unclear.

When the ICD is applied in clinical practice, there is a clear tendency to resort to the classical neurotic/psychotic dichotomy and to disregard the many other ICD codes for depression. This can be illustrated by two examples from psychiatric institutions in Vienna. First among the 27928 admissions to the Psychiatric Clinic of the University of Vienna in the 10 years from 1971 to 1980, 11% were classed as ICD-8 manic-depressive psychosis, depressed type, and 20.4% as neurotic depressive, but only 2% as reactive depressive psychosis. In the two years (1981 and 1982) after the introduction of the ICD-9 at the Psychiatric Clinic very few patients were assigned to the codes representing intermediate or new types of depression, the majority being again allocated to the two classical types of 'neurotic' and 'psychotic' depression. Of all the 3127 admissions, 15.9% were diagnosed as affective psychosis, depressed type, and 12% as neurotically depressed, but less than 1% received a diagnosis of 'other non-organic psychoses, depressive type' (298.0). Only 1.5% and 2% were classed as brief (309.0) and prolonged (309.1) depressive reactions respectively. The second example is taken from our study (Katschnig *et al.*, 1981), in which, according to the hospital ICD-8 diagnosis, 110 (62.5%) out of 176 depressed in-patients were diagnosed as suffering from a manic-depressive psychosis, depressed type (296.2), whereas 48 (27.3%) received a diagnosis of 'neurotic depression' (300.4). Only 18 diagnoses (10.2%) were ambiguous, including six with 298.0 ('reactive depressive psychosis').

In summary, although the two classical types of psychotic and neurotic depression are contained in the ICD, the provision of additional categories makes the situation rather complicated. Stressful events and their relationship to the onset of depression are given as positive inclusion criteria for at least five categories (300.4, 309.0, 309.1, 308.0, 298.0), but environmental factors may play some part also in the aetiology of 'psychotic' depression. Typically, judgments about the presence and seriousness of stressful life events and their relationship to the onset of depression are left completely to the clinician and are therefore heavily influenced by his subjective assessment of what he finds on examining the patient.

Bipolar/unipolar, psychotic/non-psychotic, and primary/secondary: popular dichotomies and their drawbacks

A number of relatively simple diagnostic dichotomies concerning depression have recently gained some popularity in psychiatric practice and research. They include the 'bipolar/unipolar', the 'psychotic/non-psychotic', and the 'primary/secondary' distinctions. These dichotomies are considered here because they are often and wrongly employed in the sense of the biological/psychosocial dichotomy. They obviously have become popular because it is relatively easy to classify depressed patients with the help of just one criterion, instead of applying complex definitions of 'endogenous' and 'neurotic'. It is characteristic of these dichotomies that *one* of the subtypes is positively defined and that a number of depressed patients readily fit the description, while the other subtype is negatively defined, i.e. as not belonging to the first type. The term 'non-psychotic' clearly reflects this concept, and it is quite logical that occasionally the term 'non-bipolar' is used instead of 'unipolar'; if one really wanted to, one could also speak of 'non-secondary' instead of primary depression. The negatively defined group may thus be quite heterogeneous, a fact which is frequently forgotten. The precise meanings of these dichotomies sometimes get lost, as the terms 'bipolar', 'psychotic', and 'primary' are frequently used as though they were synonyms for 'endogenous'. Hence, these dichotomies, although basically clear and simple, have actually served to increase the misunderstanding and confusion surrounding the subclassification of depression.

It is, for instance, relatively easy to subdivide depressed patients into those who reportedly have or have not had a manic episode, i.e. to distinguish bipolar from unipolar depressives. Although there is some plausibility to the idea that bipolar patients represent the purest form definable today (on clinical grounds) of the biological type of depression, i.e. of depressive illness (Angst, 1966; Perris, 1966), the bipolar/unipolar dichotomy does not help to distinguish a possible 'biological' from a 'psychosocial' type of depression *within the* (*much larger*) *unipolar* group. Simply comparing bipolar with unipolar depressives (see, e.g., Schildkraut, 1978) may conceal differences which in fact exist between a biological and a psychosocial form of depression, since the group of unipolar depressives may contain variable proportions of the psychosocial and the biological type. Furthermore, a subdivision based on the characteristics of the illness course may have to be revised at a later stage and thus yield a heterogeneous non-bipolar group, which also includes patients who will become manic in the future. Moreover, manic episodes are relatively rare as compared with depressive episodes; for example, in a sample of 176 depressed in-patients only 18 (10.2%) had had a previous manic episode and were thus bipolar (Katschnig *et al.*, 1981), so that nearly 90% of the patients fell into the non-bipolar group. During a two-year follow-up of the 158 'non-bipolars' eight (5.1%; 4.5% of the total sample) became manic, i.e. bipolar, and had thus been originally incorrectly assigned to the non-bipolar group.

Similar reservations apply to the psychotic/non-psychotic dichotomy. If a depressed patient reports hallucinations and delusional experiences, it is easy to label him psychotic. However, although the presence of psychotic symptoms might suggest a biological aetiology, an absence of these symptoms does not automatically signify a psychosocial aetiology. Non-psychotic depressives are probably as heterogeneous in terms of aetiology, and certainly in phenomenology, as the group of non-bipolar depressives. Moreover and again, psychotic symptoms are rather uncommon phenomena, even in more severely depressed patients: in our sample of 176 depressed in-patients we found only 17 (9.7%) with hallucinations or delusions.

The separation of 'primary' from 'secondary' depression, proposed by Robins *et al.* (1972) and incorporated into the St Louis criteria (Feighner *et al.*, 1972), has created much confusion, since these terms were and still are frequently misunderstood as synonyms for the 'biological' and the 'psychosocial' type of depression respectively, which they originally were not intended to be. On the contrary, the primary/secondary distinction was explicitly introduced as a way of classifying depression which *avoided* assumptions about aetiology. 'Secondary' is applied to those depressive disorders which occur in conjunction with a pre-existing, non-affective psychiatric illnesses, or with a life-threatening or incapacitating medical illness which precedes and co-exists with the symptoms of depression. 'Primary' refers to depressions occurring in the absence of such other illnesses (according to Spitzer, Endicott & Robins, 1978, the St Louis group no longer makes a diagnosis of secondary depression because of a pre-existing life-threatening condition). Again, when information about any additional psychiatric or somatic diseases is available, the primary/secondary distinction can easily be made. However, depressed patients may be 'misdiagnosed' as primary just because of a lack of information about preceding psychiatric illnesses. The primary/secondary distinction is very popular in research on biological markers of depression and many examples of wrongly equating primary with endogenous, or inexactly using the term primary can be found, e.g. in studies on the Dexamethasone Suppression Test (Carroll, Curtis & Mendels, 1976*a*,*b*) and on sleep architecture (Feinberg *et al.*, 1982; see also *British Medical Journal*, 1981).

It should be clear that the aforementioned dichotomies – in addition to their lack of a relationship with the biological/psychosocial dichotomy – by no means correspond to each other. While, for example, in our study (Katschnig *et al.*, 1981) by definition all 176 patients suffered from primary depression, 18 (10.2%) were diagnosed as bipolar and 17 (9.7%) as psychotic, but only three patients (1.7%) were found to be both bipolar and psychotic.

Operational diagnostic criteria: RDC, DSM-III, VRC, CATEGO classes, etc.

The publication of the St Louis criteria (Feighner *et al.*, 1972) marked the beginning of an era of research-orientated diagnostic systems, attempting to produce operational diagnostic terms which had been more implicitly than explicitly defined in the past, i.e., to write down symptomatological and other inclusion or exclusion criteria for specific traditional psychiatric concepts (such as schizophrenia or dementia). Inevitably, apart from defining existing concepts, the authors of such 'operational' diagnostic criteria also succumbed to the temptation to introduce new ones, such as the above-mentioned primary/secondary distinction of depressive disorders, thereby unfortunately creating new confusion.

The next misunderstanding was programmed when Spitzer *et al.* (1978) in their 'Research Diagnostic Criteria (RDC)' introduced the terms 'major' and 'minor' in connection with depressive disorder, referring rather to clinical severity or completeness of the clinical picture than to the factual distinction of a 'real' illness (='major') from a less 'serious' depressive reaction (= 'minor'). The usefulness of the major/minor distinction is questionable in the light of recent findings showing that less severe depressions and those with 'incomplete' clinical pictures also have biological correlates to some extent (Akiskal *et al.*, 1980). Simply equating major depressive disorder with the biological type of depression, as is frequently done, ignores the possibility provided in the RDC of subdividing 'major depressive disorder' into different subtypes, including among others an endogenous/non-endogenous, a psychotic/non-psychotic, and a situational/non-situational distinction, which can be used independently from one another. The RDC definition of 'endogenous' encompasses, among others, such traditional features as 'distinct quality of depressed mood', 'worse in the morning', 'lack of reactivity to environmental changes', and 'pervasive loss of pleasure/interest', whereas 'situational' refers to a depressive illness that 'has developed after an event or a situation that seems likely to have contributed to the appearance of the episode at that time'. However, no clear criteria are in fact given for separating situational from non-situational depressives.

The same basic considerations as for the RDC apply to the notion of 'major depressive episode' in the DSM-III, which is defined as the 'full depressive syndrome'. Here, the temptation to misinterpret the term 'major' as referring to a 'real' illness is smaller, because the term 'minor' does not exist in the DSM-III (which employs a number of other terms in order to refer to depressive disorders with only a 'partial' depressive syndrome, e.g. 'cyclothymia' or 'dysthymic disorder'). In fact, the DSM-III explicitly avoids the classical dichotomy of endogenous/neurotic. Instead it provides on a separate axis a rather ill-defined nine-point scale for 'severity of psychosocial stressors', which can be used in conjunction with any diagnosed psychiatric syndrome. On the syndromatic level both a 'psychotic' and a 'melancholic' subtype are defined. Although the definition of the 'melancholic' subtype includes 'lack of reactivity to usual pleasurable stimuli' as an obligatory item, it is principally possible also to characterise it as being the consequence of 'psychosocial stressors' in using the 'stress-axis'.

Other operational definitions include the Vienna Research Criteria (VRC) for the 'endogenomorphic cyclothymic axial syndrome' (Berner *et al.*,

1983*a*) and the CATEGO classes by Wing *et al.* (1974). Both rely exclusively on cross-sectional psychopathological symptoms. The Viennese criteria include changes in affectivity, emotional resonance, or drive following a period of habitual functioning, and biorhythmic disturbances as obligatory items. CATEGO defines a class D for psychotic and a class R for retarded depression. The latter is ambiguous in respect to the endogenous/reactive dichotomy, although it is usually lumped together with class D (e.g. Bebbington, Tennant & Hurry, 1981). CATEGO class N ('neurotic') is also defined on purely symptomatological grounds.

In a sense the subdivision proposed by Winokur *et al.* (1971) is also operational. This group uses age of onset (before and after 40) as the subdividing criterion, which they claim to have validated by familial aggregation data. 'Familial pure depressive disease' has an onset after 40 and a family history of primary depression (suggesting that it corresponds to 'true depressive illness'), whereas onset before the age of 40 qualifies for inclusion in the category of 'depression spectrum disease', with alcoholism and psychopathy more frequently found in the family history. Recently a third type, 'sporadic depressive disease', was added (Winokur, 1982).

Klein's (1974) concept of 'endogenomorphic depression' (centring on 'anhedonia') which has been recently made operational (see Davidson *et al.*, 1984*b*), the Yale definition of autonomous depression (quoted by Andreasen *et al.*, 1984) and a subscale for 'endogenomorphic depression' derived from the Hamilton scale (Kovacs *et al.*, 1981; Thase *et al.*, 1983) are further examples of 'operational' definitions of the supposedly biological type of depression, leaving the non-biological type undefined.

Diagnostic scales: the 'Newcastle Scale', the 'Depressive Category Type Scale' and the 'Michigan Discriminant Index'

The construction of a ten-item scale, the so-called 'Newcastle Scale', by Carney, Roth & Garside (1965) represents the first attempt to render the two classical clinical subtypes of depression operational. Similar 'scales' have been produced by Sandifer, Wilson & Green (1966; 'Depressive Category Type Scale') and by Feinberg & Carroll (1982; 'Michigan Discriminant Index').

All three scales contain items referring to the influence of the social environment on depression, with the intention of moving the score in the 'neurotic' direction, when such an influence is judged to be present. Thus, in the Depressive Category Type Scale a 'precipitating factor' is included as one of the 15 items on the list; in the Michigan Discriminant Index a 'precipitating event' is one of the 11 items of the scale, and in the Newcastle Scale two items are relevant: 'no adequate psychogenesis', referring to 'no psychological stress or difficulty continuing to operate after the onset of symptoms and adequate to explain the perpetuation of the illness', and the item 'blames others', which is intended to reflect the depressed person's tendency to explain his depression in terms of external social factors.

While the Depressive Category Type Scale consists of a list of 15 items (which are added together to give a total score) culled from the literature and thought to discriminate between endogenous and neurotic depression, both the Newcastle Scale and the Michigan Discriminant Index have been more systematically derived by using multivariate statistical methods. Thus, the authors of the Newcastle Scale, in order to find an algorithm for separating neurotic from endogenous depression, first collected information on 35 different items (cross-sectional psychopathological, personality, course of the illness, 'psychogenesis', etc.) in 129 depressed in-patients, whom they diagnosed as neurotic or endogenous, using their clinical judgment. A discriminant function analysis yielded 10 items which gave a satisfying separation between the two diagnostic groups. The rounded weights of these items constitute the single scores, which are added up for each patient and then used to separate the patients under study into a 'neurotic' (total score = 5 or less) and an 'endogenous' (total score = 6 or more) group.

Both in the Newcastle Scale and in the Michigan Discriminant Index psychosocial factors have the highest possible weights. In the Newcastle Scale the item 'no adequate psychogenesis' has a weight of +2 on a scale ranging from −2 to +14, with a cut-off point of 5/6 for neurotic/endogenous. Equally, in the Michigan Discriminant Index the adjusted canonical coefficient for 'precipitants present' is −0.93964, which is the highest weight among all items in the discriminant function. With a score of −6 it still has the second highest weight in the simplified 'Diagnostic Index'.

However, neither in the Newcastle Scale nor in the Michigan Discriminant Index is any provision made for reliable data collection concerning these psychosocial factors. This constitutes a major deficiency of these scales, as can be demonstrated in our sample of 176 depressed in-patients (Katschnig *et al.*, 1981). When the Newcastle Scale was applied, 108 patients were classified as neurotic and 68 as endogenous (see Figure 7.1). As can be seen in Figure 7.2 a simple change in the item 'no adequate psychogenesis' can lead to very large differences in diagnostic assignments. If a psychiatrist were to have rated all patients as having 'no adequate psychogenesis', 116 patients would have been called endogenous; if, on the other hand, a rater would have judged an 'adequate psychogenesis' to be present in all patients, only 39 would have received the 'endogenous' label. Thus, a change of response to this single, rather unreliable item could cause an avalanche of patients moving across the neurotic/endogenous border. This phenomenon has been called 'pseudoprecision' (Katschnig, 1985), in view of the fact that rating scales claim to be methodologically superior to other approaches.

On the other hand, the item 'no adequate psychogenesis' is optional, as

Figure 7.1. Depressed in-patients separated into an 'endogenous' and a 'neurotic' group according to the Newcastle Scale ($N = 176$).

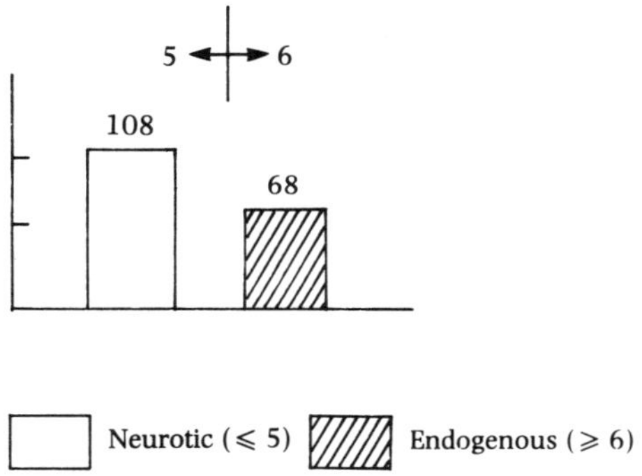

Figure 7.2. Depressed in-patients separated into an 'endogenous' and a 'neurotic' group according to the Newcastle Scale but (*a*) with the item 'no adequate psychogenesis' rated as absent and (*b*) as present, in all cases ($N = 176$).

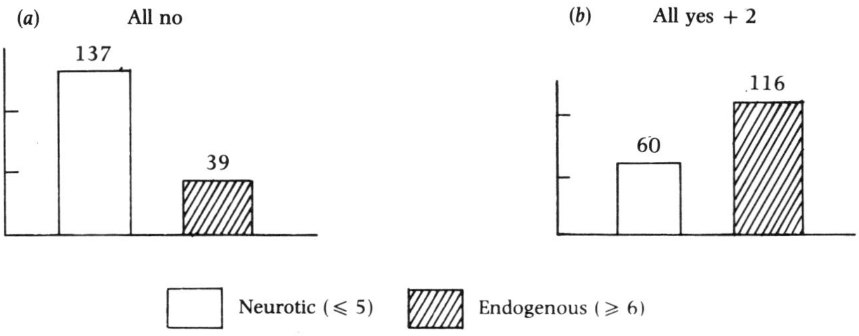

are all other items of the Newcastle Scale, since it is only the sum of scores which is important and not a constellation of specific items. In fact, among our 68 Newcastle Scale endogenous depressives, more than one third (38.2%) had an 'adequate psychogenesis', although this was significantly less than the 89.9% of the 108 neurotic patients, who were judged to have an 'adequate psychogenesis' (leaving, however, more than 10% neurotics with 'no adequate psychogenesis').

It is evident that the 'scale' approach to subtyping depressive disorders only *appears* to be objective and capable of providing replicable homogeneous groups of patients. In Tables 7.1 and 7.2 it is shown that clinical pictures which are very different from one another can belong to the same diagnostic group, whereas syndromes which are very similar to one another can belong to opposite diagnostic groups. A patient showing, e.g., a distinct quality of depression, weight loss and nihilistic delusions would be called neurotic, whereas the additional occurrence of 'guilt' would make

Table 7.1. *Newcastle Scale. Examples for composition of scores for endogenous and neurotic depression*

+1	Adequate personality	+1	Distinct quality	+1	Distinct quality
+2	No adequate psychogenesis	+2	Weight loss	+2	Weight loss
+1	Previous episode	+2	Nihilistic delusions	+2	Nihilistic delusions
+2	Depressive psychomotor activity	+1	Guilt		
Σ = 6	Endogenous	Σ = 6	Endogenous	Σ = 5	Neurotic

Table 7.2. *Newcastle Scale. Examples for composition of scores for endogenous and neurotic depression*

+1	Adequate personality	+1	Adequate personality	+1	Adequate personality
+2	No adequate psychogenesis	+2	No adequate psychogenesis	+2	No adequate psychogenesis
+2	Weight loss	+2	Weight loss	+2	Weight loss
		+1	Previous episode	+1	Previous episode
				−1	Anxiety
Σ = 5	Neurotic	Σ = 6	Endogenous	Σ = 5	Neurotic

him endogenous (Table 7.1). Similarly, a depressed patient with an 'adequate personality', 'no adequate psychogenesis' and 'weight loss' would be neurotic; if, however, he has already had a preceding depressive episode, this would make him an endogenous depressive, who again would turn into a neurotic if he showed anxiety (Table 7.2). In fact, the 68 Newcastle endogenous patients showed 39 such different symptom patterns. Obviously, the scale approach does not guarantee homogeneous samples of patients, but only suggests homogeneity to be present. The term 'pseudohomogeneity' (Katschnig, 1985) seems appropriate to characterise this phenomenon, which is in fact typical of most diagnostic formulations (see p. 227).

Depressive subtypes in research on depression

The imprecise use of diagnostic terms and concepts in research on depression

A leading article in the *British Medical Journal* on Saturday, 22 August 1981 (p. 513), announced the advent of 'the new psychiatry'. Given the increasing number of biological studies apparently showing an association between the supposedly biological subtype of depression and a range of biological markers (such as the Dexamethasone Suppression Test, the Thyrotropin-Releasing Hormone Test, urinary 3-methoxy-4-hydroxy-phenylglycol (MHPG), etc.), decisive improvements in psychiatric nosology were regarded as imminent. The diagnosis of such subtypes of depression would in the future depend not on the clinician's experience and knowledge, but rather on objective biological tests. However, a closer look at the leading article itself and at the studies quoted therein reveals a strange semantic confusion. It is, for example, astonishing to find that the terms 'primary depression' and 'endogenous depression' are used synonymously, although they have nothing in common and are quite differently defined, or to detect an equation of 'non-endogenous' with 'neurotic'. Obviously, the sophistication usually invested in research design and the measurement of 'correlates' of psychiatric disorders (e.g. abnormalities in the hypothalamic–pituitary–adrenocortical axis) is not employed in defining and naming the mental disturbances under study. On the contrary, a rather loose attitude seems to be common in this respect, and many studies are rather imprecise as far as the definition of the study population is concerned.

Two such types of imprecision in defining and naming mental disorders can be identified: a false synonymous use of terms on the one hand and a false homonymous use on the other.

The first concerns the equation of terms which originally refer to different and only partially overlapping clinical phenomena, such as 'endogenous', 'psychotic', 'major', 'primary', 'melancholic', 'endogenomorphic', to name just the most widely used terms, which are meant to refer to the biological type of depression. An example can be found in a paper by Feinberg & Carroll (1982): 'The differentiation of endogenous depression (psychotic depression, melancholia) from non-endogenous depression (reactive depression, neurotic depression) is crucial in any research involving depressed patients.' The hope to find any biological correlate for depression is obviously greater when research workers study patients diagnosed as 'endogenous', 'psychotic', etc., i.e. patients whose depression is of presumed biological origin due to a long-standing clinical assumption about a correlation between symptomatology and cause. However, since 'endogenous', 'psychotic', 'major', 'primary', 'melancholic', etc. are all differently defined – either traditionally or according to recently published operational criteria – using one of these concepts or one specific operational definition must necessarily yield a study population which is different from that of a study employing different concepts and criteria. The same holds for the terms 'non-endogenous', 'reactive', 'neurotic', 'psychogenic', etc. that are interchangeably used for referring to the non-biological type of depression. To assume, as is frequently done in review articles, that all studies using any one of these terms or concepts refer to the same phenomenon is not permissible.

The reverse phenomenon can also be found. Instead of using different terms for supposedly the same concept, the same term is used to mean many different phenomena, i.e. it is silently used as a homonym. Klerman *et al.* (1979) have shown this to be the case for the term 'neurotic depression'. They distinguished at least seven different uses of this term, which we have complemented by two further examples detected in the literature: a non-psychotic depression (defined by the absence of psychotic features), a non-endogenous depression (just lacking the common endogenous features), a form of depression showing features opposite to those of endogenous depression (such as difficulties in falling asleep or feeling worse in the evening), a depression with 'neurotic' symptoms (such as anxiety), a depression which is thought to be the expression of intrapsychic conflicts going back to the first years of life, a 'reactive depression' being the direct consequences of actual psychosocial adversities, a long-standing depression in terms of a 'characterological deformation', a less severe form of depression, and finally, a depression in out-patients as opposed to in-patients. All these uses can be found in studies employing the term neurotic and it is obvious that no cumulative body of knowledge can be built up from such investigations.

Depressive subtypes and the search for a depressive disease

The imprecise use of diagnostic terms in research will be illustrated by some of the many recent studies which have been carried out in order to identify biological markers of depression, such as the Dexamethasone Suppression Test, growth hormone stimulation, or sleep parameters. The selection of examples presented here is not comprehensive as it only serves for illustrative purposes; research on a number of other biological markers (e.g. urinary MHPG and the Thyrotropin-Releasing Hormone Test), as well as pharmacological studies, which could equally serve as illustrative examples for the imprecise use of diagnostic terms, are not considered here.

Example 1: The Dexamethasone Suppression Test and depressive subtypes

One type of study is concerned with the possible importance of a disturbance of the hypothalamic–pituitary–adrenal axis (HPA axis) for subclassifying depressive disorders. The straightforward hypothesis is that the biological form of depression is characterised by an overactivity of the HPA axis and that dexamethasone consequently does not suppress cortisol secretion, while the psychosocial form of depression and the psychiatrically healthy state are characterised by the normal functioning of this mechanism, i.e. by suppression of cortisol secretion after dexamethasone application. As opposed to this clearcut hypothesis, the actual identification of the two types of patients in Dexamethasone Suppression Test (DST) research is very inconsistent from study to study and even within the same investigation. For example, Carroll *et al.* (1976*a*, *b*), in their first attempt to show differences in DST response between these two types of depression, initially state that there is an abnormal limbic system drive on the HPA axis in 'primary depressive illness', and thereafter use the term 'endogenomorphic depression' without explaining exactly how they had separated their 42 endogenomorphic depressive patients (who showed an abnormal dexamethasone response in 57%) from the 12 patients with depressive neurosis (who showed no single abnormal dexamethasone response). They simply stated that they were using 'a complementary diagnostic classification' in primary depressive patients who had been selected according to Feighner *et al.*'s (1972) criteria. Thus, while formulating their hypothesis in terms of primary versus secondary depression, Carroll *et al.* (1976*a*, *b*) actually compared 'endogenomorphic' and 'neurotic' depression both of which were not clearly defined (although 6 years later they published a scale, the Michigan Discriminant Index, for subdividing endogenous from non-endogenous depression; Feinberg & Carroll, 1982). In 1982 Carroll summarised his work of the preceding 6 years and reached the conclusion that, for the 215 melancholic patients examined in all his studies, the DST specificity was 99% and its sensitivity 43%, when contrasted with 100 patients suffering from non-endogenous depression. The reason given by the author for now using the term melancholic instead of endogenous or endogenomorphic depression is simply that the old term had been reintroduced into clinical language by the DSM-III. However, the authors do not use the actual DSM-III definition of melancholia but simply apply the word melancholia to their own definition of the biological subtype of depression.

The results of studies of other authors are contradictory. Coryell, Gaffney & Burkhardt (1982) attempted to actually validate the DSM-III definition of melancholia by the DST but were not successful. Schatzberg *et al.* (1983) found that patients with DSM-III 'bipolar depression' or 'dysthymic-related disorders', had significantly lower cortisol levels after dexamethasone application than patients with 'major depression'. Evans, Burnett & Nemeroff (1983) found a high percentage of non-suppressors in patients with major depression according to the DSM-III, as opposed to a mixed group of patients with other diagnoses but additionally suffering from depressive symptoms (only 1 of 17 showed non-suppression in this group). Results obtained with the Newcastle Scale are contradictory: Holden (1983) reported that the endogenous subtype is associated with non-suppression, whereas Berger *et al.* (1982) could not find any DST specificity for the endogenous subtype. Berger *et al.* (1982) also applied the RDC criteria for endogenous depression without finding any DST difference between endogenous and non-endogenous depression.

Example 2: Growth hormone response and depressive subtypes

In the last 15 years it has been repeatedly reported that the normal growth hormone (GH) release reaction to various stimuli, such as hypoglycaemia, amphetamine, clonidine, or desimipramine, is blunted in depressive patients. Although there are some indications that this blunted response is specific for what various authors call endogenous depression, the evidence is so far not convincing. Laakmann (1980) found a blunted GH response after the administration of desimipramine in endogenous depressives but not in neurotic depressives. His diagnostic subdivision, however, was based on clinical diagnosis (ICD-8) provided by the doctors on the wards and not on any standardised diagnostic assignment. Similarly, Checkley, Slade & Shur (1981) found that GH response to clonidine was significantly lower in 10 drug-free patients with endogenous depression when compared with 10 normal subjects who were individually matched with the patients for age and sex. In this study a rather narrow operational definition of endogenous depression (RDC endogenous plus Newcastle Scale score of 6 or more) was used. The authors seem to confirm findings of Matussek (1978) who, however, had not employed operationalised diagnostic criteria. That comparability in subclassification may be crucial is demonstrated by the studies of Langer *et al.* (1976) and Checkley (1979) on GH response to amphetamine in endogenous depressive patients: while the first group found a reduction in GH response, this finding could not be replicated by Checkley. Although there were also other differences in research design, the different definitions of endogenous depression may be responsible for the discrepant results, since Langer *et al.*'s (1976) diagnoses were established according to the ICD-8, while Checkley used the Newcastle Scale.

Example 3: Sleep parameters and depressive subtypes

Since the introduction of standardised methods for measuring the neurophysiological correlates of sleep patterns (Rechtschaffen & Kales, 1968) efforts have been made to use such sleep patterns for the validation of subtypes of depression. Kupfer (1976) was among the first to show that primary depressives had a shortened rapid eye movement (REM) latency as compared to so-called secondary depressives, who in his study constituted a mixed group of depressives with personality disorders, anxiety neuroses, borderline schizophrenic disorders and drug abuse. In a later study (Kupfer *et al.*, 1978) REM latency and REM density discriminated between primary and secondary depression, while sleep efficiency, percentage of REM sleep, and percentage of delta sleep seemed to be able to differentiate between psychotic and non-psychotic depression. No mention of endogenous versus non-endogenous depression can be found in this paper. However, Feinberg *et al.* (1982) quote Kupfer *et al.*'s (1978) study as demonstrating a clear difference in sleep architecture between endogenous depression on the one hand and non-endogenous (neurotic) depression on the other. Feinberg *et al.* (1982) do, in fact, demonstrate that RDC endogenous and RDC non-endogenous depressives can be separated by the variables REM latency and REM density, and there would be little to criticise in this paper if it were not for the loose terminology (the authors equate non-endogenous with neurotic, which is not a term used in the RDC) and the imprecise quotation of the subclassification used by Kupfer *et al.* (1978).

In recent years, more sophistication in terms of diagnostic subclassification can be observed. For instance, Rush *et al.* (1982) used two subclassifications simultaneously: the primary/secondary and the endogenous/non-endogenous dichotomy (employing the RDC criteria). They were able to demonstrate that the sleep parameters which in Kupfer's (1976) study discriminated between primary and secondary and in Feinberg *et al.*'s (1982) study between endogenous and non-endogenous depressives did far better in discriminating between endogenous and non-endogenous than between primary and secondary depressives, when the diagnostic subgroups were formed out of the same patient sample.

These examples of biological marker studies sufficiently illustrate the confusing state of diagnostic subtyping of depression in psychiatric research, especially in terms of a lack of comparability between different studies. Given the great interest in biological markers, it has to be concluded that a polydiagnostic approach (Berner & Katschnig, 1983; Katschnig & Berner, 1985) is urgently required in this field to make better use of scarce resources and to be able to pool research results from different studies. In fact, polydiagnostic studies on the DST are already forthcoming (Davidson *et al.*, 1984*a*; Zimmerman *et al.* 1985).

Research on the subclassification of depression: the role of phenomenological and life stress variables

Although the ostensible aim of some of the biological studies quoted in the last section is the 'validation' of diagnostic subclasses of depression, the methodological emphasis of these studies is clearly on the measurement of biological markers in disease entities which are taken for granted and not on a more precise definition or even on questioning the justification of the diagnostic classes under study. In contrast, 'validation', with the specific sceptical attitude this entails, has become the central issue of a number of studies using phenomenological and life stress data to see whether or not certain ways of subclassifying depressive disorders are justified. In this section we will try to summarise the present knowledge in this field, taking our own study on 176 depressed in-patients as an additional illustrative example (Katschnig *et al.*, 1981). Other possible validating variables, such as familial aggregation or characteristics of illness course (see, e.g., Katschnig, Nutzinger & Schanda, 1986), are not examined here. We will first deal with the use of multivariate statistical methods for identifying the endogenous subtype of depression and with the application of the polydiagnostic approach, and will then summarise research on the concept of 'situational' depression. Finally, studies using life stress variables in order to validate specific diagnostic formulations of subtypes of depressive disorders will be discussed.

The search for the 'endogenous' class: cluster analysis and the polydiagnostic approach

We began this chapter by referring to Hamilton & White's (1959) factor analytic study on depression which claims to support the endogenous/reactive dichotomy. Since then, factor analytic studies have repeatedly shown an intercorrelation between variables regarded as specific for the endogenous type of depression by clinicians (Grinker *et al.*, 1961; Kiloh & Garside, 1963; Rosenthal & Klerman, 1966: Rosenthal & Gudeman, 1967; Mendels & Cochrane, 1968; Kay *et al.*, 1969; Paykel, Prusoff & Klerman, 1971; Rassaby & Paykel, 1979). However, as Maxwell (1971) has pointed out, factor analysis, being concerned with the classification of variables, is not suited to solve problems concerning the classification of patients. Maxwell recommends cluster analysis instead. In a further 'multivariate' approach, discriminant function analysis is employed for measuring the distinctness of subgroups of depressive disorders (e.g. Carney *et al.*, 1965; Kendell, 1968). However, discriminant function analysis requires the a-priori separation on clinical grounds of a group of patients into subgroups and cannot be employed for detecting a latent structure in a given patient population. Again, this can only be achieved by cluster analytic methods, whereby similarities between different patients in a large number of variables can be recognised and the patients thus grouped into homogeneous clusters. In the following sections, studies trying to identify subclasses of depression by means of cluster analysis will be summarised. An analysis of the relationship between different definitions of endogenous depression using a polydiagnostic approach will then be presented. More complex approaches using, e.g., hierarchical relationships between subtypes (Foulds, 1973) or a mixture of categorical and dimensional types (Everitt, Gourlay & Kendell, 1971) are outside the scope of this article.

Cluster analysis and endogenous depression. Cluster analysis in a sense imitates the paradigmatic form of clinical diagnosis, albeit in a replicable way. It identifies in a multi-dimensional space a 'cloud' of patients being more or less similar to the prototypical patient in the centre of the cloud. In fact one could argue that the traditional psychiatric disease entities are the result of 'intracerebral cluster analyses' of the founding fathers of modern psychiatry.

Several cluster analytic studies, which, unfortunately, have used different sets of criteria for describing depressive patients, have repeatedly identified a rather homogeneous group of patients, characterised by the classical 'endogenous' symptom pattern. However, most of these studies have failed to find a similarly homogeneous 'neurotic' group. Thus, Overall *et al.* (1966) identified a 'retarded' cluster, which responded to tricyclic antidepressants, in contrast to two other groups (an 'anxious' and a 'hostile' cluster) which did not. In a subsequent analysis of a larger sample, an additional 'agitated' type emerged which was close to 'anxious' depression (Overall, 1974). In a study on 165 depressed patients from a variety of treatment settings, Paykel (1971) found a 'psychotic' group, as opposed to several other groups, which, according to the names given to them (anxious, hostile, young depressive with personality disorder), come nearer to the concept of neurotic depression. Byrne (1978) subjected self-reported depressive symptomatology of 135 depressed in-patients to a cluster analysis: again, a cluster resembling clinical endogenous depression emerged, but no group which corresponded to neurotic depression was found. Andreasen, Grove & Maurer (1980) carried out a cluster analysis on 78 RDC 'definite major' and 8 'definite minor depressive disorder' patients and were also able to identify a clear endogenous group on the one hand, and two other clusters which could not be so easily interpreted on the other. In a replication of this study Andreasen & Grove (1982), using a larger sample of more severely depressed patients, could partly confirm these findings, but a separate 'psychotic' cluster emerged as well. Further empirical evidence favouring the concept of the existence of an 'endogenous' syndrome and refuting a corresponding 'neurotic' syndrome comes from our study (Katschnig *et al.*, 1981). A cluster analysis on 176 depressed in-patients yielded a large cluster of 100 patients who showed an endogenous symptom pattern (retardation, early morning wakening, depressive rumination, social impairment, loss of appetite, retarded thinking, depression worse in the morning). The remaining 76 patients belonged to six separate small clusters which were not easily interpretable.

While these artificially derived groupings of depression can be studied by comparing their symptom profiles – and this has in fact been done in many of the above mentioned studies in which similarities with clinical endogenous depression were found – it is also possible to compare them with existing diagnostic assignments. Thus, Overall & Zisook (1980) investigated how several operational definitions of depression (but not specifically endogenous depression) – among them the St Louis criteria for primary depression (Feighner *et al.*, 1972) and the RDC criteria for major depressive disorder (Spitzer *et al.*, 1978) – corresponded with their own cluster-analysis-derived grouping. They found that the operational criteria examined were heterogeneous in terms of the clinical syndromes as defined by their own clusters. Andreasen & Grove (1982) also studied the correspondence between their own mathematically generated clusters and the clinically derived categories of the RDC (Spitzer *et al.*, 1978). While the correspondence with the RDC categories of endogenous and psychotic depression was quite satisfying, the RDC concept of situational depression was not validated (see p. 229).

The polydiagnostic approach and endogenous depression. Studying the correspondence between different definitions of the same diagnostic concept has in itself become a promising research strategy for elucidating problems of psychiatric classification. Such simultaneous application of different definitions of the same concept to one and the same study population has been called the polydiagnostic approach (see p. 206; Berner & Katschnig, 1983; Katschnig & Berner, 1985).

Thus, Davidson *et al.* (1984*b*) specifically examined the diagnosis of melancholia and endogenous depression as defined by five different diagnostic scales and found a threefold variation in frequency and also a varying overlap between different definitions. Also in the Viennese study (Katschnig *et al.*, 1981) a more than threefold variation in frequency for eight different definitions of endogenous depression could be found for 176 depressed in-patients: while only 50 patients were diagnosed as melancholic according to the DSM-III, the RDC (Spitzer *et al.*, 1978) assigned 161 patients to the probable plus definite endogenous group. Figures for other

Table 7.3. *Numbers of patients assigned to the endogenous diagnostic group by eight different diagnostic criteria (total sample = 176 depressed in-patients)*

RDC probable plus definite endogenous	161 (91.5%)
CATEGO, Classes R or D	132 (75.0%)
RDC definite endogenous	124 (70.1%)
ICD-8 296.2	110 (62.5%)
VRC endogenomorphic cyclothymic axial syndrome	106 (60.2%)
Cluster analysis	100 (56.8%)
Newcastle Scale	68 (38.6%)
DSM-III Major depression (melancholic)	50 (28.4%)

formulations of endogenous depression lay inbetween (see Table 7.3). Moreover, in our study the overlap between different definitions of endogenous depression varied to a large extent but was on the whole rather modest (Katschnig & Seelig, 1985). The overlap – defined as the percentage of patients diagnosed as endogenous by both of two diagnostic formulations and calculated from the total of all patients diagnosed as endogenous by either one or the other of these two diagnostic formulations – ranged from 74.4% ('RDC probable plus definite endogenous' with 'CATEGO classes R or D') to 55% ('ICD-8, 296.2 with 'RDC definite endogenous') to only 35.9% ('Newcastle Scale' with 'Endogenomorphic cyclothymic axial syndrome'). In Table 7.4 these overlap percentages are presented for all combinations of diagnostic formulations.

So far we can conclude that, although artificial classification methods, such as cluster analysis, have repeatedly identified a relatively large subgroup among depressed patients resembling the clinical description of the endogenous subtype, the overlap between such clusters and published diagnostic formulations of endogenous depression, as well as the overlap between different published diagnostic formulations themselves, is, on the whole, rather modest. It is obvious that comparability must be small between results of studies which purport to be concerned with the same diagnosis but in fact use different diagnostic formulations and therefore select different study populations. It thus appears imperative for psychiatric research to use multiple diagnostic assignments, i.e. to pursue a polydiagnostic approach, whenever possible.

Apart from the application of different diagnostic algorithms for defining endogenous depression, a lack of homogeneity within one and the same definition can be an important reason for sampling different patient populations in different studies. This heterogeneity can be exemplified by analysing the 124 RDC definite endogenous patients of the Viennese study (Katschnig *et al.*, 1981) with respect to their symptom patterns (Table 7.5; see also above for similar problems concerning the Newcastle Scale, p. 217). The results of this analysis are presented here only for the four symptoms of group A (distinct quality of mood, lack of reactivity, feeling worse in the morning, pervasive loss of interest/pleasure), of which at least one is required for a definite diagnosis of endogenous depression (Spitzer *et al.*, 1978). Only 10.5% of all RDC endogenous patients presented all four symptoms. Just over 50% were characterised by three of the four symptoms, albeit in different variations. Over one third of all RDC endogenous depressives showed only two or one of these symptoms. It is interesting to note that the item 'lack of reactivity' is present in all

Table 7.4. *Percentages of overlap for cases of endogenous depression for six different diagnostic formulations*

	RDC probable plus definite endogenous	CATEGO Classes R or D	RDC definite endogenous	ICD-8 296.2	VRC endo-genomorphic cyclothymic axial syndrome	Cluster analysis
CATEGO Classes R or D	74.4					
RDC probable plus definite endogenous	77.0	64.1				
ICD-8 296.2	64.2	60.3	55.0			
VRC endogenomorphic cyclothymic axial syndrome	63.8	52.6	66.7	44.0		
Cluster analysis	58.2	46.9	61.2	45.9	47.1	
Newcastle Scale	41.4	39.9	45.5	45.9	35.9	44.8

Table 7.5. *Frequencies and patterns of group A symptoms in 124 patients with RDC definite endogenous major depressive disorder*

		Symptom patterns								
	Frequencies	Four symptoms	Three symptoms			Two symptoms				One symptom
Distinct quality	77 (62.1%)	×	×	×		×	×			
Lack of reactivity	123 (99.2%)	×	×	×	×	×		×	×	×
Worse in the morning	85 (68.5%)	×	×		×		×	×		
Pervasive loss of interest/pleasure	47 (37.9%)	×		×	×				×	
	N = 124	13	38	12	15	13	1	18	7	7
		10.5%	52.4%			31.5%				5.6%

but one of the RDC endogenous depressives. Apart from this item, however, the constellation of symptoms is rather diverse. Altogether nine different symptom patterns can be identified within the four symptoms of group A. When the additional six symptoms of group B are included, the picture becomes much more complicated in that 49 different symptom patterns emerge, documenting a high degree of heterogeneity.

Discrepancies between studies using an identical design may therefore even arise when identical diagnostic algorithms are used, since smaller or larger proportions of a specific symptom pattern could be responsible for a smaller or larger correlation with specific external variables. An uncritical reliance on 'operational' definitions and diagnostic algorithms without taking the symptomatological infrastructure of the study population into account may therefore be very misleading.

Defining situational depression

In the RDC (Spitzer *et al.*, 1978), depressive illness that 'has developed after an event or a situation that seems likely to have contributed to the appearance of the episode at that time' is called 'situational' depression. Certainly, the provision of the situational/non-situational dichotomy as an additional dimension which can be simultaneously used with other dichotomies – such as endogenous/non-endogenous, psychotic/non-psychotic – constitutes considerable progress. Using this approach of multiple assignment to different dichotomies, Endicott & Spitzer (1979) could, for instance, demonstrate that 42% of RDC situational depressives were also diagnosed as having endogenous depression, and that 37% of endogenous patients were also situational, i.e., that these two classifications were largely independent from each other. Prusoff *et al.* (1980) observed the same phenomenon in a therapeutic study and could also show that the RDC endogenous/non-endogenous and situational/non-situational dimensions were independent from each other in terms of therapeutic responsiveness.

Apart from the advantage which a multiaxial approach in itself constitutes the definition of situational depression in the RDC is very problematic. It is not 'operational' in any sense, and it is already clear from the definition that this diagnostic assignment must be rather unreliable. To judge whether 'an event or a situation... *seems* likely to have contributed to the appearance of the episode at that time' is a highly arbitrary process depending both on the patient's and on the diagnostician's theories and attributional styles with all the implications of selective perception of reality. Thus, Hirschfeld (1981; Hirschfeld *et al.*, 1984) could not validate the clinical RDC diagnosis of situational depression when preceding life stress was also measured independently by a more rigorous life event methodology, and Nelson & Charney (1980) showed that different raters disagreed about the presence of a precipitating event and therefore also about the inclusion of a depressed patient in a 'reactive' group. It is clear that diagnostic formulations which include a clinical judgment about reactivity without providing rigorous methodological guidelines of how to collect the relevant information suffer from a built-in lack of reliability. For the Newcastle Scale we have shown above how influential a single reactivity item can be for dramatic changes in diagnostic assignments.

In the Viennese study on depression, several ways of defining situational depression were applied simultaneously. When 'reactive' was defined by the 'presence of at least one life event in the week before onset' as measured by the method of Brown (1974), among the 176 in-patients only 23 patients (13.1%) could be classed as reactive depressives, whereas as many as 79 (44.9%) were classed as reactive depressives when the patient's judgment that either an acute or a chronic psychosocial stress was responsible for the outbreak of his depression was used as a definition (see Table 7.6). The percentages of 'reactive cases' according to other definitions range between these two extremes. The overlap between these different objective and subjective definitions of situational depression is even smaller (around 25%) than that shown for endogenous depression.

As the studies by Hirschfeld *et al.* (1984) and Nelson & Charney (1980) and our own results show it is clearly not enough to just have a clinician make a judgment about whether a psychological disorder is reactive or not. In some sense, it is easier to collect clinically symptomatological data than life event data and the inclusion of the latter into a diagnostic algorithm – as

Table 7.6. *Numbers of patients assigned to the reactive diagnostic group by five different formulations (total sample = 176 depressed in-patients)*

At least one life event in week before onset (researcher's judgment)	23 (13.1%)
At least one life event in four weeks before onset (researcher's judgment)	50 (28.4%)
'Chronic psychosocial stress responsible for onset' (patient's judgment)	53 (30.1%)
'Acute psychosocial stress responsible for onset' (patient's judgment)	58 (33.0%)
'Acute or/and chronic psychosocial stress responsible for onset' (patient's judgment)	79 (44.9%)

is the case in the Newcastle Scale and in the Michigan Discriminant Index – may introduce a significant element of unreliability in these diagnostic instruments (see also the chapter by Katschnig, p. 74, this volume).

Life stress as a validating criterion for phenomenologically defined depressive subtypes

Only few studies have so far explicitly tested the classical assumption of a relationship between phenomenologically defined diagnostic subgroups and life stress. Unfortunately, nearly all of these studies use different methodologies both for diagnostic assignment and for eliciting life stress and cannot easily be compared. We will consider first a handful of early studies, together with some recent ones which have used an inadequate life event methodology, but to which reference is sometimes made in the literature. In a second part studies using a more rigorous life event methodology will be analysed.

Studies using less rigorous life event methodologies. In an early study using an operational definition of endogenous (a positive score on four of the five symptoms: retardation, diurnal variation, early morning wakening, impaired concentration, ideas of guilt), Forrest, Fraser & Priest (1965) could not find a difference between an endogenous and a neurotic group of depressives in the 'incidence of pre-admission social stress factors' (elicited by a simple checklist covering the three previous years). Equally, Thomson & Hendrie (1972) found no difference in preceding life stress (as measured by the Social Readjustment Rating Scale of Holmes & Rahe, 1967) between endogenous and neurotic depressives. However, given the drawbacks both of Holmes & Rahe's life event methodology (see Katschnig, p. 74, this volume) and the use of clinical diagnosis for separating endogenous from neurotic depressives, the general applicability of this finding must remain doubtful. In a retrospective interview study covering several decades, Matussek & Neuner (1981) found that 'significantly more neurotic depressives than endogenous depressives had experienced the loss of a close person in the year before a depression. When the loss experiences were divided up, however, it became clear that the difference was due only to separations, and in particular to separations from an important partner.'

Two studies have used diagnostic distinctions, which are not directly referring to the endogenous/reactive dichotomy, although given the imprecise use of concepts discussed earlier in this chapter, they are of some relevance to the problem discussed here. Cadoret *et al.* (1972) compared patients whose depressive illness started before the age of 40 with later-onset depressives. After excluding brief reactions by loss through deaths they were able to demonstrate a significantly higher incidence of real or threatened personal losses in the early-onset than in the late-onset depressives, arguing that this result was in agreement with the separation of depressive disorders into 'depressive spectrum disease' and 'pure depressive disease' according to Winokur *et al.* (1971). The study by Patrick, Dunner & Fieve (1978) also has some relevance to this question. Using a life event questionnaire, the authors found no significant differences in life stress among patients classified as bipolar and unipolar; furthermore they were unable to show a decreased familial load for affective disorders in relatives of patients with 'reactive' primary affective illness.

Although when taken as a whole the results of these studies contradict the classical clinical assumption of endogenous depression being unprecipitated and neurotic depression being a consequence of life stress, the lack of methodological comparability prevents one from drawing any definite conclusion.

*Studies using more rigorous life event methodologies**. Brown, Ní Brolcháin & Harris (1979), Bebbington *et al.* (1981) and Katschnig *et al.* (1981) addressed the problem of validating the classical endogenous/reactive dichotomy by using the rigorous and laborious life event methodology developed by Brown (1974) for eliciting life stress. The results should thus be to some extent comparable, although a number of caveats are necessary (see below). Paykel (1971) and Benjaminsen (1981), when examining the question of a relationship between diagnostic subtypes and life stress, also used a sufficiently sophisticated and differentiated life event methodology (Paykel, 1983).

Bebbington and his colleagues (1981) found in their combined data on depressed community cases and psychiatric out-patients in London 'that syndromes typified by pathological guilt, retardation, or agitation, in comparison with syndromes without these symptoms, occurred in people who were relatively unlikely to have experienced adversity in the preceding three months'. This finding clearly supports the dualistic view of depression postulating two separate classes, a disease class and a distress class. However, the studies by Paykel (1971), Brown *et al.* (1979), Benjaminsen (1981) and Katschnig *et al.* (1981) suggest that there is no significant difference in preceding life stress between psychotic/endogenous and neurotic/reactive depression.

* This section is partly based on an article published by Katschnig (1984*a*).

A superficial look at the methodological sections of these five studies reveals a situation well known to authors trying to review a given scientific field. The studies are not comparable because different definitions of the same variables were used. In the studies quoted, this objection concerns both the ways of subclassifying depression and measuring life stress, although the instruments used were the same in some of the studies. Thus, whereas each of the five studies is more or less methodologically sound, this in itself does not help to create a cumulative body of knowledge.

For example, Brown *et al.* (1979), Bebbington *et al.* (1981) and Katschnig *et al.* (1981) used the same method for rating the severity of threat of a *single* life event (Brown, 1974); however, they constructed different indices for measuring the *total amount* of life stress experienced by a person before the onset of depression. Bebbington *et al.* (1981) used both a different cut-off point on the threat scale and a different time period from the study of Brown *et al.* (1979); Katschnig *et al.* (1981) used the same cut-off point as Brown *et al.* (1979), but took a different time period before onset. Brown & Harris (p. 108, this volume) are right to point out that these changes in definition undermine comparability.

As far as diagnostic subclassification is concerned, comparability is also not guaranteed. Paykel (1971) used a cluster-analysis-derived grouping; Brown *et al.* (1979) relied on clinical judgment; Bebbington *et al.* (1981) separated their cases in CATEGO classes 'N' (neurotic) and 'R or D' (retarded or psychotic) according to the Present State Examination (PSE)/CATEGO system (Wing *et al.*, 1974); Benjaminsen (1981) applied five dichotomies (among them endogenous/non-endogenous according to a private definition); and Katschnig *et al.* (1981), in their study on depressed in-patients, used several subclassifications which are not comparable with those of other groups. All authors, however, seem to equate their definitions of subclasses with the classical dichotomy of endogenous versus neurotic depression.

Comparisons between these five studies are therefore not possible and it is problematic for Bebbington (1984) to quote the Vienna study as showing conflicting evidence to his own data (Bebbington *et al.*, 1981), since neither the same life stress index nor the same subclassification of depression were used. Since the two studies are not comparable with respect to the main variables, contrasting them is pointless. We were, however, in the fortunate position to be able to reformulate both our diagnostic and life stress variables in order to render the two studies comparable (Katschnig, 1984*a*).

The main purpose of the Viennese study had been to determine to what extent different ways of subclassifying depression are valid in terms of preceding life stress. To realise this objective, we developed a comprehensive data collection instrument – based on the PSE by Wing *et al.* (1974) – containing all elements of information necessary to subdivide depressive disorders in as many ways as possible into subgroups defined in the literature, i.e. we have used a polydiagnostic approach (Berner & Katschnig, 1983; Katschnig & Berner, 1985). Among the diagnostic formulations used were the RDC definitions of endogenous versus non-endogenous depression (Spitzer *et al.*, 1978), the Viennese Research Criteria for the 'Endogenomorphic cyclothymic axial syndrome' (Berner *et al.*, 1983*a*), the DSM-III (American Psychiatric Association, 1980) and the ICD (WHO, 1967). A cluster analysis of symptoms yielded a clearcut endogenous cluster which could be set off from the rest of the patient population. Since the PSE was used, we were also able to replicate Bebbington *et al.*'s (1981) subdivision of CATEGO classes 'R or D' versus 'N'.

In contrast to Bebbington *et al.*'s (1981) results, no significant difference

Table 7.7. *Percentage of depressive patients with at least one life event in month before onset (only patients with complete psychological health in month before onset)*

	Endogenous	Non-endogenous	Test for comparing proportions (Fienberg, 1977)
RDC probable plus definite endogenous versus non-endogenous	36.6	50.0	ns
RDC definite endogenous versus non-endogenous	33.3	50.0	ns
ICD-8 296.2 versus 300.4	25.7	60.0	$P \leqslant 0.001$
Endogenomorphic cyclothymic axial syndrome (Vienna) versus rest	36.2	40.5	ns
Cluster analysis endogenous versus rest	34.7	42.6	ns
CATEGO class 'R or D' versus 'N'	37.8	40.7	ns
DSM-III Major depression (melancholic) versus rest	32.4	40.0	ns

in preceding life stress could be found for any of the subdivisions used. This held for a large number of different life stress indices based on the method of Brown (1974) – including the one employed by Bebbington *et al.* (1981) – and for different time periods as well. The only exception (to be discussed below) is the hospital ICD-8 diagnosis which showed the classical pattern of higher stress in neurotic depressives. In Tables 7.7 to 7.10 the results are presented for two such life stress indices covering the periods of 1 month and 6 months respectively before onset. Only patients with complete psychological health during the 1 month or the 6 months before onset were taken into consideration. Since the discrepancies between the London and the Vienna studies remain, even though identical diagnostic and stress definitions are used (Katschnig, 1984*a*), the conclusion is that Bebbington *et al.*'s data from London support the disease/distress dichotomy, whereas ours do not. We have to look therefore for other methodological differences which could explain these discrepant results.

If, as was the case in Bebbington *et al.*'s (1981) study, the same

Table 7.8. *Percentage of depressive patients with at least one severe life event in month before onset (only patients with complete psychological health in month before onset)*

	Endogenous	Non-endogenous	Test for comparing proportions (Fienberg, 1977)
RDC probable plus definite endogenous versus non-endogenous	10.7	30.0	ns
RDC definite endogenous versus non-endogenous	10.3	30.0	ns
ICD-8 296.2 versus 300.4	5.4	28.6	$P \leqslant 0.001$
Endogenomorphic cyclothymic axial syndrome (Vienna) versus rest	12.5	11.9	ns
Cluster analysis endogenous versus rest	10.7	14.9	ns
CATEGO class 'R or D' versus 'N'	11.1	18.5	ns
DSM-III Major depression (melancholic) versus rest	8.1	14.1	ns

interviewer elicits both symptomatological and life event information, the possibility cannot be ruled out that a correlation between neurotic depression and life stress on the one hand, and the lack of such a correlation with retarded/psychotic depression on the other, reflects the preconceived opinion of the interviewer. In our own study such a contamination is practically impossible, since two independent teams of interviewers elicited psychopathological and life stress information, and the life event interview was only carried out after the depressive episode had receded. A further possible explanation may be found in the different treatment status of the two samples. In London a community sample and out-patients were studied, as opposed to in-patients in Vienna. It is possible that illness behaviour factors bring relatively more class R/D cases than class N cases with preceding life stress into hospital treatment and thus level out possible life stress differences which may actually exist between the two diagnostic groups.

One further discrepancy remains to be explained, namely that within our

Table 7.9. *Percentage of depressive patients with at least one life event in the 6 months before onset (only patients with complete psychological health in the 6 months before onset)*

	Endogenous	Non-endogenous	Test for comparing proportions (Fienberg, 1977)
RDC probable plus definite endogenous versus non-endogenous	62.0	85.7	ns
RDC definite endogenous versus non-endogenous	60.0	85.7	ns
ICD-8 296.2 versus 300.4	46.0	93.3	$P \leqslant 0.001$
Endogenomorphic cyclothymic axial syndrome (Vienna) versus rest	60.8	68.6	ns
Cluster analysis endogenous versus rest	62.7	65.7	ns
CATEGO class 'R or D' versus 'N'	60.3	75.0	ns
DSM-III Major depression (melancholic) versus rest	53.6	69.0	ns

own data. In Tables 7.7 to 7.10 one diagnostic formulation, that of the ICD as employed by the doctors on the ward, consistently shows an association between the neurotic form of depression and life stress. From what has been discussed above (p. 207) it is, however, clear that the definitions of the ICD belong to the classical paradigmatic type of diagnosis and include not only symptomatological criteria, but also aetiological and other factors, thus leaving it to the clinician to decide on more or less subjective grounds whether a patient should or should not be placed in a particular diagnostic class. It is conceivable that the clinician's decision whether to diagnose a neurotic or an endogenous depression is mainly guided by the fact that he learns of some pre-existing life stress when interviewing the patient and is not based on symptomatology.

In order to examine this possibility a discriminant function analysis was carried out, using the same psychopathological symptoms which were employed in the cluster analysis (see p. 225). It turned out that ICD endogenous and ICD neurotic depressives did not differ in terms of these

Table 7.10. *Percentage of depressive patients with at least one severe life event in the 6 months before onset (only patients with complete psychological health in the 6 months before onset)*

	Endogenous	Non-endogenous	Test for comparing proportions (Fienberg, 1977)
RDC probable plus definite endogenous versus non-endogenous	21.5	28.6	ns
RDC definite endogenous versus non-endogenous	18.3	28.6	ns
ICD-8 296.2 versus 300.4	10.0	40.0	$P \leqslant 0.01$
Endogenomorphic cyclothymic axial syndrome (Vienna) versus rest	21.6	22.9	ns
Cluster analysis endogenous versus rest	21.6	22.9	ns
CATEGO class 'R or D' versus 'N'	17.5	30.0	ns
DSM-III Major depression (melancholic) versus rest	14.3	25.9	ns

psychopathological symptoms. In fact, the proportion of variance in psychopathology explained by the ICD classification was only 9%. When the patient's subjective judgment about a relationship between some form of acute or chronic psychosocial stress and the outbreak of his depressive episode was analysed, 69% of patients with ICD neurotic and 32% of those with ICD endogenous depression attributed the onset of their episode to external social stress. These rates differ significantly (see Table 7.11). Taken together, these findings favour the above mentioned hypothesis that at least the Viennese clinicians, when applying the paradigmatic ICD categories of endogenous and neurotic depression, are mainly influenced by the patient's reports about the presence or absence of psychosocial stressors and not by specific psychopathological features. The difference in preceding life stress found in our study between ICD neurotic and ICD endogenous can thus be easily explained as a tautological phenomenon.

Conclusion

The empirical evidence presented in this chapter suggests that the currently used arbitrary definitions of depressive subtypes are still lacking validity. There is, at least, no clear evidence that phenomenologically defined subtypes of depression are differently associated with life stress. The same holds for other validating criteria such as biological markers or illness course. The only more or less consistent finding is that cluster analytic studies using phenomenological data have repeatedly identified a rather homogenous endogenous cluster of depressive patients but not a neurotic one.

This inconclusiveness of present research on depressive subtypes results from a number of methodological deficiencies, which have been repeatedly demonstrated in this chapter. Among these are the confusion surrounding

Table 7.11. *Proportions of patients attributing the onset of their depression to life stress for ICD neurotic and ICD psychotic depression*

	ICD-8 neurotic 300.4	ICD-8 psychotic 296.2	
Either acute or chronic psychosocial stress responsible for onset (patient's judgment)	33/48 = 69%	35/110 = 32%	$P < 0.001$

the terminology of depressive subtypes, the nearly exclusive reliance on a categorical approach to classification, the use of different definitions of the same diagnostic concept in different studies, and the frequent denial of the difficulties of reliably assessing life stress. If a cumulative body of knowledge on the subclassification of depression is to be obtained, it is necessary to make up for these deficiencies in future research (see also Chapter 8, p. 246, this volume). First, terminological questions have to be taken more seriously and operational definitions may be a great help for that purpose, although they obviously do not guarantee homogenous patient populations. Given the heterogeneity of even operationally defined patient samples, additional data analyses on the symptom level are required in order not to miss specific aetiological relationships. Furthermore, in order to avoid artificial correlations between the phenomenological and the aetiological level, i.e. between psychopathological symptoms and life stress, the categorical approach to psychiatric diagnosis must be supplemented, or even replaced by a multiaxial approach with as independent an assessment of the different axes as possible. Using alternative theoretical models, such as hierarchical or dimensional ones, as opposed to the sole reliance on the 'pigeonhole' model, should also be taken into consideration. Furthermore, the simultaneous use of different diagnostic formulations in one and the same research project, i.e. pursuing a polydiagnostic approach, also seems necessary, in order to improve comparability between different studies. Finally, more rigorous life event methods, which are available but rarely used nowadays, would have to replace the frequent commonsense judgments usually relied on even by seemingly serious researchers. Even when the burden on a research project is considerably increased, it is imperative that life event data be collected with all the sophistication possible today. Unfortunately, there is no short and simple way to disentangling complex relationships in the field of psychopathology and those who continue to go the easy way are bound to fail.

References

Akiskal, H. S., Rosenthal, T. L., Haykal, R. F., Lemmi, H., Rosenthal, R. H. & Scott-Strauss, A. (1980). Characterological depressions. Clinical and sleep EEG findings separating 'subaffective dysthymias' from 'Character spectrum disorders'. *Archives of General Psychiatry*, **37**, 777–83.

American Psychiatric Association (1980). *Diagnostic and statistical manual of mental disorders*, 3rd edition, *DSM-III*. Washington: American Psychiatric Association.

Andreasen, N. C. & Grove, W. (1982). The classification of depression: traditional versus mathematical approaches. *American Journal of Psychiatry*, **139**, 45–52.

Andreasen, N. C., Grove, W. M. & Maurer, R. (1980). Cluster analysis and the classification of depression. *British Journal of Psychiatry*, **137**, 256–65.

Andreasen, N. C., Reich, T., Scheftner, W., Hirschfeld, R. M A. & Coryell, W. (1984). Endogenous versus nonendogenous depression: validation through family studies. In *Clinical neuropharmacology*, vol. 7, suppl. 1, ed. G. Racagni, R. Paoletti & P. Kielholz, pp. 708–9. New York: Raven Press.

Angst, J. (1966). *Zur Atiologie und Nosologie endogener depressiver Psychosen*. Berlin: Springer.

Bebbington, P. E., Tennant, C. & Hurry, J. (1981). Adversity and the nature of psychiatric disorder in the community. *Journal of Affective Disorders*, **3**, 345–66.

Benjaminsen, S. (1981). Stressful life events preceding the onset of neurotic depression. *Psychological Medicine*, **11**, 369–78.

Berger, M., Doerr, P., Lund, R., Bronisch, T. & von Zerssen, D. (1982). Neuroendocrinological and neurophysiological studies in major depressive disorders: are there biological markers for the endogenous subtype? *Biological Psychiatry*, **17**, 1217–42.

Berner, P., Gabriel, E., Katschnig, H., Kieffer, W., Koehler, K., Lenz, G. & Simhandl, Ch. (1983*a*). *Diagnostic criteria for schizophrenic and affective disorders*. Washington: American Psychiatric Press.

Berner, P. & Katschnig, H. (1983). Principles of 'multiaxial' classification in psychiatry as a basis of modern methodology. In *Evaluation of psychiatric treatment*, ed. T. Helgason, pp. 71–9. Cambridge University Press.

Berner, P., Katschnig, H. & Lenz, G. (1983*b*). DSM-III in German speaking countries. In *International perspectives on DSM*-III, ed. R. L. Spitzer, J. B. W. Williams & A. E. Skodol, pp. 109–25. Washington: American Psychiatric Press.

British Medical Journal (1981). The new psychiatry. 283, 513–14.

Brockington, I. F., Kendell, R. E. & Leff, J. P. (1978). Definitions of schizophrenia: concordance and prediction of outcome. *Psychological Medicine*, **8**, 387–98.

Brown, G. W. (1974). Meaning, measurement and stress of life events. In *Stressful life events: their nature and effects*, ed. B. S. Dohrenwend & B. P. Dohrenwend, pp. 217–43. New York: John Wiley.

Brown, G. W., Ní Bhrolcháin, M. & Harris, T. O. (1979). Psychotic and neurotic depression. *Journal of Affective Disorders*, **1**, 195–211.

Byrne, D. G. (1978). Cluster analysis applied to self-reported depressive symptomatology. *Acta Psychiatrica Scandinavica*, **57**, 1–10.

Cadoret, R. J., Winokur, G., Dorzab, J. & Baker, M. (1972). Depressive disease: life events and onset of illness. *Archives of General Psychiatry*, **26**, 133–6.

Carney, M. W. P., Roth, M. & Garside, R. F. (1965). The diagnosis of depressive syndromes and the prediction of ECT response. *British Journal of Psychiatry*, **111**, 659–74.

Carroll, B. J. (1982). The dexamethasone suppression test for melancholia. *British Journal of Psychiatry*, **140**, 292–304.

Carroll, B. J., Curtis, G. C. & Mendels, J. (1976*a*). Neuroendocrine regulation in depression. I. Limbic system–adrenocortical dysfunction. *Archives of General Psychiatry*, **33**, 1039–44.

Carroll, B. J., Curtis, G. C. & Mendels, J. (1976*b*). Neuroendocrine regulation in depression. II. Discrimination of depressed from nondepressed patients. *Archives of General Psychiatry*, **33**, 1051–8.

Carroll, B. J., Martin, F. I. R. & Davies, B. M. (1968). Resistance to suppression by dexamethasone of plasma 11-OHCS levels in severe depressive illness. *British Medical Journal*, **111**, 285–7.

Checkley, S. A. (1979). Corticosteroid and growth hormone responses to methylamphetamine in depressive illness. *Psychological Medicine*, **9**, 107–15.

Checkley, S. A., Slade, A. P. & Shur, E. (1981). Growth hormone and other responses to clonidine in patients with endogenous depression. *British Journal of Psychiatry*, **138**, 51–5.

Coryell, W., Gaffney, G. & Burkhardt, P. E. (1982). DSM-III melancholia and the primary–secondary-distinction: a comparison of concurrent validity means of the dexamethasone suppression test. *American Journal of Psychiatry*, **139**, 120–2.

Davidson, J., Lipper, S., Zung, W. W. K., Strickland, R., Krishnan, R. & Mahorney, S. (1984*a*). Validation of four definitions of melancholia by the dexamethasone suppression test. *American Journal of Psychiatry*, **141**, 1220–3.

Davidson, J., Turnbull, C., Strickland, R. & Belyea, M. (1984*b*). Comparative diagnostic criteria for melancholia and endogenous depression. *Archives of General Psychiatry*, **41**, 506–11.

Endicott, J. & Spitzer, R. L. (1979). Use of the research diagnostic criteria and the schedule for affective disorders and schizophrenia to study affective disorders. *American Journal of Psychiatry*, **163**, 52–6.

Essen-Möller, E. & Wohlfahrt, S. (1947). Suggestions for the amendment of the official Swedish classification of mental disorders. *Acta Psychiatrica Scandinavia Supplement*, **47**, 555.

Evans, D. L., Burnett, G. B. & Nemeroff, C. B. (1983). The dexamethasone suppression test in the clinical setting. *American Journal of Psychiatry*, **140**, 586–9.

Everitt, B. S., Gourlay, A. J. & Kendell, R. E. (1971). An attempt at validation of traditional psychiatric syndromes by cluster analysis. *British Journal of Psychiatry*, **119**, 399–412.

Eysenck, H. J. (1970). The classification of depressive illnesses. *British Journal of Psychiatry*, **117**, 241–50.

Feighner, J. P., Robins, E., Guze, S. B., Woodruff, R. A., Winokur, G. & Munoz, R. (1972). Diagnostic criteria for use in psychiatric research. *Archives of General Psychiatry*, **26**, 57–63.

Feinberg, M. & Carroll, B. J. (1982). Separation of subtypes of depression using discriminant analysis. I. Separation of unipolar endogenous depression from non-endogenous depression. *British Journal of Psychiatry*, **140**, 384–91.

Feinberg, M., Gillin, J. Ch., Carroll, B. J., Greden, J. F. & Zis, A. P. (1982). EEG studies of sleep in the diagnosis of depression. *Biological Psychiatry*, **17**, 305–16.

Fienberg, S. E. (1977). The analysis of cross-clarified categorical data. Cambridge, Mass.: MIT Press.

Forrest, A. D., Fraser, R. H. & Priest, R. G. (1965). Environmental factors in depressive illness. *British Journal of Psychiatry*, **111**, 243–53.

Foulds, G. A. (1973). The relationship between the depressive illnesses. *British Journal of Psychiatry*, **122**, 531–3.

Grinker, R. R., Miller, J., Sabshin, M., Nunn, R. & Nunnaly, J. C. (1961). *The phenomena of depressions*. New York: P. Hoeber.

Hamilton, M. & White, J. M. (1959). Clinical syndromes in depressive states. *Journal of Mental Science*, **105**, 985–98.

Hirschfeld, R. M. A. (1981). Situational depression: validity of the concept. *British Journal of Psychiatry*, **139**, 297–305.

Hirschfeld, R. M. A., Klerman, G. L., Keller, M. B., Andreasen, N. & Clayton, P. J. (1984). The validity of situational/reactive major depressive disorder. *Clinical Neuropharmacology*, **7**, Supplement 1, 710–11.

Hofmann, G., Katschnig, H., Kremser, M. & Schultes, H. (1971). Längsschnittverläufe rezidivierender endoger Depressionen und Psychopharmaka. *Pharmacopsychiatry Neuro-Psychopharmakologie*, **4**, 285–90.

Holden, N. L. (1983). Depression and the Newcastle Scale. Their relationship to the dexamethasone suppression test. *British Journal of Psychiatry*, **142**, 505–7.

Holmes, Th. H. & Rahe, R. H. (1967). The Social Readjustment Rating Scale. *Journal of Psychosomatic Research*, **11**, 213–18.

Katschnig, H. (1984*a*). Inferring causes: some constraints in the social psychiatry of depression. Commentary to the article by P. E. Bebbington. *Integrative Psychiatry*, **2**, 77–9.

Katschnig, H. (1984*b*). Der polydiagnostische Ansatz in der psychiatrischen Forschung. In *Forschungen zur biologischen Psychiatrie*, ed. A. Hopf & H. Beckmann, pp. 63–78. Berlin, Heidelberg & New York: Springer.

Katschnig, H. (1985). Problems in the use of global scores of rating scales in psychiatric research. In *Psychiatry – the state of the art*, vol. 1, *Proceedings of the 7th world congress of psychiatry*, ed. P. Berner, pp. 241–28. New York: Plenum Press.

Katschnig, H. & Berner, P. (1985). The polydiagnostic approach in psychiatric research. In *Mental disorders, alcohol and drug related problems: international perspectives on their diagnosis and classification*, ed. Alcohol, Drug and Mental Health Administration/WHO. Amsterdam: Elsevier.

Katschnig, H., Brandl-Nebehay, A., Fuchs-Robetin, G., Seelig, P., Eichberger, G., Strobl, R. & Sint, P. P. (1981). *Lebensverändernde Ereignisse, psychosoziale Dispositionen und depressive Verstimmungszustände*. Psychiatrische Universitätsklinik Wien: Abteilung für Sozialpsychiatrie und Dokumentation.

Katschnig, H., Nutzinger, D. & Schanda, H. (1986). Validating depressive subtypes. In *New results in depression research*, ed. H. Hippius, G. Klerman & N. Matussek, pp. 36–44. Heidelberg: Springer.

Katschnig, H. & Seelig, P. (1985). The polydiagnostic approach in psychiatric research on depression. In *Psychiatry – the state of the art*, vol. 1, *Proceedings of the 7th world congress of psychiatry*, ed. P. Berner, pp. 109–14. New York: Plenum Press.

Kay, D. W. K., Garside, R. F., Beamish, P. & Roy, J. R. (1969). Endogenous and neurotic syndromes of depression: a factor analytic study of 104 cases. Clinical features. *British Journal of Psychiatry*, **115**, 377–88.

Kendell, R. E. (1968). *The classification of depressive illnesses*. Maudsley Monograph No. 18. London: Oxford University Press.

Kendell, R. E. (1976). The classification of depression: a review of contemporary confusion. *British Journal of Psychiatry*, **129**, 15–27.

Kiloh, L. G. & Garside, R. F. (1963). The independence of neurotic depression and endogenous depression. *British Journal of Psychiatry*, **109**, 451–63.

Klein, D. F. (1974). Endogenomorphic depression: a conceptual and terminological revision. *Archives of General Psychiatry*, **31**, 447–54.

Klerman, G. L., Endicott, J., Spitzer, D. R. & Hirschfeld, R. M. A. (1979). Neurotic depressions: a systematic analysis of multiple criteria and meanings. *American Journal of Psychiatry*, **136**, 57–61.

Kovacs, M., Rush, A. J., Beck, A. T. & Hollon, S. D. (1981). Depressed outpatients treated with cognitive therapy or pharmacotherapy – a one-year follow-up. *Archives of General Psychiatry*, **38**, 33–9.

Kraepelin, E. (1904). *Psychiatrie*, 7th edition. Leipzig: Barth.

Kraepelin, E. (1913). *Psychiatrie*, 8th edition. Vol. III. Leipzig: Barth. (English edition: *Manic depressive insanity and paranoia*, trans. R. M. Barclay from the 8th edition of *Psychiatrie*. Edinburgh, 1921: Livingstone.)

Kupfer, D. J. (1976). REM latency: a psychobiological marker for primary depressive disease. *Biological Psychiatry*, **11**, 159–74.

Kupfer, D. J., Foster, F. G., Coble, P., McPartland, R. J. & Ulrich, R. F. (1978). The application of EEG sleep for the differential diagnosis of affective disorders. *American Journal of Psychiatry*, **135**, 69–74.

Laakmann, G. (1980). Beeinflussung der Hypophysenvorderlappen-Hormon-sekretion durch Antidepressiva bei gesunden Probanden, neurotisch und endogen depressiven Patienten. *Nervenarzt*, **51**, 725–32.

Langer, G., Henze, G., Reim, B. & Matussek, N. (1976). Reduced growth hormone responses to amphetamine in 'endogenous' depressive patients. Studies in normal, 'reactive' and 'endogenous depressive', schizophrenic, and chronic alcoholic subjects. *Archives of General Psychiatry*, **33**, 107–15.

Lewis, A. (1971). 'Endogenous' and 'exogenous': a useful dichotomy? *Psychological Medicine*, **1**, 191–6.

Matussek, N. (1978). Neuroendokrinologische Untersuchungen bei depressiven Syndromen. *Nervenarzt*, **49**, 569–75.

Matussek, P. & Neuner, R. (1981). Loss events preceding endogenous and neurotic depressions. *Acta Psychiatric Scandinavica*, **64**, 340–50.

Maxwell, A. E. (1971). Multivariate statistical methods and classification problems. *British Journal of Psychiatry*, **119**, 121–7.

Mendels, J. & Cochrane, C. (1968). The nosology of depression. 1. Some points of method. *American Journal of Psychiatry*, **124**, supplement, 1–11.

Mezzich, J. E. (1979). Patterns and issues in multiaxial psychiatric diagnosis. *Psychological Medicine*, **9**, 125–37.

Mezzich, J. E., Fabrega, H. & Mezzich, A. C. (1985). An international consultation on multiaxial diagnosis. In *Psychiatry – the state of the art, Proceedings of the 7th world congress of psychiatry*, ed. P. Berner, pp. 51–6. New York: Plenum Press.

Nelson, J. G. & Charney, D. S. (1980). Primary affective disorder criteria and the endogenous-reactive distinction. *Archives of General Psychiatry*, **37**, 787–93.

Overall, J. E. (1974). The brief psychiatric rating scale in psychopharmacology research. In *Modern problems in pharmacopsychiatry*, vol. 1, ed. P. Pichot, pp. 67–78. Basel: Karger.

Overall, J. E., Hollister, L. E., Johnson, M. & Pennington, V. (1966). Nosology of depression and differential response to drugs. *Journal of the American Medical Association*, **195**, 946–8.

Overall, J. E. & Zisook, S. (1980). Diagnosis and the phenomenology of depressive disorders. *Journal of Consulting and Clinical Psychology*, **48**, 626–34.

Patrick, V., Dunner, D. L. & Fieve, R. R. (1978). Life events and primary affective illness. *Acta Psychiatrica Scandinavica*, **58**, 48–55.

Paykel, E. S. (1971). Classification of depressed patients: a cluster analysis derived grouping. *British Journal of Psychiatry*, **118**, 275–88.

Paykel, E. S. (1983). Methodological aspects of life event research. *Journal of Psychosomatic Research*, **27**, 341–52.

Paykel, E. S., Prusoff, B. & Klerman, G. L. (1971). The endogenous–neurotic continuum in depression: rater independence and factor distributions. *Journal of Psychiatric Research*, **8**, 73–90.

Perris, C. (1966). A study of bipolar and unipolar recurrent depressive psychoses. *Acta Psychiatrica Scandinavica*, supplement 194.

Prusoff, B. A., Weissman, M. M., Klerman, G. L. & Rounsaville, B. J. (1980). Research diagnostic criteria subtypes of depression. Their role as predictors of differential response to psychotherapy and drug treatment. *Archives of General Psychiatry*, **37**, 796–801.

Rassaby, E. & Paykel, E. S. (1979). Factor patterns in depression. A replication study. *Journal of Affective Disorders*, **1**, 187–94.

Rechtschaffen, A. & Kales, A. (eds.) (1968). *A manual of standardized terminology, techniques and scoring system for sleep stages of human subjects*. National Institute of Health Publication 204. Washington: US Government Printing Office.

Robins, E., Munoz, R. A., Martin, S. & Gentry, K. A. (1972). Primary and secondary affective disorders. In *Disorders of mood*, ed. J. Zubin & F. Freyhan, pp. 33–45. Baltimore & London: The Johns Hopkins Press.

Rosenthal, S. & Gudeman, J. E. (1967). The endogenous depressive pattern: an empirical investigation. *Archives of General Psychiatry*, **16**, 241–9.

Rosenthal, S. H. & Klerman, G. L. (1966). Content and consistency in the endogenous depressive pattern. *British Journal of Psychiatry*, **112**, 471–84.

Rush, A. J., Giles, D. E., Roffwarg, H. P. & Parker, C. R. (1982). Sleep EEG and dexamethasone suppression test findings in outpatients with unipolar major depressive disorders. *Biological Psychiatry*, **17**, 327–41.

Sandifer, M. G., Wilson, I. C. & Green, L. (1966). The two-type thesis of depressive disorders. *American Journal of Psychiatry*, **123**, 93–7.

Schatzberg, A. F., Rothschild, A. J., Stahl, J. B., Bond, T. C., Rosenbaum, A. H., Lofgren, S. B., MacLaughlin, R. A., Sullivan, M. A. & Cole, O. J. (1983). The dexamethasone suppression test: identification of subtypes of depression. *American Journal of Psychiatry*, **140**, 88–91.

Schildkraut, J. J. (1978). The current status of the catecholamine hypothesis of affective disorders. In *Psychopharmacology: a generation of progress*, ed. M. Lipton, A. DiMascio & K. Killam, pp. 1223–34. New York: Raven Press.

Schneider, K. (1959). *Clinical psychopathology*. New York: Grune & Stratton.

Spitzer, R. L., Endicott, J. & Robins, E. (1978). Research diagnostic criteria: rationale and reliability. *Archives of General Psychiatry*, **35**, 773–82.

Thase, M. E., Hersen, M., Bellack, A. S., Himmelhoch, J. M. & Kupfer, D. J. (1983). Validation of a Hamilton subscale for endogenomorphic depression. *Journal of Affective Disorders*, **5**, 267–78.

Thomson, K. C. & Hendrie, H. C. (1972). Environmental stress in primary depressive illness. *Archives of General Psychiatry*, **26**, 130–2.

Wing, J. K., Cooper, J. E. & Sartorius, N. (1974). *The measurement and classification of psychiatric symptoms*. Cambridge University Press.

Winokur, G. (1982). The development and validity of familial subtypes in primary unipolar depression. *Pharmacopsychiatry*, **15**, 142–6.

Winokur, G., Cadoret, R., Dorzab, J. & Baker, M. (1971). Depressive disease: a genetic study. *Archives of General Psychiatry*, **24**, 135–44.

World Health Organisation (1967). *International classification of diseases*, 8th revision, Chapter V (1965 revision). Geneva: WHO.

World Health Organisation (1978). *Mental disorders: glossary and guide to their classification in accordance with the ninth revision of the International Classification of Diseases*. Geneva: WHO.

Zimmermann, M., Coryell, W., Pfohl, B. & Stangl, D. (1985). Four definitions of endogenous depression and the dexamethasone suppression test. *Journal of Affective Disorders*, **8**, 37–45.

8

Prospects for future research

HEINZ KATSCHNIG

Introduction

The degree of enthusiasm expressed about the results of life event research by different authors in this book varies, and repeatedly scepticism has arisen: is it useful to pursue the life event approach further, if the amount of variance in psychopathology explained by life events is so modest? Is it worthwhile to continue doing life event research on supposed disease entities, such as depressive subtypes, given all the unsolved problems of psychiatric diagnosis? What about the pitfalls in life event methodology which may seriously invalidate research results? Recently, even most available research results on a positive relationship between life event stress and the outbreak of a schizophrenic episode have been questioned (Tennant, 1985).

Since, however, research has the essential function of introducing an element of control in our attempts to understand reality, these and similar questions should, as I see it, be understood as challenges and lead to improving research strategies and methods rather than to abandoning the field. The more so, as sophisticated and solid research is especially needed in psychiatry, where ideological prejudices are frequent and where irreconciliable biological and psychosocial positions are often irrationally opposed to each other. It may therefore be useful to present some guidelines as to how future research into the relationship between life stress and psychiatric illness can be made more effective.

Since it is clear from the existing evidence that a one to one relationship between simply defined life stress and a simply defined mental illness is the least one can expect to find, future research projects will undoubtedly become more complicated and more cumbersome. Among the aspects of life event and illness studies which will need closer attention, at least five seem to me to be of primary importance: (1) increasing the precision in the phenomenological description of mental disorders; (2) increasing the precision in measuring life stress; (3) studying the process of coping with life events and its relationship to moderating factors (such as personality and social network variables); (4) studying the interplay between psychosocial and biological variables; and (5) utilizing multiple methods of data analysis. Each of these aspects will be dealt with in turn.

Increasing the precision in the phenomenological description of mental disorders

If the ultimate aim of psychiatric research is to find adequate therapeutic and prophylactic strategies for our patients, stress research cannot be confined to animal experiments and laboratory studies of healthy subjects, but has to be continued in psychiatrically ill populations. It is therefore of utmost importance to increase the precision in the phenomenological description of functional mental disorders in order to help reduce current misunderstandings and improve comparability between different studies. A number of recommendations can be formulated in this respect.

First, paradigmatical definitions of mental disorders, such as those included in the 'International Classification of Diseases' of the World Health Organisation, should no longer be used for research purposes, since they cannot guarantee that identical study populations are identified in different investigations (see Chapter 7, p. 207, this volume). There is no doubt that for the purpose of psychiatric research the use of operational diagnostic criteria constitutes in itself a considerable advance over the traditional paradigmatical approach. However, it has to be borne in mind that providing a diagnostic algorithm as such does not yet constitute an 'operational' definition in the proper sense; it must also be ascertained that the elements of information composing the algorithm are collected in an operational, i.e. in a reliable and valid, way. This does not only refer to psychopathological symptoms but also to other areas of information, such as course characteristics and triggering events, which are often methodologically neglected. The reliable collection of information about life stress and reactivity is of special importance in the field of operationally defining depressive subtypes. A further problem concerns the implicit assumption that operational diagnostic criteria provide homogeneous study populations. Since it could be shown that operational criteria may still produce considerable heterogeneity (see chapter 7, pp. 217 and 227, this volume), it is of great importance to retain the information on the individual items composing an algorithm and also carry out analyses on the symptom level in addition to overall diagnostic analyses (see e.g. Paykel, Rao & Taylor, 1984). Furthermore, 'multiaxial' diagnostic approaches – i.e. keeping several areas of information separate from each other, when classifying a psychiatric patient – should be given preference in future studies. In the context of the topic of this book this especially refers to information concerning phenomenological variables, i.e. the psychopathological syndrome and its course characteristics, on the one hand, and information about psychosocial stressors, i.e. on 'reactivity', on the other, which should be collected and documented independently from each other.

Finally, considering the still hypothetical character of all – both operational and non-operational – diagnostic formulations of functional mental disorders, one definition must be regarded to be as good as the other. From this follows the recommendation not to carry out studies which simply rely on one diagnostic definition, but which utilize several such definitions simultaneously. Such a 'polydiagnostic approach', as opposed to the usual 'monodiagnostic' approach of just employing one diagnostic formulation, should become standard in future research (Katschnig & Berner, 1985). Moreover, a fundamental shift in emphasis seems necessary in respect to psychiatric diagnosis, in the sense that the concept of 'validation' should become more prominent in research on functional mental disorders. Using this concept represents a completely different research paradigm from the traditional approach. Instead of, for example, 'proving' that 'endogenous' depression is not triggered by life stress, whereas 'neurotic' depression is, the question is asked, whether a symptomatological definition of endogenous depression can be 'validated' by the absence of life stress, with the opposite applying to neurotic depression. The same would apply to other variables such as biological markers, course characteristics, and even to responsiveness to specific therapeutic agents and procedures (e.g. Rickels, Feighner & Smith, 1985). This new paradigm implies that a specific diagnostic formulation is not taken for granted but that the question should be asked whether this specific diagnostic definition is justified at all.

Increasing the precision in measuring life stress

There is ample evidence to assume that self-rating inventories of the kind of the 'Schedule of Recent Experience' (SRE) (Holmes & Rahe, 1967) seriously distort the representation of people's actual life experiences and should no longer be used. The only way of reliably collecting life event information is to carry out a semi-standardized interview, which not only permits adherence to definitional standards but also makes a precise dating of life events possible. The London 'Life Event and Difficulty Schedule' (LEDS) by Brown & Harris (1978) seems to be the most suitable of the available life event methods. Since this method is rather cumbersome, similar but shorter methods (e.g. Paykel, 1983) have been proposed, while Miller & Salter (1984) maintain that there are no short cuts.

In any case, bearing in mind that different stress indices are used in different studies, life event data should be collected in such a way that specific 'stress indices' used by published studies can be easily reconstructed. We have demonstrated in reconstructing the index used in the study by Bebbington, Tennant & Hurry (1981) that this can easily be done (see Chapter 7, p. 235, this volume). One principal difference between such stress indices concerns the question of whether an additive model (the sum of individual life event stresses in a specific time period) or a threshold model (at least one stressful life event in a specific time period) is chosen. Another important difference concerns the length and number of periods into which the time before disease onset is broken down. If the conclusion resulting from a specific life event study is that life stress increases before the onset of illness, the term 'before' can have many different meanings and it may have a considerable influence on the results obtained whether 6-month or 3-week periods are chosen for studying a possible rise in life stress before disease onset. Since there is a complete lack of standardization in this respect, data should be collected in such a way, i.e. by dating life events exactly, that any time period may be chosen for the statistical analyses. This would make post-hoc comparisons with other studies possible, as was also shown in Chapter 7. Also the application of more sophisticated models, such as a 'dissipation model' (Surtees & Ingham, 1980) would become possible.

To collect life event information in as much detail as possible is also relevant for the post-hoc categorization of life events into the different subtypes proposed and used by different research workers. Paykel *et al.*'s (1969) proposition of dividing life events into desirable and undesirable ones, or exit and entrance events, is relevant here, as well as the suggestion by Dohrenwend & Dohrenwend (1981) to keep at least three populations of life events distinct (physical illnesses and injuries to the subject; events possibly confounded with the physical health and the psychiatric condition of the subject; and, finally, events which are independent of health problems). Miller & Ingham's (1983) 'dimensions of experience' (choice of action, uncertainty of outcome, personal loss, hopeless situation, antisocial act) are a further example.

With regard to increasing the precision of measuring life stress also the distinction between an actual life *change* event and a *long standing* difficulty is imperative. Most life event studies, however, are astonishingly inconsistent in this respect: although they theoretically start with the concept of an acutely stressful life change event, they eventually lose sight of their original starting point. For instance, in the SRE, clearcut life changes (death of a spouse, gain of a new family member) are listed alongside problematic life situations which may be of considerable duration and need not necessarily have begun recently (e.g. sexual difficulties, problems with the in-laws). On the other hand, although the London LEDS collects information on life events and chronic difficulties separately, Brown & Harris (1978) eventually construct a composite stress index of 'at least one severe life event *or* one major difficulty', which makes it impossible to evaluate the relative contribution of life change stress and of chronic difficulties to the onset of depression. This is problematic, since chronic difficulties may themselves act as 'vulnerability factors', i.e. they may amplify the negative influences of stressful life events. Whether or not this is so is a question for research, which can only be answered if the two parameters are kept separate right from the beginning of a study until its end. How complicated the measurement of life stress is and how important the detailed collection of life event data may be was recently shown by Miller & Ingham (1985) who demonstrated that life events which cause each other were less pathogenic than those which occurred independently of each other.

Studying the process of coping with life events and its relationship to moderating factors

While there is an extensive psychological literature on the coping process in normal subjects (e.g. Lazarus, 1966; Meichenbaum, Turk & Burstein, 1975; Haan, 1977), little work has been carried out in relation to mental illness. Among the few studies which have investigated the influence of social factors on the life event–coping–disease process the more important have studied personality factors and social network characteristics. In the study by Henderson, Byrne & Duncan-Jones (1981), personality factors were found to be much more important than social support for determining the outcome of life event stress with regard to psychiatric disorders and it was concluded 'that it is not so much the social environment which is important as how individuals construe it, particularly under adversity' (Henderson, 1983). It is also important to consider that individuals, due to personality characteristics, may avoid, search out or even create their specific social environments, some of which may be connected with a higher or a lower probability of occurrence of life events. Risk-taking personalities may choose to live in circumstances with a high probability of permanent changes, whereas timid personalities may withdraw from stressful environments, thus regulating the amount of stress with which they can cope. It is evident that much more attention must be paid to personality variables in future studies on life event stress and psychiatric disorders. However, the concept of 'personality' is a difficult one, and its use in psychiatric research is beset by many pitfalls. One of the most common problems is that personality inventories may not pick up personality traits but just measure state variables. There are, however, methods available for making personality assessment more valid, such as assessing the personality of psychiatric patients only after the disease episode has receded, or relying on external sources of information, such as relatives or friends. As far as the relationship between the coping process and an individual's social network is concerned it is both commonsense knowledge and seems to be scientifically proven that social support has a buffering effect in the presence of life stress (Clayton, Halikas & Maurice, 1972; Brown & Harris, 1978). The full range of possible relationships between the personal social network of an individual affected by life events and psychiatric disorders has, however, not yet been explored (Mueller, 1980; Canton & Fraccon, 1985; Monroe & Steiner, 1986). Social relationships may not only buffer stress effects but may also create stress, since a large social network also increases the probability that life events occur. Life events may themselves be regarded as a 'network rupture', and Zubin (1979) has pointed out that 37 of the 42 events of the SRE correspond to a 'reduction or disruption in the network relationships of the affected individual'. Thus, 'network rupture' can be regarded as an important aspect of the possible pathogenic effect of life events.

Another important issue in relation to coping is the individual's help-seeking behaviour after the occurrence of a life event. The organization of crisis intervention services (see Cooper, 1979; Katschnig & Cooper, 1986) has to take such 'help-seeking behaviour factors' into consideration. It is a reasonable hypothesis to assume that whenever people are unable to cope with life events by making use of their immediate environmental network, the probability of their contacting health, psychiatric and social services increases. In some respect professional helpers may be regarded as temporary network surrogates when a person's social network is non-existent or fails to be of sufficient help. But crisis intervention workers and psychiatric emergency services must also take into consideration that the person's social environment may be overtaxed or not willing and motivated to help and therefore try to delegate the problem to an institution. These mechanisms are not only important for the organization of crisis intervention and psychiatric emergency services but have also to be taken into consideration as selection factors in clinical life event studies.

Studying the interplay between psychosocial and biological variables

Although it has become increasingly fashionable to speak of a 'multifactorial aetiology' of mental disorders, very little research encompassing both psychosocial and biological variables in fact exists. This is especially true for life event research where studies have mainly been undertaken by research workers interested in the psychosocial and social psychiatric aspects of mental disorders and not in the biological ones. On the other hand, researchers interested in the biological aspects of mental disorders have not tackled the question of a possible interplay between biological and psychosocial variables. However, studies on psychiatric patients focusing on the interplay between biological and psychosocial variables are now beginning to appear (Zimmerman, Coryell & Corenthal, 1984; Dolan *et al.*, 1985).

As far as the possible pathogenetic process in the development of functional mental disorders is concerned, a rather complex interplay between both specific and non-specific psychological and biological mechanisms must be assumed. It must also be borne in mind that aetiology, symptom presentation and failure to recover may each have a separate set of factors upon which these phenomena depend (Gilbert, 1984). A complex 'vulnerability' model seems most appropriate to understand these processes, assuming a set of specific psychological and biological vulnerabilities which constitute points of weakness in a complex pathogenetic chain. Specific psychological 'vulnerabilities' may contribute to an event being evaluated as uncontrollable by some persons, but not by others, and it is conceivable, though not necessarily so, that only those events which are not 'filtered' out lead to a set of biological stress reactions including unspecific changes. Examples are the activation of the hypothalamic–pituitary–adrenocortical axis through stress, changes in lymphocyte function which have been found in bereaved persons (Stein, Keller & Schleifer, 1981; Bartrop *et al.*, 1977), and the alteration of central acetylcholine availability through stress, postulated by Janowsky & Risch (1985). Subsequently, specific biological vulnerabilities to such general biological stress reactions may be activated and lead to specific psychopathological symptoms. For instance, Zubin & Spring (1977) and Ciompi (1982) propose vulnerability models for schizophrenia and the vulnerability concept is also inherent in Wing's (1978) metaphor of schizophrenia corresponding to a walk on a tightrope between understimulation and overstimulation.

In view of the increasing evidence that psychological and biological variables are intimately connected in the aetiology of mental disorders, simple classifications relying on a mind–body dichotomy, such as the neurotic–endogenous distinction of depression, must be regarded as obsolete. Therefore, assuming that there is, for instance, a class of depression which is purely biological and a different class which is purely psychological can no longer be a serious approach. It is conceivable that specific aetiological factors which are amenable to empirical research – such as life events and biological markers – may be less intimately connected with diagnostic classes than with specific pathogenetic mechanisms and specific phenomenological expressions of a disease process. It might therefore be more appropriate to look for correlations of such factors with specific symptoms than with hypothetical disease entities (see also above, p. 247).

How complicated research on the relationships between psychological, biological and phenomenological variables may be can be demonstrated by recent findings on the Dexamethasone Suppression Test (DST), originally believed to be a biological marker for 'endogenous' depression. Since a positive DST has been shown to arise also when people fast, correlations between a positive DST and specific types of depression become problematic, because many endogenous depressive patients are anorectic and lose weight. In the Dahlem conference on 'the origins of depression' (Angst, 1983) a long list of such variables – including among others hospitalization and drug withdrawal – possibly intervening in a positive DST test was drawn up. These considerations do not only tentatively invalidate existing findings about the DST but, again, point to the relationship between psychosocial and biological variables, since a positive DST may obviously just be the consequence of unspecific psychosocial stress factors.

Utilizing multiple methods of data analysis

Two final recommendations concern data analysis. First, certainly more complex methods of data analysis have to be employed, if the relationships between the many possible independent, intervening and dependent variables are to be better understood. For instance, Dohrenwend & Dohrenwend (1981) have outlined six possible hypotheses about the 'life stress process' and Golden & Dohrenwend (1981) have suggested the use of the statistical technique of path analysis to test these hypotheses. Secondly, insufficient attention has so far been paid to the influence of the use of specific methods of data analysis on the kind of results obtained. This question was raised by Tennant & Bebbington (1978) in their discussion of Brown & Harris' (1978) work on the 'origins of depression'. They showed that using a different method for analysing Brown & Harris' data, namely log-linear analysis, yielded results differing from those in the original publication. Everitt & Smith (1979), in summing up the discussions on this topic, suggested that no decision could yet be made as to which type of data analysis would be more correct, Brown & Harris' comparison of proportions or log-linear analysis. They concluded therefore that it would be best to apply several methods of data analysis simultaneously, an opinion which must certainly be supported.

Final comment

One final comment seems appropriate, although it may be somehow far reaching. Whereas in terms of practical research and data collection a division between psychosocial and biological variables is unavoidable, it seems important that future controversies in life event research do not focus on the traditional Cartesian mind–body dichotomy. While life events are clearly of a psychosocial nature, pathogenetic processes can certainly not be attributed to *either* one *or* the other of the two once artificially formed and now reified spheres of reality, the *psychosocial* and the *biological* realm. Future controversies should rather centre around the postulation of *specific 'life stress-vulnerability' risk constellations* and *specific pathogenetic processes*, regardless of whether biological or psychosocial factors are involved. A strict dichotomy between mind and body may, in fact, turn out to be a decisive obstacle to increasing our knowledge (Ryle, 1949; Engel, 1985).

References

Angst, J. (ed.) (1983). *The origins of depression: current concepts and approaches*. Berlin, Heidelberg, New York & Tokyo: Springer.

Bartrop, R. W., Lazarus, L., Luckherst, E. & Kiloh, L. H. (1977). Depressed lymphocyte function after bereavement. *The Lancet*, **1**, 834–6.

Bebbington, P. E., Tennant, C. & Hurry, J. (1981). Adversity and the nature of psychiatric disorder in the community. *Journal of Affective Disorders*, **3**, 345–66.

Brown, G. W. & Harris, T. O. (1978). *Social origins of depression: a study of psychiatric disorder in women*. London: Tavistock Publications. New York: Free Press.

Canton, G. & Fraccon, I. G. (1985). Life events and schizophrenia. A replication. *Acta Psychiatrica Scandinavica*, **71**, 211–16.

Ciompi, L. (1982). *Affektlogik. Uber die Struktur der Psyche und ihre Entwicklung. Ein Beitrag zur Schizophrenieforschung*. Stuttgart: Klett-Cotta.

Clayton, P. J., Halikas, J. A. & Maurice, W. L. (1972). The depression of widowhood. *British Journal of Psychiatry*, **120**, 71–8.

Cooper, J. E. (1979). *Crisis admission units and emergency psychiatric services*. Public Health in Europe, 11. Copenhagen: Regional Office for Europe, World Health Organisation.

Dohrenwend, B. S. & Dohrenwend, B. P. (1981). Life stress and illness: formulation of the issues. In *Stressful life events and their contexts*, ed. B. S. Dohrenwend & B. P. Dohrenwend, pp. 1–47. New York: Prodist.

Dolan, R. J., Calloway, S. P., Fonagy, P., De Souza, F. V. A. & Wakeling, A. (1985). Life events, depression and hypothalamic–pituitary–adrenal axis function. *British Journal of Psychiatry*, **147**, 429–33.

Engel, G. L. (1985). Misapplication of a scientific paradigm. *Integrative Psychiatry*, **3**, 9–11.

Everitt, B. S. & Smith, A. M. R. (1979). Interactions in contingency tables: a brief discussion of alternative definitions. *Psychological Medicine*, **9**, 581–3.

Gilbert, P. (1984). *Depression: from psychology to brain state*. London: Lawrence Erlbaum Associates.

Golden, R. R. & Dohrenwend, B. S. (1981). A path analytic method for testing causal hypotheses about the life stress process. In *Stressful life events and their contexts*, ed. B. S. Dohrenwend & B. P. Dohrenwend, pp. 258–87. New York: Prodist.

Haan, N. (1977). *Coping and defending. Processes of self-environment organization*. New York: Academic Press.

Henderson, A. S. (1983). Vulnerability to depression: the lack of social support does not cause depression. In *The origins of depression: current concepts and approaches*, ed. J. Angst, pp. 107–19. Berlin: Springer.

Henderson, A. S., Byrne, D. G. & Duncan-Jones, P. (1981). *Neurosis and the social environment*. Sydney: Academic Press.

Holmes, Th. H. & Rahe, R. H. (1967). The Social Readjustment Rating Scale. *Journal of Psychosomatic Research*, **11**, 213–18.

Janowsky, D. S. & Risch, S. C. (1985). An acetylcholine hypothesis of stress modulation. *Integrative Psychiatry*, **3**, 3–16.

Katschnig, H. & Berner, P. (1985). The polydiagnostic approach in psychiatric research. In *ADAMHA/WHO: Mental disorders, alcohol and drug-related problems: international perspectives on their diagnosis and classification*, pp. 113–20. Amsterdam: Elsevier Scientific Publishers.

Katschnig, H. & Cooper, J. (1986). Crisis intervention and emergency services. In *Community psychiatry*, ed. D. Bennett & H. Freeman. London: Churchill Livingstone.

Lazarus, R. S. (1966). *Psychological stress and the coping process*. New York: McGraw-Hill.

Meichenbaum, D., Turk, D. & Burstein, S. (1975). The nature of coping with stress. In *Stress and anxiety*, vol. 2, ed. I. G. Sarason & C. D. Spielberger, pp. 337–58. New York: Wiley.

Miller, P. McC. & Ingham, J. G. (1983). Dimensions of experience. *Psychological Medicine*, **13**, 417–29.

Miller, P. McC. & Ingham, J. G. (1985). Are life events which cause each other additive in their effects? *Social Psychiatry*, **20**, 31–41.

Miller, P. McC. & Salter, D. P. (1984). Is there a short-cut? An investigation into the life event interview. *Acta Psychiatrica Scandinavica*, **70**, 417–27.

Monroe, S. M. & Steiner, C. (1986). Social support and psychopathology: Interrelations with preexisting disorder, stress, and personality. *Journal of Abnormal Psychology*, **95**, 29–39.

Mueller, D. P. (1980). Social networks: a promising direction for research on the relationship of the social environment to psychiatric disorder. *Social Science & Medicine*, **14A**, 147–61.

Paykel, E. S. (1983). Methodological aspects of life events research. *Journal of Psychosomatic Research*, **27**, 341–52.

Paykel, E. S., Myers, J. K., Dienelt, M. N., Klerman, G. L., Lindenthal, J. J. & Pepper, M. P. (1969). Life events and depression. A controlled study. *Archives of General Psychiatry*, **21**, 753–60.

Paykel, E. S., Rao, B. M. & Taylor, C. N. (1984). Life stress and symptom pattern in out-patient depression. *Psychological Medicine*, **14**, 559–68.

Rickels, K., Feighner, J. P. & Smith, W. T. (1985). Alprazolam, amitriptyline, doxepin, and placebo in the treatment of depression. *Archives of General Psychiatry*, **42**, 134–41.

Ryle, G. (1949). *The concept of mind*. London: Hutchinson & Co.

Stein, M., Keller, S. & Schleifer, S. (1981). The hypothalamus and the immune response. In *Brain, behaviour and bodily disease*, ed. H. Weiner, M. A. Hofer & A. J. Stunkard, pp. 45–65. New York: Raven Press.

Surtees, P. G. & Ingham, J. G. (1980). Life stress and depressive outcome: application of a dissipation model to life events. *Social Psychiatry*, **15**, 21–31.

Tennant, C. (1985). Stress and schizophrenia: a review. *Integrative Psychiatry*, **3**, 248–55.

Tennant, C. & Bebbington, P. (1978). The social causation of depression: a critique of the work of Brown and his colleagues. *Psychological Medicine*, **8**, 565–75.

Wing, J. (1978). *Schizophrenia. Towards a new synthesis*. London: Academic Press.

Zimmerman, M., Coryell, W. & Corenthal, C. (1984). Attribution style, the Dexamethasone Suppression Test, and the diagnosis of melancholia in depressed inpatients. *Journal of Abnormal Psychology*, **4**, 373–7.

Zubin, J. (1979). Discussion, part IV, and overview. In *Stress and mental disorder*, ed. J. E. Barrett, R. M. Rose & G. L. Klerman, pp. 279–89. New York: Raven Press.

Zubin, J. & Spring, B. (1977). Vulnerability: a new view of schizophrenia. *Journal of Abnormal Psychology*, **86**, 103–23.

INDEX